HEALTH

CARE ETHICS

Critical Issues for the 21st Century

Second Edition

Eileen E. Morrison, EdD, MPH, CHES

Professor, School of Health Administration
Texas State University San Marcos
San Marcos, Texas

World Headquarters
Jones and Bartlett Publishers
40 Tall Pine Drive
Sudbury, MA 01776
978-443-5000
info@jbpub.com
www.jbpub.com

Jones and Bartlett Publishers Canada
6339 Ormindale Way
Mississauga, Ontario L5V 1J2
Canada

Jones and Bartlett Publishers International
Barb House, Barb Mews
London W6 7PA
United Kingdom

Jones and Bartlett's books and products are available through most bookstores and online booksellers. To contact Jones and Bartlett Publishers directly, call 800-832-0034, fax 978-443-8000, or visit our website www.jbpub.com.

Substantial discounts on bulk quantities of Jones and Bartlett's publications are available to corporations, professional associations, and other qualified organizations. For details and specific discount information, contact the special sales department at Jones and Bartlett via the above contact information or send an email to specialsales@jbpub.com.

This publication is designed to provide accurate and authoritative information in regard to the Subject Matter covered. It is sold with the understanding that the publisher is not engaged in rendering legal, accounting, or other professional service. If legal advice or other expert assistance is required, the service of a competent professional person should be sought.

Production Credits
Publisher: Michael Brown
Production Director: Amy Rose
Associate Editor: Katey Birtcher
Production Editor: Tracey Chapman
Production Assistant: Roya Millard
Marketing Manager: Sophie Fleck
Manufacturing and Inventory Control Supervisor: Amy Bacus
Composition: Cape Cod Compositors, Inc.
Cover Design: Kate Ternullo
Cover Image: © Morgan Lane Photography/ShutterStock, Inc.
Printing and Binding: Malloy, Inc.
Cover Printing: Malloy, Inc.

Library of Congress Cataloging-in-Publication Data
Health care ethics : critical issues for the 21st century / [edited by] Eileen E. Morrison.—2nd ed.
    p. ; cm.
    Rev. ed. of: Health care ethics / John F. Monagle, David C. Thomasma.
    Includes bibliographical references and index.
    ISBN-13: 978-0-7637-4526-4 (pbk.)
    ISBN-10: 0-7637-4526-X (pbk.)
    1. Medical ethics.   I. Morrison, Eileen E.   II. Monagle, John F. Health care ethics.
  [DNLM: 1. Bioethical Issues.   2. Ethics, Clinical. WB 60 H4337 2008]
  R724.M66 2008
  174.2—dc22

                           2007044093

6048
Printed in the United States of America
13 12 11 10 09 10 9 8 7 6 5 4 3 2

Writing is a solitary task, and yet no one really writes alone. Writers are accompanied by those who believe in and support them in their tasks. The second edition of Health Care Ethics: Critical Issues for the 21st Century *is dedicated to all those who contributed their time and talent to update existing chapters or develop new ones.*

On a personal level, I would like to dedicate the second edition of this text to those who have provided both inspiration and advice. First and foremost, there is always my son, Grant Edward, who believes that Mom can do the impossible—it just takes longer. There are also my colleagues and friends—you each know how much you have meant to me during this process. Finally, there are my publisher, Michael Brown and my editors, Katey Birtcher and Tracey Chapman, whose knowledge, guidance, and patience made major contributions to the quality and integrity of this work.

Contents

Contributors

George J. Agich, PhD
Professor of Philosophy
Director of BGeXperience Program
Bowling Green State University
Bowling Green, Kentucky

Karen J. Bawel-Brinkley, RN, PhD
Associate Professor
School of Nursing
San Jose University
San Jose, California

Melissa F. Brandon, RN, MS, FACHE
Project Safety Specialist
Post Market Safety Surveillance
Research and Development
Alcon Laboratories
Ft. Worth, Texas

Sidney Callahan, PhD
Distinguished Scholar
The Hastings Center
Garrison, New York

Bryon Chell, JD
Executive Director
California Medical Assistance
  Counsel (ret.)
Sacramento, California

David B. Clarke, DMin, JD, MPH
Director, Massachusetts Health
  Decisions
Sharon, Massachusetts

Kevin T. Fitzgerald, SJ, PhD
Research Associate Professor
Georgetown University
Washington, D.C.

Dexter Freeman, DSW
Assistant Professor of Social Work
Texas State University
  San Marcos
San Marcos, Texas

Janet Gardner-Ray, EdD
Chief Executive Officer
Country Home Healthcare Inc.
Charlottesville, Indiana

Glenn C. Graber, PhD
Professor of Philosophy
University of Tennessee
Knoxville, Tennessee

Chris Hackler, PhD
Director, Division of Medical
  Humanities
University of Arkansas for Medical
  Sciences
Little Rock, Arkansas

T. Patrick Hill, PhD
Senior Policy Fellow
Edward J. Bloustein School of
  Planning and Public Policy
Rutgers University
New Brunswick, New Jersey

Kenneth V. Iserson, MD, MBA
Professor of Emergency Medicine
Director of the Arizona Bioethics
  Program
University of Arizona
Tucson, Arizona

Nicholas King, PhD
Assistant Professor
Departments of Bioethics and
  History
School of Medicine
Case Western Reserve University
Cleveland, Ohio

**John F. Monagle, MA, Phd,
D.A.S.H.R.M**
President, American Institute of
  Medical Ethics
Davis, California

Jessica Moore, DHCE, MA
Research Associate
Case Western Reserve University
Cleveland, Ohio

Eileen E. Morrison, EdD, MPH
Professor, School of Health
  Administration
Texas State University at San
  Marcos
San Marcos, Texas

James Lindemann Nelson, PhD
Professor of Philosophy, Faculty
  Associate
Center for Ethics and Humanities in
  the Life Sciences
Michigan State University
East Lansing, Michigan

**Carol Petrozella, RN, MSN,
MSED, EdD**
Professor and Director of the
  Institute of Ethics in Healthcare
Miami Dade College
Miami, Florida

Barbara Supanich, RSM, MD
Medical Director
Palliative Medicine and Senior Care
Holy Cross Hospital
Silver Spring, Maryland

Jim Summers, PhD
Professor, School of Health
  Administration
Texas State University
  San Marcos
San Marcos, Texas

Carole Warshaw
Executive Director, Domestic
  Violence & Mental Health
  Policy Initiative
Director, National Center on
  Domestic Violence, Trauma &
  Mental Health
Chicago, Illinois

Michael P. West, EdD, FACHE
Executive Director
Fort Worth Center
University of Texas at Arlington
Arlington, Texas

Carrie S. Zoubul, JD, MA
Borchard Fellow
Center for Health Science and
  Public Policy
Brooklyn Law School
Brooklyn, New York

About the Author

Eileen E. Morrison is a professor in the School of Health Administration at Texas State University San Marcos. Her academic background includes a doctorate from Vanderbilt University and a Master of Public Health Degree from the University of Tennessee. In addition, she holds a clinical degree in dental hygiene.

Dr. Morrison has taught graduate and undergraduate ethics courses and provided professional workshops on ethics to physicians, nurses, clinical laboratory professionals, dental professionals, and counselors. She has authored articles and chapters on ethics for a variety of publications. In addition, she is the author of *Ethics in Health Administration: A Practical Approach for Decision Makers*, published by Jones and Bartlett.

Preface

Important works often are created by walking in the footsteps of giants. This aphorism is especially true when considering this new edition of *Health Care Ethics: Critical Issues for the 21st Century*. In the first edition, giants in the field of bioethics, Monagle and Thomasma, used their wisdom and forward thinking to coordinate the writings of influential writers in bioethics and ethical theory. They envisioned challenges to be faced in the continuing evolution of the healthcare system that are still germane today. In creating the first edition, they assisted readers' understanding of what the future might hold for health care. The first edition raised both consciousness and conscience for healthcare professionals.

Many changes and challenges have occurred in health care since the publication of the first edition. In light of these changes, it became necessary to revisit some of the areas raised in the previous edition. Contributors updated their chapters with current examples and introduced new thought-provoking concepts. Additional experts in bioethics, long-term care, health administration, and other areas also added new content to existing chapters. New authors provided chapters on areas of concern such as the ethics of spirituality and of disaster response.

When studying complex issues such as those that arise in healthcare ethics, it is often helpful to have an organizational model. For this new edition, the model of a Greek or Roman temple was used in homage to some of the early ethics writers (see Figure 1).

Notice that the foundation of the temple is ethics theory and principles that will be the first part of this new edition. Not only does this section provide a theoretical framework, it also facilitates the analysis of issues presented in subsequent chapters.

The rest of the text is organized around the three main pillars of the model: individual, organizational, and societal issues. An introduction to each part provides an overview of the issues to be discussed in the chapters that follow. Each chapter within the area has its own overview to better acquaint the reader with key chapter concepts. At the end of each chapter, discussion questions provide

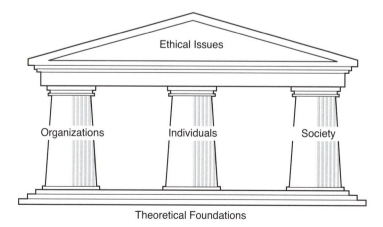

Figure 1 Health Care Ethics Organizational Model

the opportunity for thoughtful analysis and application of the issues raised in the chapter.

Although it is not possible to know all of what the future of health care holds, the expectation for this new edition of *Health Care Ethics: Critical Issues for the 21st Century* is that it will challenge the reader to think beyond the existing system of medicine. It is also hoped that many of the issues will spark curiosity and lead to future exploration and thought. However, the overall intent of this new edition is to increase awareness of future ethical issues and enhance the ability to formulate professional or organizational responses to these issues.

PART I

Foundations in Theory

Healthcare professionals face many issues in dealing with the complexities of both patient treatment and the larger healthcare system. Addressing these issues requires a firm foundation of knowledge and skills in order to provide services that will positively affect patient treatment and organizational outcomes. Certainly, the community expects professionals to have a thorough understanding of the foundation in their professions before they can practice. In short, you are supposed to "know your stuff" if you want to be considered a professional in healthcare.

The same is true with the study of ethics. Ethics in health care is not just about doing the right thing. The issues faced often are exceedingly complex and far from black and white. In addition, society and the health professions themselves often have stringent ethics expectations. In light of these challenges, it seems logical that one must have a solid foundation in the theory and principles of ethics in order to make appropriate professional decisions. The first section of the new edition of *Health Care Ethics: Critical Issues for the 21st Century* begins with two chapters that will provide this foundation.

The foundation in ethics theory and principles provided in these chapters also will give you practical tools for analyzing ethics-related issues that you will encounter in the future. Without an ethics foundation, it would be difficult to develop plausible solutions to the thorny issues that will emerge. Thus, a foundation in theory, principles, and decision making will enhance your ability to reason through whatever problems are presented.

As you face ethics dilemmas in the future, you could ask, "What theory or theories best apply here?" or "If I take this position, what principles will I support or violate?" or "What is the price of not being ethical?" Because ethical issues are usually broader in scope than they appear, you could also think about their affect on individuals, your organization, or on the society in which you live. This type of thinking is and will continue to be necessary in the healthcare environment, where even the smallest issue may have a large impact on professionals and the institutions in which they work.

In an immediate sense, a foundation in ethics theory and principles will be useful to you as a student of this subject matter. The principles and theories explained in this section will frequently be used in subsequent chapters to examine the issues presented. In addition, at the end of each chapter questions are provided to encourage you to take your intellect beyond what you have read. Many of these questions relate directly to the application of a particular theory or principle. By answering these questions, you will enhance the depth of your understanding not only of the specific issue, but also of the application of ethical theory and/or principles.

In Chapter 1, Dr. Summers presents a well-researched overview of the theories commonly used in healthcare ethics. He begins with a model so that you can see where ethics fits into the study of philosophy. Following that, he reviews ethics theories that might not have as much relevance to healthcare practice as other theories, including authority-based ethics, egoism, and ethical relativism. He then presents the most commonly held ethics theories that are applied in healthcare practice. These include natural law, deontology, utilitarianism, and virtue ethics. In his discussions, he uses examples to help you better understand how these theories apply to your professional practice. In fact, he refers to them as part of your *ethics toolbox*.

In Chapter 2, Dr. Summers continues his scholarly discussion of ethics by presenting the four most commonly used principles: nonmaleficence, beneficence, autonomy, and justice. Because justice is the most complex of the four, he provides additional material about the types of justice. He also provides information on how you can decide what is just. At the end of Chapter 2, Summers presents a decision-making model called the *reflective equilibrium model*. This model demonstrates the application of ethics theory and principles in the practice of making clinical and business decisions.

If you read these chapters thoroughly and think about their content, you should be well prepared to discuss the issues presented in this book in a rational way. Many of the issues presented in this text are emotional in nature, but emotional decisions might not be the best ones. Consequently, using the knowledge gleaned from these two chapters should be useful to you as a student and as a professional.

CHAPTER 1

Theory of Healthcare Ethics

Jim Summers

OVERVIEW

In this chapter, Summers presents a scholarly account of the main theories that are applied to the ethics of healthcare situations. Why bother with such a discourse? The answer is that without a foundation, you are left to make decisions without a structure to support them. You would not have the wisdom of the theorists to defend your decisions if you need to do so. In addition, you would not have a knowledge base to analyze the many issues that you will face in health care in the twenty-first century. Therefore, this chapter and the one on the principles of ethics, which follows, will serve as your ethics toolbox.

ETHICS AND HEALTH CARE

From the earliest days of philosophy in ancient Greece, people have sought to apply reason in determining the right course of action for a particular situation and in explaining why it is right. Such discourse is the topic of *normative ethics*. In the twenty-first century, issues resulting from technological advances in medicine and science will continue to provide challenges that will necessitate similar reasoning. Healthcare resource allocations will become more global and more vexing as new diseases threaten, global climate change continues apace, and ever more people around the world find their lives increasingly desperate as disease and poverty overtake them. Managers of healthcare organizations will find the resources to carry out their charge increasingly constrained by lack of money and labor shortages. A foundation in ethics theory and ethical decision-making tools can help in assessing the choices to be made in these vexing circumstances.

Knowledge of ethics can also be valuable when working with other healthcare professionals, patients and their families, and policy makers. In this sense, ethical understanding, particularly of alternative views, becomes a form of cultural competence.[1] However, this chapter is confined to a discussion of normative ethics and metaethics. By definition, *normative ethics* is the study of what is right and wrong; *metaethics* is the study of ethical concepts. Normative ethics examines ethical theories and their application to various disciplines, such as health care. In health care, ethical concepts derived from normative theories, such as autonomy, beneficence, justice, and nonmaleficence, often are used to guide decision making.[2] These concepts and principles are discussed in Chapter 2.

As one might suspect, when normative ethics seeks to determine the moral views or rules that are appropriate or correct and explain why they are correct, major disagreements in the interpretation often result. Those disagreements influence the application of views in many areas of moral inquiry, including health care, business, warfare, environmental protection, sports, and engineering. Figure 1–1 lists the most common normative ethical theories. Each of these theories will be considered in the text. Although no single theory has generated consensus in the ethics community, there is no cause for despair.

The best way to interpret these various ethical theories, some of which overlap, is as a toolbox. Each of these theories teaches something and provides tools that can assist with decision making. The choice of tools in the ethics toolbox depends significantly on our professional role in health care. One advantage of the toolbox approach is that you will not find it necessary to choose one ethical theory over another for all situations. You can choose the best theory for the task, according to the requirements of the role and the circumstances. Trained philosophers will find flaws with this approach, but hopefully, the practical advantages will suffice to overcome these critiques.

All of the theories presented have a value in the toolbox, although like any tool, some are more valuable than others; for example, I shall argue that virtue ethics has much more value for healthcare applications. Before explaining why this chapter has chosen to present particular theories, a quick overview is in order:

- Authority-based theories can be faith based, such as Christian, Muslim, Hindu, or Buddhist ethics. They could also be purely ideological, such as those based on the writings of Karl Marx (1818–1883) or on capitalism. Essentially, authority-based theories determine the right thing to do based on what some authority has said. The job of the ethicist is to determine what that authority would decree for the situation at hand.

- Natural law theory, as considered here, will use the tradition of St. Thomas Aquinas (1224–1274) as the starting point of interpretation. The key idea behind natural law is that nature is ordered rationally and providentially. The right thing to do is that which is in accord with the providentially ordered nature of the world. In health care, natural law theories are important, owing to the influence of the Roman Catholic Church and Aquinas as an early writer in the field of ethics. Several important debates, such as those surrounding abortion, euthanasia, and social justice, draw upon concepts with roots in natural law theory.

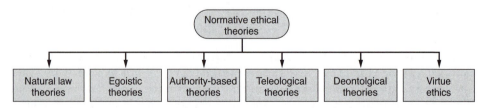

Figure 1–1 Normative ethical theories.

- Teleological theories consider the ethics of a decision to be dependent on the consequences of the action. Thus, these theories are more commonly known as *consequentialism*. The basic idea is to maximize the good of a situation. The originators of the theory, Jeremy Bentham (1748–1832) and John Stuart Mill (1806–1873), called this maximization of good *utility*, thus this theory is most often referred to as *utilitarianism*.

- Deontological theories are usually traced to Immanuel Kant (1724–1804). The term *deon* is from the Greek and means "duty." Thus, deontology could be called the science of determining our duties. Most authors place Kant in extreme opposition to consequentialism, because he argued that the consequences themselves are not relevant in determining what is right. Thus, doing the right thing might not always lead to an increase in the good.[3]

- Virtue ethics has the longest tenure among all of these views, except for authority-based theories. Its roots can be traced to Plato (427–347 BCE) and to Aristotle (384–322 BCE). The key idea behind virtue ethics is to find the proper end for humans and then to seek that end. In this sense, people seek their perfection or excellence. Virtue ethics comes into play as people seek to live virtuous lives, developing their potential for excellence to the best of their ability. Thus, virtue ethics addresses issues any thinking person should consider, such as "What sort of person should I be?" and "How should we live together?" Virtue ethics can contribute to several of the other theories in a positive way, particularly in the understanding of professional ethics and in the training necessary to produce ethical professionals.

- Egoistic theories argue that what is right is that which maximizes a person's self-interests. Such theories are of considerable interest in contemporary society due to their relationship to capitalism. However, the ethical approach of all healthcare professions is to put the interests of the patient above the practitioners' personal interests. Even when patients are not directly involved, such as with healthcare managers, the role is described as a *fiduciary relationship*, meaning that patients can trust that their interests come before those of the practitioners. Egoistic theories are so at odds with the value systems of nearly all healthcare practitioners that it is not necessary to take them up in any depth.

Before exploring any of these ethical theory tools in depth, it is first necessary to confront the relativist argument, which denies that ethics really means anything.

ETHICAL RELATIVISM

Those who deal with ethical issues, whether in everyday life or in practice, will inevitably hear the phrase "It is all relative." Given that the purpose of this text is to help healthcare professionals deal with real-world ethical issues, it is important to determine what this phrase means and the appropriate course of action. No satisfactory ethical theory has been developed that covers every situation. In fact, philosophers are expert at finding flaws in any theory, thus no theory will be infallible. It is also well known that different cultures and different groups have varying opinions about what is right and wrong and how to behave in certain situations.[4]

Does the fact that people's views differ mean that any view is acceptable? This appears to be what is meant by statements such as "It is all relative." In that sense, deciding that something is right or wrong, or good or bad, has no more significance than choices of style or culinary preferences. Thus, ethical decision making and practice is a matter of aesthetics or preferences, with no foundation to ground it. This view makes a normative claim that there is no real right or wrong or good or bad.

One could equally say that there is no truth in science, because scientists disagree about the facts and nothing is ever proven, only falsified by experiment.[5] However, the intrinsic lack of final certainty in the empirical sciences does not render them simply subjective. As one commentator on the rapid changes in scientific knowledge put it, these changes reveal "the extraordinary intellectual and imaginative yields that a self-critical, self-evaluating, self-testing, experimental search for understanding can generate over time."[6] Why should we expect any better of ethics?

Sometimes the claim is made that because there are many perspectives, there cannot be a universal truth about ethics. Therefore, we are essentially on our own. A very helpful essay by Hugh LaFollettee showed a way out of these issues.[7] LaFollettee argued that the lack of an agreed-upon standard or the inability to generalize an ethical theory does not render ethical reasoning valueless. Rather, the purpose of ethical theories is to help people decide the right course of action when they are faced with troubling decisions. Some ethical theories work better in some situations than others. The theories themselves provide standards, akin to grammar and spelling rules, as to when something is properly executed using that theory.

Thus, even though ethics might not produce final answers, we are still called upon to make decisions. Ethics theories and principles are tools to help us in that necessary endeavor. The lack of absoluteness in ethical theory also does not eliminate rationality. Often, we simply must apply our rationality without knowing if we are correct. The better our understanding of ethics, the more likely it is that the decision we reach will be appropriate.

ETHICAL THEORIES

Let's begin to examine the tools in the toolbox, knowing that we are fallible, but also that we are rational, too.[8] The first tool has little application to healthcare ethics; however, it is widely believed, and therefore it must be addressed. It involves the idea of egoism in ethics.

Egoism

Egoism operates from the premise that people either should (a normative claim) seek to advance solely their own self-interests or that (psychologically) this is what actually people do. The normative version, *ethical egoism*, sets as its goal the benefit, pleasure, or greatest good of the self alone.[9] In modern times, the theory of ethical egoism has become popularized through the writings of Ayn Rand[10] and her theory of *objectivism*.[11] For example, Rand said, "The pursuit of his own rational self-interest and of his own happiness is the highest moral purpose of his life."[12] This is a normative statement, and a reasonable description of ethical egoism.

Although this theory has importance to the larger study of ethics, it is less important in healthcare ethics, because the healing ethic itself requires a sublimation of self-interests to those of the patient. A healthcare professional who fails to do this is essentially not a healthcare professional. No codes of ethics in the healthcare professions declare the interests of the person in the professional role to be superior to those of the patient.

> A healthcare professional who does not understand the need to sublimate his or her own interests to those of the patient or his or her role has not yet become a health professional.

Although occasionally healthcare professionals do not put the patient's best interest first, it is not a goal of the profession. Thus, we leave egoism of any form behind.

Authority-Based Ethical Theories

Most teaching of ethics ignores religion-based ethical theories, much to the chagrin of those with deep religious convictions. The use of religion-based ethics in healthcare practice should be avoided for several reasons. These include:

Which Authority Is the Correct One?

Authority-based approaches, whether based on a religion or an ideology, such as communism or capitalism, are flawed relative to the criteria needed to qualify as a normative ethical theory. Each of the authority-based approaches claims to be normative relative to everyone. Because many of these authority-based approaches conflict, there is no way to sort them out other than by an appeal to reason. There are other philosophical issues in addition to the difficulty of finding a way to agree on which of the opposing inerrant authorities is correct. For example, religious theories add an unnecessary layer of complexity to the argument and, at the same time, make defense of their claims more difficult. When faced with two competing theories that each seem to adequately explain the phenomenon, the appropriate choice is to choose the simpler explanation.

Religions and Health Care

All religions provide explanations of the cause or the meaning of disease and suffering. Many theologies also encourage believers to take steps to remove or ameliorate causes of disease and suffering. Over the millennia, some of these religions have even formalized their positions by becoming involved with health care.

In addition, patients often have religious views that help them to understand and cope with their conditions. Understanding a person's faith can help the clinician provide health care that is more patient focused.[13] For some patients, an ethical issue arises if their faith or lack of a faith practice is neither recognized nor respected.

Beyond direct patient care, a second reason to understand the authority-based philosophies common in the healthcare environment is their affect on healthcare policy. The role of authority-based ethical positions appears to be gaining importance in the twenty-first century. To be effective working within the health policy arena, whether at the institutional, local, regional, state, federal, or international level, an understanding of the influence of the religious views of those involved in the debates and negotiations can only serve to strengthen your ability to reason with them. Proper engagement in healthcare debates or negotiations requires an understanding of the fundamental importance of health and the role of religion and philosophy in healthcare policy. In other words, it is important to understand the "common" morality of those engaged in the debate. The more diversity in beliefs and reasoning, the more important the need for understanding of what those beliefs and reasoning might be.

Religion also plays an important role in the creation of healthcare policy because religions have provided a multiplicity of philosophical answers to questions about the nature and truth of the world and how we should act in it. They explain what is considered right or wrong and why it is right or wrong. They also help people define who they are, their role in the world, and how they should relate to one another. Religions explain the nature of the world relative to our place in it.

Thus, as a tool, understanding authority-based philosophical systems has value because it can help in the treatment of patients. It also increases your understanding about the positions of persons who may be involved in debates over healthcare issues, such as resource allocations, or clinical issues, such as abortion. In addition, it is important to understand authority-based philosophical systems relative to yourself. As a healthcare professional, your role requirements dictate that you do not impose your religious views on patients. At the same time, it is not part of the role for you to accept the imposition of another's values, even those of a patient.

These complex issues relate to professional ethics and are not part of the scope of this chapter. However, it does seem incumbent on all healthcare professionals to evaluate their own faith and to recognize the extent to which they might impose it on others. From the earliest tradition of Hippocrates, the charge was to heal the illness and the patient. More recently, the Declaration of Geneva from the World Medical Association (1983) stated that members of the medical profession would agree to the statement: "I will not permit considerations of religion, nationality, race, party politics, or social standing to intervene between my duty and my patient."[14]

Let's now turn our attention to the oldest non-authority-based ethical theory—virtue ethics.

Virtue Ethics

Virtue ethics traces its roots most especially to Aristotle (384–322 BCE). Aristotle sought to elucidate the highest good for humans. Bringing the potential of that good to actualization requires significant character development. The concept of character development falls into the area of virtue ethics, because its goal is the development of those virtues in the person and the populace.

Aristotle's ethics derived from both his physics and metaphysics. He viewed everything in existence as moving from potentiality to actuality. This is an organic view of the world, in the sense that an acorn seeks to become an oak tree. Thus, your full actuality is potentially within you. As your highest good, your potential actuality is already inherent, because it is part of your nature; it only needs development, nurture, and perfecting. This idea is still with us in many respects as part of the common morality.

Finding Our Highest Good

Just what did Aristotle conclude was our final cause or our highest good? The term Aristotle uses for this is *eudaimonia*. The typical translation is "happiness." However, this translation is inadequate and many scholars have suggested enhancements. Many prefer to use the translation "flourishing." However, any organic entity can flourish, such as a cactus, so the term is not an adequate synonym.

The major complaint about translating *eudaimonia* as "happiness" is that our modern view of happiness would render it subjective. No one can know if you are happy or not; you are the final arbiter. Aristotle thought *eudaimonia* applied only to humans, because it required rationality that goes beyond mere happiness. In addition, *eudaimonia* includes a strong moral component that is lacking from our modern understanding of happiness. In this sense, "happiness" would necessarily include doing the right thing, being virtuous. Others could readily judge if you were living a virtuous or "happy" life by observing your actions. For Aristotle, happiness is not a disposition, as in "he is a happy sort."

Eudaimonia is an activity. Indeed, children and other animals, unable to engage self-consciously in rational and virtuous activities cannot yet be in the state translated as "happy."[15] Because it is commonplace to describe children as being "happy," this is clearly not an adequate translation. Given these translation problems, I shall use the term *eudaimonia* rather than its translations of "happiness" or "flourishing." Essentially, *eudaimonia* is best understood as a perfection of character nurtured by engaging in virtuous acts over a life of experience.

> Essentially, *eudaimonia* is best understood as a perfection of character nurtured by engaging in virtuous acts over a life of experience.

The most important element of *eudaimonia* is the consideration of what it takes to be a person of good character. Such a person seeks to develop excellence in himself or herself. To be excellent, what sort of person should I be? Because Aristotle recognized the essential social and political nature of humans, the answer to this question would necessarily have to include consideration of how we should live together.

Developing a Professional as a Person of Character

Consider what it takes to develop a competent and ethical healthcare professional. The process involves a course of study at an accredited university taught by persons with credentials and experience in the field. It also includes various field experiences, such as clerkships, internships, and residencies or clinical experiences with patients. Part of the education includes coming to an understanding of what behaviors are appropriate for the role, which is often called *professional socialization*.

For all healthcare professions, the educational process includes a substantial dose of the healing ethic by specific instruction or by observation of role models. The most fundamental idea behind this healing ethic as a form of role formation is the healthcare professional's sublimation of his or her self-interests to the needs of the patient. This education also includes recognition of the idea that the healing ethic means first do no harm and that whatever actions are taken should provide a benefit.[16]

The Character of a Physician

The goal of professional education and socialization is to produce healthcare professionals of high character. Many professional ethics codes describe the character traits that define high character. These traits might also be considered virtues.[17] For example, the 2001 American Medical Association statement of the principles of medical ethics states that the principles are "standards of conduct which define the essentials of honorable behavior for the physician."[18] Essentially, the principles define the appropriate character traits or virtues for a physician.

Relative to virtue ethics, these traits or virtues combine to create not only a good physician, but also a person of good character. Like Aristotle's person of virtue, engaging in the activities of *eudaimonia* (clearly the translation "happiness" does not fit here) produces practical wisdom. "Moral virtue comes about as a result of habit."[19] The virtues come into being in us because "we are adapted by nature to receive them, and they are made perfect by habit."[20]

Not only is practice required, but the moral component is indispensable. Good physicians are not merely technically competent; they are persons of good character. How do we know this? Their actions coalesce to reveal integrity. In addition, a physician or any other person of good character does not undertake to do what is right simply to appear ethical. In a modern sense, the properly socialized physician or person has internalized the ethical expectations. To do the right things is part of their identity.[21]

To use Aristotle's term, physicians have become persons of practical wisdom. The mere fact that inculcation of such character traits is so important in all healthcare professions indicates the extent to which these ancient teachings are part of the common morality, or at least the professional morality within the healthcare professions. It is part of our cultural competence. In short, persons of virtue nurture *eudaimonia* because they believe it is the right way to live and "[w]ith the presence of practical wisdom will be given all the virtues."[22] Good physicians are living excellent lives; perfecting themselves is part of their self-identity.[23] These persons will, as a matter of course, act on the ethical principles that form the core of their identification of themselves with their role. In health care, principles function as virtues.

Principles of Biomedical Ethics as Virtues

The authors Tom Beauchamp and James Childress have popularized what they call the "principles of biomedical ethics" in texts that have gone through five editions, from 1978 to 2001.[24] These well-known principles are provided in the following list along with brief definitions (an extended discussion of these principles is provided in Chapter 2):

- *Autonomy* is the ability to decide for oneself. The word derives from the Greek word for "self" (*auto*) and "rule" (*nomos*). It means that people are free to make their own decisions. The failure to respect the personhood of others, making decisions for them without their consent, is *paternalism*.

- *Beneficence* is from the Latin root *bene*, meaning "to do well." More specifically, it derives from the Latin term *benefacere*, meaning "to do a kindness, provide a benefit." It is the practice of doing the good thing. Health care has clearly valued beneficence from its early Hippocratic origins. It is the second part of the dictum "first do no harm, benefit only." Professionalism requires healthcare practitioners to put the patients' interests before their own. When combined with beneficence, healthcare professionals hold dear the value, norm, or virtue of altruism.

- *Nonmaleficence* derives from the Latin *mal*, meaning "bad." A *malevolent* person wishes ill of someone. Thus, nonmaleficence means to *NOT* do wrong toward another. Clearly, this captures the first part of the Hippocratic dictum: "first do no harm . . ."

- *Justice* is a concept with a vast history and multiple interpretations. The etymology is Latin, and suggests more than just fairness. The terms *just* and *justice* include elements of righteousness ("she is a just person"), equity ("she received her just due"), and lawfulness ("to bring to justice").[25] A just person is fair, lawful, reasonable, correct, and honest.[26] Most writers in ethics discuss two kinds of justice: distributive and procedural. *Distributive justice* determines if burdens and benefits are shared properly. *Procedural justice* determines if the rules were applied properly in the hearing of a case. Because of the importance of justice in resource allocations, this topic will be discussed at length in Chapter 2.

I agree with Beauchamp and Childress that these concepts are foundational principles of healthcare ethics.[27] A person having these virtues as part of his or her character structure, self-definition, and actions would be considered to be a person of good character. In healthcare terms, such a person would be walking the talk of the healing ethic and would be a person of practical wisdom.

Elitism

A person who seeks to nurture *eudaimonia* through his or her actions achieves this goal after long practice of Aristotle's practical wisdom. Such a person also sets the standard for the right action in a particular situation. Thus, virtue ethics has the problem of being elitist. Aristotle was quite aware of this elitism, but it did not pose a problem to him 2300 years ago. He thought that some people were simply not capable of maximizing their potential to reach the highest good, owing to his view of the hierarchical nature of reality.[28]

Aristotle noted the difficulty of encouraging many to a character of virtue; a life of nobility and goodness.[29] Aristotle believed that most people are motivated by fear, living by emotions, and pursuing pleasures. They lack even a conception of the noble and truly pleasant, having never known it. Aristotle seemed to despair that once these bad traits have long been in place, they are impossible to remove. He concluded, "we must be content if, when all the influences by which we are thought to be good are present, we get some tincture of virtue."[30] The person of practical wisdom becomes the standard for ethical decision making. This leads to an understanding of how virtue ethics can facilitate the management of ethical conflicts.

Balancing Obligations from the Virtue Ethics Perspective

It is not possible to practice in the healthcare profession for long without encountering some kind of ethical dilemma because different principles of ethics or different virtues conflict. For example, some treatments involve harm yet provide a benefit. An experienced healthcare professional must be able to explain the relative benefits and risks and gain the cooperation of the patient for such treatments.

Sometimes one principle might create conflict. For example, physicians must know how to tell the truth to patients. Even though information can be regarded as therapy, information delivered at the wrong time or in the wrong way can be devastating. Information not delivered at the right time or never delivered at all could mean that the physician is not being honest and is guilty of paternalism. Learning how to deal with these issues effectively takes experience and theoretical knowledge.

A major component of the patient–clinician relationship is the patients' trust that their caregivers have their best interests at heart and that they are competent. If patients perceive caregivers as persons of integrity, virtue, or practical wisdom, their confidence in their caregivers will increase. That increase in the patients' confidence has documented effects on enhancing the placebo effect.[31] How caregivers communicate, and even how they carry themselves, will do much to influence these perceptions.[32] The caregiver who knows how to do these things, who is an exemplar of the character traits and the virtues in the AMA's Principles of Medical Ethics, is a person of practical wisdom, at least when it comes to medical practice.

Caregivers with practical wisdom, which by necessity includes being of good character or virtuous, will be able to make appropriate decisions about the means to ends. This has significant implications for healthcare ethics. When faced with ethical challenges in medical care, such caregivers will have the practical wisdom to know how to weigh the various issues and concerns and form a conclusion. Because wise and good people can, and do, come to different conclusions about the ethically appropriate choice of action, persons of practical wisdom should consult with one another.

Healthcare organizations have sought to institutionalize this approach by using ethics committees. Those with practical wisdom in health care are far ahead in having a decades-long tradition of ethics committees, ethics consultations, institutional review boards, and the like. These administrative mechanisms make it easier to manage disagreement. The key here is that persons of good character, pursuing virtuous ends, are much more likely to make an appropriate choice than those without such experience or such character. These choices would appear to refute one of the usual criticisms levied against virtue ethics: that there is no clear way on how to resolve disputes when those who have practical wisdom disagree about the correct course of action.

Virtue ethics thus leads to the conclusion that, within health care at least, the probability is good that persons socialized to put the patient's interests first will come up with the ethically correct ranking of options. They will also respect the patient's wishes, even if they do not agree with those wishes. Of course, this depiction makes the situation sound much better than it is. Persons well trained in the healing ethic take unethical actions everyday. Is that a fault of the education or the person? Aristotle would fault the person. In Aristotle's view, some people, by nature, are unable to control their passions, their desires, and their emotions. Others are unable to act rationally. Some are just wicked.[33] Yes, the theory results in a form of elitism. However, it seems fair to say that health care has a major advantage over many other fields in that it has a strong educational and socialization process for developing the right character. In a sense, the purpose of the educational process is to develop a cadre of elite professionals. In doing so, they should become persons of high character.

Ethical Theories and Professional Roles

A knowledge of virtue ethics offers one further advantage. A person of practical wisdom should be better prepared to know when to use a particular ethical theory, depending on the role in which they find themselves. Again,

take physicians as an example. Although physicians have a primary obligation to their patients, it is not their only role. Consider the following physician roles, none of which involves patients directly: conducting scientific
studies; negotiating with vendors selling equipment and supplies; and hiring, firing, and supervising employees. In addition, physicians might be
negotiating with third-party payers, lobbying on behalf of health policy
issues, and conducting peer review of other physicians. They might also be
involved in the management of healthcare organizations and participate on
various advisory and regulatory agency boards. Many other non-patient-
related tasks could be listed, such as working with community groups or
serving as faculty as needed.

Some of the ethical theories work better in these roles than others. How do
physicians choose the appropriate theory? The socialization process develops
caregivers who are persons seeking the highest good, at least in health care.
This foundational process should develop persons of integrity and practical
wisdom who can manage the inevitable ethical dilemmas and make the best
ethics decisions in any role. They can apply reason to the situation and make
the best possible decision within their respective role.

Natural Law

The theory of natural law owes a great debt to Aristotle. Natural law also is
important to Roman Catholic theology, given its origins with St. Thomas
Aquinas. Many texts on ethics and medical ethics leave out natural law or
give it short shrift. Some authors consider the theory a version of moderate
deontology, defining *deontology* as having a different view from consequentialism . . . .[34] In the realm of healthcare ethics, such an approach appears overly
limiting. As a tool in the ethical theory toolbox, there are a number of good
reasons to know natural law theory. Even if philosophically this theory can be
reduced to another, natural law is sufficiently definitive and important to consider on its own merits.[35]

One key to understanding natural law is its assumption that nature is
rational and orderly. This theory goes back to the ancient Greeks, who
believed that the cosmos was essentially unchanging in its order. Aristotle certainly believed in this.[36] This is now a statement of physics—a statement
about the nature of the world—rather than a statement about ethics.

Natural Law's Relationship to Aristotle, St. Thomas Aquinas, and the Catholic Church

Aquinas' beliefs gained prominence in the Catholic Church at the Council
of Trent (1545–1563) when Catholic reformers used his works to draft their
decrees. In 1879, Pope Leo XIII declared Thomism (Aquinas' theology) to be
eternally valid.[37] Nearly all writers recognize St. Thomas Aquinas as setting
the standard for natural law theory, just as Aristotle is recognized as the
standard bearer for virtue ethics.[38] Aquinas developed his theory in his work
entitled *Summa Theologica*, meaning the "highest theology." The work is
structured in the form of a series of questions, which St. Thomas answers. He
also answers the criticisms of the questions to develop his theology. The

major treatment of natural law occurs in what is called the treatise on law, or question 94, although there are many other relevant passages in other sections as well.[39]

The Thomistic conception of *natural law* proceeds as follows: "All things subject to Divine providence are ruled and measured by the eternal law" (ST IaIIae 91, 2). "The rational creature is subject to Divine providence in the most excellent way. . . . Wherefore it has a share of the Eternal Reason, whereby it has a natural inclination to its proper act and end: and this participation of the eternal law in the rational creature is called the natural law" (ST IaIIae 91, 2). This establishes that natural law is given by God and thus authoritative over all humans.

Aquinas went on to argue that all humans, as rational animals, can potentially know this law. "The light of natural reason, whereby we discern what is good and what is evil, which is the function of the natural law, is nothing else than an imprint on us of the Divine light. It is therefore evident that the natural law is nothing else than the rational creature's participation of the eternal law" (ST IaIIae 91, 2). Not only can we know the law, as rational and moral creatures we can violate it.

Recall Aristotle's concept of practical wisdom; Aquinas uses the same concept. In fact, he calls Aristotle "the Philosopher" and cites him as frequently as Scripture. The importance of practical reason, how it works, its similarity to Aristotle's conception of it, and the most concise statement of what the natural law compels are all found in the following quote:

> "Good" is the first thing that falls under the apprehension of the practical reason, which is directed to action: since every agent acts for an end under the aspect of good. Consequently the first principle of practical reason is one founded on the notion of good, viz. that "good" is that which all things seek after." Hence, this is the first precept of law, that good is to be done and pursued, and evil is to be avoided." All other precepts of the natural law are based upon this: so that whatever the practical reason naturally apprehends as man's good (or evil) belongs to the precepts of the natural law as something to be done or avoided (ST IaIIae 94, 2).

Unfortunately, some have stopped at this quote and simply say that natural law means to "do the good and avoid the evil."[40] Because this lacks clarity about what the good might be or any decision rule by which to decide what to do when goods conflict or when rankings are required, this statement alone does not constitute an ethical theory. It sells the theory short.[41]

Aquinas also drew on Aristotle's idea of potentiality moving to actuality and states that in the realm of what is good "all desire their own perfection" (ST Ia 5, 1). Only the fully actual would have full perfection, but anything that exists even in a relative way has some perfection (ST Ia 5, 1).[42] Again following Aristotle's lead, Aquinas notes that when it comes to practical reason, the rules might be clear, but their application might not be. In short, the details make the principle more difficult to apply (ST IaIIae 94, 4).

St. Thomas then offers an excellent example that shows the difficulty at hand. Everyone would agree that in general "goods entrusted to another should be restored to their owner," (ST IaIIae 94, 4). However, he noted that "it may happen in a particular case that it would be injurious, and therefore unreasonable, to restore goods held in trust; for instance, if they are claimed for the purpose of fighting against one's country. And this principle will be found to fail the more, according as we descend further into detail" (ST IaIIae 94, 4). Taking this practical wisdom approach even further, he generalized that "the greater the number of conditions added, the greater the number of ways in which the principle may fail" (ST IaIIae 94, 4).

Aquinas even went so far as to note that, although all are governed by the natural law, all might not know it or act upon it: "In some the reason is perverted by passion, or evil habit, or an evil disposition of nature" (ST IaIIae 94, 4).[43] This seems to add a quandary. All decisions are specific and the details will change, so how do we know what to do?

At this point, scholars disagree on exactly how Aquinas resolves the quandary, and we do not need to follow them in those debates. However, a decision principle is still needed for when there are disputes among the various actions that can be taken. The one most closely associated with natural law theory is discussed next.

Principle of Double Effect

The first principle that proposes to distinguish between the good and the evil is the *theory of double effect*. Derived from *Summa Theologica*, the principle has four key points:

- That we do not wish the evil effects, but make all reasonable efforts to avoid them;
- That the immediate effect be good in itself;
- That the evil is not made a means to obtain the good effect; for this would be to do evil that good might come of it—a procedure never allowed; the end cannot justify the mean;
- That the good effect be as important at least as the evil effect.[44]

The theory of double effect has use in applied ethics, such as medical ethics, when dealing with abortion, euthanasia, and other decisions where there is a conflict between a good and an evil. For example, abortion is an evil, but saving the life of a mother is a good. Euthanasia is an evil, but relieving pain by use of morphine is a good. If the person dies, and it was not intended, then is it acceptable? Major issues arise in the application of the theory concerning how to determine a person's intent. We know that not everyone is a person of practical wisdom who only has a good intent. However, how would we know this?[45]

At the policy-making level, is it acceptable to cut taxes for the rich at the expense of the poor? What good comes of it? Because there are few rich and many poor, does the good of the rich count more than the good lost by the poor? Note that the further we delve into these types of questions, the more important consequences seem to become, until natural law becomes a form of consequentialism, perhaps rule consequentialism.[46] It is not necessary to resolve these disputes here, because the purpose is to understand the theories for the purposes of making appropriate decisions in health care. Relative to that end, a second decision rule for natural law is available.

Entitlement to Maximize Your Potential

In seeking a principle to determine what is good and what is bad, it was not difficult to find specific behaviors listed in Aquinas. However, an excellent philosophical overview of natural law by Michael Murphy concluded that there are no obvious master principles, but plenty examples of flawed acts.[47] A lengthy article on ethics in the *Catholic Encyclopedia* suggests a goodly number of things that would be wrong or right under the dictum to always do good and avoid harm, but nothing about how to resolve conflicts among these requirements.[48]

The key to understanding this proposed decision rule relates to metaphysics: "Ethics especially is impossible without metaphysics, since it is according to the metaphysical view we take of the world that ethics shapes itself."[49] The Thomistic ethic draws heavily on the Aristotelian metaphysics that describes the world as a hierarchy of being, with all entities in it striving to reach their own complete state of actualization of their potential. This means that it is a part of the natural order for all entities to strive to maximize their potential. To deny something its ability to actualize its potential is to violate its very nature. Such a violation causes harm to the entity and would be a violation of its nature and the natural law to avoid harm. Thus, natural law proscribes any activities that would violate an entity's potential.[50] Concerns about termination of potential, at least for rational creatures, are evident in several contemporary healthcare issues.

Abortion, Euthanasia, and Social Justice

The ethics of natural law ethics are based on pursing perfection (the ability to know God), using God's providence that gives us the desire to move from potentiality to actuality, and having an obligation to do the good and avoid the evil. Once you understand the metaphysics and the meaning of the natural laws that flow from this theory, it is easy to understand why adherents of natural law would be opposed to several kinds of activity. For example, under natural law

- Abortion is clearly wrong, because it terminates the potential of a being ensouled at conception. The dead have no further potential to actualize, and life is the *sine qua non*[51] of having a potential to actualize.
- Arguments against birth control are similar to those used against abortion.
- Euthanasia is not quite so clear a violation of natural law, because medical technology is extending life and dying beyond anything imaginable to the theory's founders as being natural. Nonetheless, to take a life early, even to relieve suffering (*active euthanasia*), is to terminate a life ahead of its time. This cuts short what the life could have been. *Passive euthanasia* means simply allowing the person to die without doing anything to hasten the death. This includes not doing anything heroic to intervene. The definition of *heroic* changes as medical technology advances. Considerable discussion about the duty to alleviate

suffering, what it means to "play God," and whether that is avoidable occupy medical ethics.[52] The double-effect theory plays a major role in these discussions.

- Suicide is directly opposed because a person's life is not his or her own; it belongs to God. According to natural law, it is wrong to undermine the right God has to your person.[53] Obviously, suicide terminates the person's potential as well.

Many religions and social activists place a considerable emphasis on social and political factors that prevent humans from actualizing their potential. These groups often are at the forefront of social justice movements addressing poverty, ignorance, unhealthy living conditions, and slavelike working conditions. Clearly, healthcare professionals need to understand natural law theory when working with patients who believe in its tenets and with those who advocate social justice. This might include those who are working to improve public health, social conditions, and/or human rights. Now let us look at another common ethical theory, deontology.

Deontology

The term *deontology* is derived from the Greek word *deon*, which means "duty." Thus, deontology is concerned with behaving ethically by meeting our duties. The ethical theory of deontology originates with the German philosopher Immanuel Kant (1724–1804).[54] Although, Kant's influence on deontology is significant, many other thinkers are part of the deontological tradition as well.[55] Nonetheless, just as we relied on Aristotle for virtue ethics and on Aquinas for natural law, Kant sets the standard for deontology. Before exploring the usefulness of Kant's theory, a detailed explanation of the theory is required. Note that Kant is one of the more difficult of philosophers to follow.

Kant's Metaphysics and Epistemology Ground His Ethics

Kant is most well known for his work in metaphysics and epistemology, the *Critique of Pure Reason*,[56] but he also did groundbreaking work in ethics. Kant's writings on ethics appear in several different volumes, with titles such as *Groundwork of the Metaphysics of Morals*[57] and *Critique of Practical Reason*,[58] among others.

The concept of honoring commitments clearly did not start with Kant, but his approach to the issue led to the identification of his ethical theory with deontology. Kant's work in metaphysics and epistemology had a significant influence on this approach and his ethical views. In what he called a "Copernican revolution for philosophy," Kant concluded that the belief that perception represented the world was incorrect, or at least incomplete. Instead, the structure of consciousness processes sense data through the means of categories of thought and two forms of intuition: space and time.

Of these categories of thought, the one that relates most directly to ethics is causality. All experiences are subject to causation, which in Kant's view undermines free will. In fact, he finds free will to be essential for ethics. If a person's every act is determined, how can he or she be held responsible for his or her choices?

At the same time, Kant's reasoning inexorably leads him to conclude that we cannot know what the world is like in and of itself. It is beyond knowing, because we cannot experience anything without use of the categories and forms of intuition. He thus divided the realm of being into the *phenomenal world* of experience and the *noumenal world*. We can think about the noumenal world, but we cannot directly experience it. Thus, we have "an unavoidable ignorance of things in themselves and all that we can theoretically *know* are mere appearances" (B xxix).[59] Relative to ethics, it should be clear from Kant's perspective that the metaphysical issue of whether free will is possible is foundational.[60]

Relative to morality, Kant argued that knowledge of the sensible world was insufficient for knowing the moral law.[61] Yet Kant argued that free will makes ethics possible. Free will is the precondition of ethics. If all things are determined by natural causes—causality is one of the categories—then our supposed ethical choices are specious, an illusion. The human as a natural phenomenon is determined by natural laws; causality applies to all natural phenomena. However, the self, in and of itself (the soul), is free from those laws.[62]

Kant recognized that this puts morality beyond the pale of empirical science, and indeed the question about free will is beyond such testing. However, Kant believed that he left a crack in the door that is wide enough to allow for morality. He does this by arguing that the concept of freedom, although not knowable in a scientific way, is something we can think about without contradiction: "Morality does not, indeed, require that freedom should be understood, but only that it should not contradict itself, and so should at least allow of being thought" (B xxix).[63] In this sense, Kant redefines humans as partaking in two kinds of reality: the phenomenal and the noumenal. According to Kant, "There is no contradiction in supposing that one and the same will is, in the appearance, that is, in its visible acts, necessarily subject to the law of nature, and so far *not free*, while yet, as belonging to a thing in itself, is not subject to that law, and is therefore *free*" (B xxviii).[64]

Freedom of the Will

Like Aristotle and Aquinas, Kant certainly thought good character was laudable. However, he was concerned that the properties that constitute good character, without a good will to correct them, could lead to bad outcomes. For example, courage and perseverance can be misused without the direction of good will.[65] Kant would go so far as to argue that one should act on the duty of obligation to the moral law regardless of any relationship that might have an outcome such as *eudaimonia*:[66] "A good will is good not because of what it performs or effects, not by its aptness for the attainment of some proposed end, but simply by virtue of its volition, that is, it is good in and of itself" (AK 4:394).[67] In other words, good will is good because it wills properly. Thus, Kant set a high standard. Some of his language even suggests that the true test of a good will is if the person continues to act out of duty and reverence for the moral law even when it has no personal benefit and might "involve many a disappointment to the ends of inclination" (AK 4:396).[68]

Reason, Autonomy, the Moral Law, and the Will

Kant is distinctive relative to his predecessors in seeking to ground our duties in a self-governing will. This is an appeal to reason itself being autonomous, meaning we are free to choose, and that if we choose according to reason, we shall conform to the moral law: "If reason completely determined the will, the action would without exception take place according to the rule" (AK 5:20).[69] One can see the extremely prominent principle of autonomy coming into play here.

Typically, an autonomous agent is one who makes his or her own rules and is responsible for his or her actions.[70] To violate that autonomy is to violate a person's innermost selfhood, something Kant develops as one form of the categorical imperative. Thus, the foundation of ethics is sought not in the development of a person of good character seeking to actualize his or her intrinsic nature, seeking the end of *eudaimonia*.[71] Instead, the subject matter of ethics is not character, but rather the nature and the content of the principles that determine a rational will. The free will is determined by moral principles that cohere with the categorical imperative. This abstruse approach, for many, simply disconnects the moral law and free will from real life.

The idea of autonomy here is not the view that individuals make their own laws. It means the laws that bind you in some sense derive from your own making, your own self.[72] For Kant, the will is free in the sense that it chooses to be bound by those principles of reason. This capacity to make such a choice is what makes humans members of what he called the "kingdom of ends." The person has chosen freely to bind him or herself to the constraints of the categorical imperative and the dictates of reason.

The requirement of the duty to obey the moral law to express a good will brings the notion of intent into the discussion. Why a person acts in such a way as to conform to the moral law is an important component of ethical evaluation in the Kantian scheme. Let us turn to what Kant thought would count as rational principles that would ground ethics or the moral law.

Kant attempted to discover the rational principle that would ground all other ethical judgments. He called this principle the *categorical imperative*. The categorical imperative is not so much a rule as a criterion for determination of what ethical principles meet the test of reason.[73] The imperative would have to be categorical rather than hypothetical, or conditional, because true morality should not depend on individual likes and dislikes or on abilities and opportunities. These are historical "accidents." Any ultimate principle of ethics must transcend them in order to meet the conditions of fairness. Kant developed several formulations of the categorical imperative. The most commonly presented ones follow:[74]

- Always act in such a way that you can also will that the maxim of your action should become a universal law (AK 4:421).[75] This principle often is caricatured as the Golden Rule: Do unto others as you would have them do unto you.[76] This does not capture the full meaning of what Kant had in mind, and may indeed miss the essence of his teachings, as he specifically disavowed that this was his intended meaning (AK 4:430).[77]

- Act so that you treat humanity, both in your own person and in that of another, always as an end and never merely as a means (AK 4:429).[78] Kant spoke of the good society as a place that was a kingdom of ends (AK 4:433–434).[79]

The Categorical Imperative as a Formal Decision Criterion

Although Kant believed that these two statements of the categorical imperative were formally equivalent, the first illustrates the need for moral principles to be applied universally. That a principle be logically consistent was important to Kant. The second formulation points to the radical distinction to be made between things and persons and emphasizes the necessity of respect for persons.

Kant's theory evaluates morality by examining the nature of actions and the will of agents rather than goals achieved. Therefore, a deontological theory looks at intentions rather than outcomes. You have done the right thing when you act out of your obligation to the moral law, not simply because you act in accordance with it. One reason for the emphasis on duties in Kant's deontology is that we are praised or blamed for actions within our control, and that includes our willing, not our achieving. Most people think that there is something wrong with saying that people are good when they do not have a good will and their good outcomes were merely happenstance. Kant *did* care about the outcomes of our actions, but he thought that, as far as the moral evaluation of actions was concerned, consequences did not matter. As Kant pointed out, this total removal of consequences "is strange enough and has no parallel in the remainder of practical knowledge" (AK 5:31).[80] Let us now look at the second version of the categorical imperative, which is much easier to understand and which is foundational in healthcare ethics.

The Categorical Imperative as Respect for Persons

The second version of the categorical imperative emphasizes respect for persons. According to Kant, you should "[s]o act as to treat humanity, whither in thine own person or in that of any other, in every case as an end withal, never as means only" (AK 4:429).[81] People, unlike things, ought never to be merely used. Their value is never a means to our ends; they are ends in themselves. Of course, a person might be useful as a means, but that person must always be treated with respect. Kant holds this view because of his belief that people are rational and that this bestows them with absolute worth: Our "rational nature exists as an end in itself" (AK 4:428).[82] This makes people unique in the natural world. In this sense, it is our duty to give every person consideration, respect, and dignity. Individual human rights are acknowledged and inviolable in a deontological system. The major emphasis on autonomy in health care springs from these considerations and others like it. Although most people who defend autonomy and treating people as ends and not merely as means do not use these formalistic Kantian reasons, this principle of autonomy is foundational in healthcare ethics. It is part of health care's common morality.

The Categorical Imperative and the Golden Rule

According to the categorical imperative, if the maxim or the rule governing an action is not capable of being universalized, then it is unacceptable. Note that universalizability is not the same as universality. Kant's point is not that we would all agree on some rule. Instead, we must logically be able to will that it be made universal. This is why the concept seems very much like the Golden Rule: Do unto others as you would have them do unto you.[83] If you cannot will that everyone follow the same rule, your rule is not a moral one. As indicated earlier, many think Kant's first formulation of the categorical imperative implies or even is a restatement of the Golden Rule. However, Kant specifically repudiates the Golden Rule interpretation (AK 4:430, note 13).[84]

Kant does not believe the Golden Rule properly describes his views. Like most others, he saw the justification for the Golden Rule in terms of consequences and fairness. If it is fair for me to do something, then it should be fair for everyone. Alternatively, in consequential terms, we typically hear officials, merchants, managers, and parents, when exceptions to policy are being sought, say that if I do X for you I have to do X for everyone. If exceptions were made, then the consequences would be bad and unfair.

Kant wanted to get beyond such issues. He wanted to know whether an act was performed out of duty to moral law and thus expressed the good will. He stipulated that the moral agent acting solely out of the good will should ignore empirical considerations such as consequences, fairness, inclinations, and preferences. For Kant, an act carried out from an inclination, no matter how noble, is not an act of morality (AK 4:398).[85] Indeed, he went so far as to say that the less we benefit from acting on the moral law, the more sublime and dignified it is (AK 4:425).[86] He did favor such acts, but resisted calling them "moral."

Acts take on moral worth if the person acts solely from duty to the moral law, absent any emotional inclinations or tangible benefits. This sets up the very difficult standard that we can only know if persons are morally worthy or obeying the moral law when there is nothing in it for them. Their actions would be opposed to their desires, inclinations, even their self-interest. Taking such an extreme position essentially disconnects Kant from the real world of where people live and make ethical judgments.

Virtue Ethics and Kant's Moral Law

Although likely controversial, it seems, for purposes of healthcare ethics, that the best way to make sense of Kant is to conceive of the person of good will in a manner akin to Aristotle's virtue ethics. Thus, to make Kantian deontology useful, you could say that a person of good will also is a person of practical wisdom as described by Aristotle. Does this inclusion of Aristotle reject Kant's work? No, but a critical analysis and comparison to virtue ethics is warranted.

Although Kant's theory suffers from being disconnected from any normal motivational structure in human life, it still has applications in healthcare ethics.[87] The deontological theory emphasizes the attention to duty found in all codes of ethics in health care. Kant put into sharp relief the ethical idea that it is wrong for someone to claim they can follow a principle or maxim that suits their interests, but would not want others to do the same. This analysis is the underpinning of the critique of ethical egoism and relativistic arguments. Most importantly for health care is the recognition of human dignity and autonomy. To use people solely as means to an end, whether as teaching material in medical schools, prisoners in research experiments, or slaves, is fundamentally a violation of all being. Now, having looked at Kant as the representative of deontology, some common critiques of deontology are merited.

Deontology poses two problems that lead many to reject it. First, the statement of categorical imperatives, maxims, duties, rules, or commandments yields only absolutes. Kant really has only one absolute. His absolute is that your action must be motivated solely by a good will, a reverence for, and an obligation to the moral law formalized by the categorical imperative. However, the lack of prescriptive content leaves many unsatisfied. Actions either pass or fail with no allowance for a "gray area." Virtue ethics handles the gray areas by depending on the wisdom of the person of practical wisdom. This is one reason why as an ethical tool virtue ethics enables us to handle the problems of healthcare ethics more robustly.

The inability to make distinctions between lesser evils or greater goods is the other problem. Moral dilemmas are created when duties come into conflict and there is no mechanism for resolving them. Kant, with his very limited description of only one ethical duty—to obey the moral law—can claim to escape this problem within his philosophy. He used the radical view that such decisions are outside the bounds of morality if they are to be based on inclinations or consequences. Defining the real world of ethics in this radical way does not help much when you are faced with decisions that involve your inclinations and the weighing of consequences. Even if you have, as Kant seemed to think, only one duty, it is a formal one, and its various manifestations could conflict.

Virtue ethics and the natural law theory face this problem of conflicting duties as well. For example, whereas abortion is clearly wrong under the natural law theory, the outcome of unwanted children, starving children, child abuse, overcrowding, malnutrition, and so on also have moral bearing. Duties often conflict in healthcare situations. For example, if I tell the truth in some situation, it may lead to someone getting hurt, when a lie could have prevented it. My duty is both not to lie and not to do things that lead others to harm. No matter what I do, a duty is violated. Pure deontology theory does not allow for a theoretically satisfying means of ranking conflicting duties. However, most duty-driven people are not going to be so caught up with the theory of deontology that they find themselves unable to rank conflicting duties. Virtue ethics offers the guidance of a person of practical wisdom using the available tools of considered judgments, common morality, ethical theories, and ethical principles to resolve the difficulty and move on.

Of the theories presented so far, virtue ethics offers a much more useful and helpful approach in achieving ethical processes and ethical outcomes in the realm of healthcare. Virtue ethics is more interested in the development of ethical persons than in the development of maxims and imperatives. The normal understanding of the Golden Rule works perfectly well in ethical decision making within the framework of virtue ethics, even if Kant himself disavowed it.

The policy implications for deontology are significant because of the emphasis on duty and the training of most healthcare professionals in the duties incumbent upon them. The emphasis on duty leads most clinicians to consider themselves deontologists. However, most would balk at the pure Kantian version of duty and would more readily assent to the duties experienced by a person of practical wisdom, following the virtue ethics tradition. Duty-driven clinical staff can walk into a meeting and know in advance what the right thing to do is: to maximize the benefit to their patients. This is their duty, which is usually codified in their professional code of ethics. If they had to rank their duties, they would be patient first, their profession second, other clinical professionals third, with maybe their employing organization a distant fourth.

Having such a clear sense of their duties and having only a few duties on the list makes it very easy for clinicians to talk about their obligations to patient care. In contrast, healthcare managers and officials who make policy have a much more difficult ethical chore. They must balance competing claims among many groups. Their loyalty is not simply to one group, such as patients. For healthcare managers, even if their loyalty is only to patients, that loyalty to them is in the aggregate. Managers represent the organization, whereas clinicians represent the patients. The ethical obligations of managers are much more complex; if the organization fails, the clinicians will not be able to help the patients. Let us now examine the ethical theory that describes how most managers work, consequentialism.[88]

Consequentialism

Consequentialist moral theories evaluate the morality of actions in terms of progress toward a goal or end. The consequences of the action are what matter, not their intent. This is in contrast to previously noted theories (e.g., deontology, virtue ethics, and natural law) that take intent into account. Consequentialism is sometimes called *teleology*, using the Greek term *telos*, which refers to "ends." Thus, the goal of consequentialism is often stated as the greatest good for the greatest number. Consequentialism has several versions, the best known of which is utilitarianism. *Utilitarianism* defines morality in terms of the maximization of the net utility expected for all parties affected by a decision or action. For the purposes of discussion, consequentialism and utilitarianism are used as synonyms.

For the consequentialist, the person's intentions are irrelevant to the ethical evaluation of whether the deed is right or wrong. Outcomes are all that matter. The consequentialist will agree that intentions do matter, but only to the evaluation of a person's character, not the evaluation of the morality of his or her acts. Remember that in natural law, virtue ethics, and deontology, part of the ethical assessment concerns the person's intention. The consequentialist would say that intention simply confuses two issues: (1) whether the act itself is leading to good or bad outcomes and (2) whether the person carrying out the act should be praised for it or not. Consequentialists consider the second issue to be independent of moral consideration relative to the act. It is relevant to the evaluation of the person's moral character. Of course, to leave out intentions completely seems to violate a deep sense of our understanding about what it means to be ethical. Most people find something wrong with saying an act is ethical if it happened by accident.

Types of Consequentialism

The two major types of consequentialism are as follows:[89]

- **Classical utilitarianism (or act consequentialism).** Each act is considered based on its net benefit. This version of utilitarianism has received the most criticism and is not supported by modern ethicists. Nonetheless, it makes a convenient target for those who dislike consequentialism.
- **Rule consequentialism.** The decision maker develops the rules that will have the greatest net benefit.[90] The development of rules to guide conduct is clearly similar to the actions of managers who develop policies.

In organizational healthcare settings, policymaking is an important component of the work, and consequentialism often is used. For example, a diversity policy could readily be construed as being justified by rule consequentialism, as could policies to further informed consent. Lawmakers and administrators who set health policies at the national level also use consequential arguments to justify decisions, such as requirements to provide indigent care or emergency services.

Classical Utilitarianism

Classical utilitarians spoke of maximization of pleasure or happiness. Classical utilitarianism is most often associated with the British philosopher John Stuart Mill (1806–1873). He developed the theory from a pleasure-maximizing version put forward by his mentor Jeremy Bentham (1748–1832). As clearly stated by Mill, the basic principle of utilitarianism is that actions are right to the degree that they tend to promote the greatest good for the greatest number.[91]

Of course, it is unclear what constitutes "the greatest good." For Bentham, it was simply the tendency to augment or diminish happiness or pleasure. Bentham, being a hedonist in theory, did not try to make distinctions about whether one form of pleasure or happiness was better than another.

For Mill, however, not all pleasures were equally worthy. He defined "the good" in terms of well-being and distinguished it not just quantitatively, but also qualitatively, between various forms of pleasure.[92] Mill would be closer to the virtue theory idea of *eudaimonia* as a goal by specifying qualitative distinctions rather than simply adding up units of happiness or pleasure.[93] Indeed, Mill said that one is duty bound to perform some acts, even if they do not maximize utility.[94] In the case of Bentham and Mill, a conception of what is the appropriate aim of human activity is presupposed. Thus, consequentialists would differ from Kant in terms of defining the proper human good because Kant thought the good will was the precondition for deserving happiness. He would not have thought happiness-seeking acts were moral acts, because they derive from inclination.

A defining characteristic of any type of consequentialism is that the evaluation of whether an outcome is good or bad should be, in some sense, measurable, or that the outcomes should be within the realm of predictability. Thus, in the realm of consequentialism, ethical theory attempts to become objective, seeking a foundation that is akin to the sciences. This principle is enshrined in the world of commerce, trade, management, and administration as the *cost-benefit analysis approach*.

As a theory, consequentialism is not tied as closely to its founder as were the previous three theories. Thus, rather than probing the depths of Mill's writing, a more free-ranging approach is used and various versions of consequentialism that are in play today are presented. This approach will avoid the considerable controversies surrounding what Mill meant by his theories[95] and draw out of consequentialism tools that are useful to persons dealing with issues in healthcare ethics.

Relative to what the consequentialism means, Bentham insisted that "the greatest number" included all who were affected by the action in question with "each to count as one, and no one as more than one."[96] Thus, in Bentham's version of the theory the various intrinsic goods that counted as utility would have an equal value, such that one unit of happiness for you is not worth more than one unit of happiness for me. Quite clearly, to talk about units of "happiness" is far-fetched, and indeed that is one of the criticisms of the theory.[97] However, numerous correctives to the theory have been advanced over the years, and some of these are helpful.

Unlike deontology and natural law with conflicting absolutes, consequentialism of any form allows for degrees of right and wrong. If the consequences can be predicted and their utility calculated, then in such situations the choice between actions is clear-cut: Always choose those actions that have the greatest utility. For this reason, the theory has had great appeal in economic and business circles. However, in healthcare decision making the economic view of utility is not fully satisfactory. For example, how do you compute the suffering of someone whose spouse has been disabled? Although attorneys do calculate the monetary value of life years lost when a person is injured, whether monetary settlements can really compensate for a lost livelihood or a broken future is debatable.

In spite of this objection, managers of healthcare organizations, including clinical managers, must often think in terms of the aggregate when evaluating their decisions. Persons taking the tack of a deontologist and trying to fulfill their duty can readily say that their obligation is to the patient. Managers have to consider the patients in the aggregate, the organization, the larger community, and their employees in their decision making. Managers' divided duties and obligations are part of their job descriptions, as opposed to the single obligation to the patient that clinicians enjoy. Managers also are trained to consider their decisions in terms of maximization—the best outcome for the resources expended is the greatest good[98]—or as managers say, the "biggest bang for the buck." Of course, in management, as in ethics, problems arise:

- It is not always clear what the outcome of an action will be, nor is it always possible to determine who will be affected by it.
- The calculation required to determine the right decision is both complicated and time consuming.
- Because the greatest good for the greatest number is described in aggregate terms, the good might be achieved under conditions that are harmful to some, so long as that harm is balanced by a greater good. This leads to the attack that consequentialism means that "the end justifies the means."[99]

The theory fails to acknowledge any individual rights that could be violated for the sake of the greatest good, which is sometimes called the "tyranny of the majority." Indeed, even the murder of an innocent person would seem to be condoned if it served the greater number. This complaint is similar to the prior complaint, but notes that consequentialism ignores the existence of basic rights and ethical principles such as autonomy and beneficence. The fact that Mill would categorically deny this by saying some acts are wrong, regardless of the consequences, is held as a violation of his own stated philosophy. Of course, we are not seeking doctrinal purity, but useful tools to help us in healthcare ethics.

Lastly, who has time to run endless computations every time a decision is needed? "Analysis paralysis" would be the predicted outcome, which would not maximize any version of utility. In any case, because of these problems few philosophers today subscribe to consequentialism.[100] The proposed improvement to several of these problems is rule consequentialism.

Rule Consequentialism

The idea behind rule consequentialism is that behavior is evaluated by rules that would lead to the greatest good for the greatest number. At this point, the theory begins to tie in more clearly to virtue ethics and to the person who has achieved practical wisdom. It takes a person of some experience to know how to develop rules that will likely lead to the greatest good for the greatest number. Managers and government officials would call these rules *policies*. Now, once the policy is developed, presumably by evaluation of the likely outcomes, then the person who needs to make a decision refers to the applicable policy instead of having to make endless evaluations and calculations. Indeed, a person of practical wisdom might well conclude that long-term utility is undermined by acts of injustice. He or she would then develop a policy that recognizes and respects autonomy. Rule utilitarianism thus could use the utility principle to justify rules establishing human rights and the universal prohibition of certain harms. They would codify the wisdom of experience and preclude the need for constant calculation.

Rule consequentialism looks like the very same activity in which managers and policymakers engage when they make policies and procedures. A policy is a general statement meant to cover any number of situations. The person creating it makes the decision that following the policy is the best way to achieve the organization's goals. Procedures are then used as the means to carry out the created policies. Managers and government officials have been using this process for a long time. Overall, it works well, even though rules or policies do not work fairly in every situation.

Indeed, the failure of the rules to fit every situation is one of the reasons to have humans in charge instead of machines. At this point, the inclusion of a person of practical wisdom, from the virtue ethics tradition, comes into play. Managers or clinicians (persons of practical wisdom) can decide if the special circumstances warrant making an exception to the rule when judgments need to be made. If so, the rule could be modified to consider these special circumstances. In this way, fairness is preserved.

These exceptions might be justified by such material reasons as need, merit, potential, or past achievement. However, the manager or policymaker will also have to recognize, and be willing to accept, that sometimes the enforcement of a rule will lead to unfair outcomes. However, the principle is still sound and much better than the chaos of trying to evaluate the probable consequences of a situation each time a decision is required.[101]

Rule consequentialism can also incorporate the goals of negative consequentialism. The idea behind *negative consequentialism* is that alleviation of suffering is more important than the maximization of pleasure. Further, to have as a goal alleviation of suffering incorporates into the goal the protection of the powerless, the weak, and the worse off. Thus, from a social policy point of view, rules that operate as safety nets can accomplish this goal. Allowing access to emergency treatment regardless of ability to pay is an obvious healthcare example. Now let us look at the last version of consequentialism, preference consequentialism.

Preference Consequentialism

Preference consequentialism argues that the good is the fulfillment of preferences and the bad is frustration of desires or preferences. People in this sense are not seen as having preferences for pleasure or happiness per se; their preferences are left to them. Thus, autonomy becomes a bedrock value. For example, persons preferring to suffer great sacrifices to get into medical school are seeking to fulfill their preferences.

In another example, a patient could have termination of treatment as a preference, even if it leads to their early death. It is hard to imagine how that leads to happiness or pleasure when the person is not alive to experience such states. Other preferences could be losing weight, making a new friend, or rearing a healthy child. Note the similarity of this point of view to the emphasis in health care of respecting peoples' wishes that forms part of the general attack on paternalism. The theme here is to find out a person's expectations and then to seek to meet them. Within preference consequentialism, any number of states or conditions might be preferred, owing to the vast variability among people's desires. Consequentialism of this form is compatible with many different theories about which things are good or valuable.

How can someone know another person's preferences when making decisions that involve that person? Health care has developed clearly enunciated procedures in the area of informed consent to answer this question. One can also speak of *substituted judgment*, when the preferences of a person who is now incompetent are known.[102] In cases where the person has not communicated his or her preferences, we are forced to fall back on what is called the "best interests standard," or, more commonly, the "reasonable person standard." What would a reasonable person want in the circumstances at hand?[103] Healthcare ethicists have done a decent job in trying to discern what the preferences are of an individual who has become incompetent. However, policy-making decisions have an impact on large groups of people, most of whom will be personally unknown to the decision makers. Development of the tools to ascertain the preferences of a large aggregate of individuals is a much different task.[104] The tack that seems to occur is that the decision maker applies the "reasonable person standard" to the aggregate. However, considerable evidence suggests that such a standard may fall considerably short of meeting that person's actual preferences, whether it is what a reasonable person would want or not.[105] Simply put, the preferences humans have are so diverse and so changeable that it might not even make sense to use them as a standard for maximization.

Evaluation of Consequentialism

One of the most common criticisms of consequentialism is that it appears to allow some to suffer mightily if the net outcome is an improvement for a greater number. This argument is specious. The concept of respect for autonomy appears to be presupposed by the very statement that the good sought is the greatest good for the greatest number. Although consequentialists might talk about utility, the good in mind has to include respect for the personhood of the others as a minimum requirement. If not, why would they even be included in the prescription? If respect for the other is not presupposed, then it seems the theory would really devolve into a form of egoism. Thus, respect for the wants, preferences, hopes, and choices of others must be implicit for the theory to remain intact. Lacking this foundational component, many seem to think that the theory means that the ends justify the means, as noted earlier. Such a view is off base relative to the intent of the theory.

Mill himself stated this quite clearly in his classic essay, "On Liberty." He said, "the only freedom which deserves the name is that of pursuing our own good in our own way, so long as we do not attempt to deprive others of theirs, or impede their efforts to obtain it."[106] It is difficult to think of a more obvious reference to the respect for the autonomy of others and their liberty to pursue it. Some argue that this meant that Mill was really a deontologist. However, such arguments seem arcane, academic, and irrelevant to our purposes. Thus, I consider it a compliment to Mill that he recognized the need to temper his "greatest good for the greatest number" with respect for basic principles of autonomy and freedom.

ETHICAL THEORIES AND THEIR VALUE TO HEALTHCARE PROFESSIONALS

Over thousands of years, no ethical principle or theory has survived criticism by trained philosophers without serious flaws emerging. Nonetheless, healthcare professionals cannot throw up their hands. Decisions must be made, and reasons must be given for those decisions. Leadership often means choosing a course that you know some will not support.[107] Healthcare professionals understand the need for picking and choosing among the theories to work with the circumstances at hand.[108] This is why the person of practical wisdom, from the virtue ethics tradition, serves as the best model and is the model person the various healthcare professions have sought to produce. In the case of physicians, the tradition goes back for millennia. For other healthcare professions, the time period for development of a sense of professionalism, for production of persons of practical wisdom, is much shorter.[109]

The clinician and the healthcare manager will use their practical wisdom to advance the interests of specific patients, patients in the aggregate, the community, and the organization by drawing upon principles and theories as necessary to advance these interests. For managers, having rules that tend to provide the greatest good for the greatest number over the long term functions as a guiding principle in the same way that duties do for the clinician. Both clinicians and managers can come to the table with some clear ideas about what is appropriate to do in a given situation. The clinician has the emotional upper hand, because most people respond better to appeals that are directed toward helping a specific individual rather than protecting a policy. Nonetheless, the manager is well equipped by understanding the proper role of rules or policies.

For people in the policy-making arena, the evaluation of the behavior or motivations of various stakeholders will be enhanced if they determine the ethical system these stakeholders are likely to be using. Clinicians are likely to take a deontological approach, because their training makes their primary duty to the individual patient. They will not be as concerned with the external consequences of the decision (e.g., costs, inconvenience to the family, etc.) as they are with whether the right thing is done for the patient's medical care. The right thing is that which allows them to meet their duty and therefore uphold their sense of themselves as upholding the integrity of the profession. In other words, they want to uphold their sense of themselves as virtuous persons, persons of practical wisdom in the field of medicine or health care, doing the right thing for their patients. The right thing includes not only meeting their duty, but also evaluating the consequences of their decisions on the patients and their families.

Managers are in a more difficult position, because they have obligations to many stakeholders, not just to the individual patient. Those obligations are often unequal, sometimes conflicting. Sometimes their best strategy is to recognize that they lack the luxury of having obligations that are so pure and easily defined. Instead, they have to think of multiple and conflicting stakeholders and try to develop a solution that will generate the greatest good for the greatest number. All the while, they must respect the principles of autonomy, justice, beneficence, and nonmaleficence.[110] In their experience, the rules they adhere to have had those positive results; therefore, they suggest them in the current case. It is clear to see that the ethical challenge for a healthcare manager is more difficult than for those working from a strictly clinical perspective.

SUMMARY

This chapter makes it clear that no one ethics theory is sufficient for all healthcare decision making. However, a review of the principle features of main ethics theories used in health care provides a toolbox for decision making. After a brief explanation of authority-based ethics, a discussion of the features and use of natural law theory is provided. This is followed by two prominent ethics theories used in health care: utilitarianism and deontology. Finally, there is a discussion on the merits of considering virtue ethics as a healthcare professional.

The twenty-first century promises challenging healthcare ethics issues for individuals, organizations, and society. Therefore, a deeper understanding and the ability to apply ethics theory will be even more necessary for appropriate responses to these challenges. As you noticed in this chapter, ethical theory has not been developed in a vacuum. Each theorist studied the works of those who went before him and provided his own wisdom. Similarly, theories form the basis for the main ethical principles used in healthcare practice and decision making. You will find a discussion of these principles in Chapter 2. In addition, subsequent chapters will apply the both theories and principles to current and future healthcare challenges.

QUESTIONS FOR DISCUSSION

1. Why should you have a foundation in ethics if you are involved in health care? Are you not already a good person?

2. How can you use the tenants of natural law in your practice of health care?

3. What are the key features or points to remember about virtue ethics?

4. Why is deontology still important in contemporary healthcare practice? How can you use the categorical imperative to make decisions in today's healthcare practice?

5. How does utilitarianism affect healthcare decision making? Do you think this theory will be useful for making decisions about future issues?

NOTES

1. For a good overview of the value of cultural competence in health care, see J. R. Betancourt, A. R. Green, and J. E. Carillo, *Cultural Competence in Health Care: Emerging Frameworks and Practical Approaches* (The Commonwealth Fund, 2002). Available at www.cmwf .org/usr_doc/betancourt_culturalcompetence_576.pdf. Accessed October 14, 2006.

2. T. L. Beauchamp and J. F. Childress, *Principles of Biomedical Ethics*, 5th ed. (New York: Oxford University Press, 2001). Oxford University Press popularized these four concepts, starting with the first edition in 1979. The concepts, or "principles," as these authors call them, are examined later. The authors consider the principles to be more valuable than the

theories (Chapter 9). For purposes of clinical medical ethics, this ordering may be appropriate. It seems less suitable for the more general category of healthcare ethics, which includes policymaking well beyond the bedside.

3. Some authors distinguish deontology from consequentialism solely by the fact that it places total or some limits on the relevance of the consequences in the deliberations. See T. A. Mappes and J. S. Zembaty, *Biomedical Ethics*, 2nd ed. (New York: McGraw Hill, 1981), 4.

4. R. Benedict, "A Defense of Moral Relativism," *Journal of General Psychology* 10 (1934): 59–82. This work is one of the most influential and most reprinted contemporary defenses of ethical relativism, which was written by a leading figure in twentieth-century anthropology. It is reprinted in numerous anthologies, including *Everyday Life*, 3rd ed., edited by C. Sommers and F. Sommers (San Diego: Harcourt, Brace and Jovanovich, 1992). This reference was found at http://ethics.acusd.edu/theories/relativism/. Accessed June 15, 2006. The source contains an excellent bibliography on this subject and many other ethical issues, as well as videos, Internet accessible articles, and PowerPoint presentations. It is maintained by L. M. Hinman, Professor of Philosophy and Director of the Values Institute at the University of San Diego.

5. See K. Popper, *The Logic of Scientific Discovery* (New York: Basic Books, 1959), for the defense of falsifiability as a criterion of scientific knowledge.

6. V. Klingenborg, "On the Recentness of What We Know," *New York Times*, August 9, 2006. Available at http://nytimes.com/2006/08/09/opinion/09talkingpoints.html. Accessed August 13, 2006.

7. H. LaFollettee, "The Truth in Relativism," *Journal of Social Philosophy* (1991): 146–154. Available at www.stpt.usf.edu/hhl/papers/relative.htm. Accessed June 15, 2006.

8. The lack of certainty and infallibility disturbs many. See M. J. Slick, "Ethical Relativism" (Christian Apologetics and Research Ministry, 2003). Available at www.carm.org/relativism/ethical.htm. Accessed June 15, 2006. This organization renounced relativism because "right and wrong are not absolute and must be determined in society by a combination of observation, logic, social preferences and patterns, experience, emotions, and 'rules' that seem to bring the most benefit." According to this group, this messy process was improved by reliance on Scripture.

9. In an introductory chapter, a complete account is not possible. However, for an extensive bibliography see L. M. Hinman, "A Survey of Selected Internet Resources on Ethical Egoism," *Ethics Updates* (2004). Available at http://ethics.acusd.edu/theories/egoism/. Accessed June 13, 2006.

10. See, for example, A. Rand, *Virtue of Selfishness* (New York: Signet, 1964).

11. The Ayn Rand Institute Web site recommends L. Peikoff, *Objectivism: The Philosophy of Ayn Rand* (London: Meridian, 1993). Available at www.aynrand.org/site/PageServer?page name=objectivism_intro. Accessed June 15, 2006.

12. A. Rand, *Introducing Objectivism* (Ayn Rand Institute, 1962). Available at www.aynrand .org/site/PageServer?pagename=objectivism_intro. Accessed June 15, 2006.

13. The spiritual dimension is one of the nine elements of the patient-centered care model championed by the Planetree model. See S. B. Frampton, L. Gilpin, and P. A. Charmel, *Putting Patients First: Designing and Practicing Patient-Centered Care* (San Francisco: Jossey-Bass, 2003). Available at www.planetree.org/about/components.htm. Accessed June 5, 2006. See also B. Justice, *Who Gets Sick: How Beliefs, Moods and Thoughts Affect Your Health*, 2nd ed. (Houston: Peak Press, 2000). This book provides an overview of the scientific literature relative to how mental states, including spiritual states, influence healing. For more recent articles, see L. Guterman, "Duping the Brain Into Healing the Body," *Chronicle of Higher Education* 52, no. 15 (2005): A12; H. Koneig, "Meeting the spiritual needs of patients," *The Satisfaction Monitor* (July-August 2003). Available at www.pressganey.com/products_services/readings_findings/satmon/print_article.php?article_id=94. Accessed June 16, 2006.

14. World Medical Association, "The Declaration of Geneva" (World Medical Association, 1983). Available at www.phrusa.org/research/methics/methicsint.html. Accessed June 16, 2006.

The URL includes several other organizational statements relating to medical ethics, mostly in the form of codes of medical ethics.

15. Following the tradition, the references used to locate the passage are cited by the name of the work and the particular line number. See *Nicomachean Ethics*, Bk I, Chp 9, 1099b32-1100a5. The actual version used is R. McKeon, *Basic Works of Aristotle* (New York: Random House, 1971).

16. Very substantial arguments arise over just what *harm* and *benefit* mean, but those are not necessary to consider here. The exact words noted do not occur in the Hippocratic Corpus. However, it is clearly stated in *Of the Epidemics*, Bk. I, section II, part 5: "The physician must . . . have two special objects in view with regard to disease, namely, to do good or to do no harm." Available at http://classics.mit.edu/Hippocrates/epidemics.html, an online collection of the Hippocratic Corpus. Accessed June 7, 2006.

17. There is a considerable discussion about what virtues are, which ones are important, and the like. I shall have to leave that debate aside and simply hope the reader has an ordinary conception of what a virtue is.

18. See American Medical Association, *Principles of Medical Ethics* (Chicago: American Medical Association, 2001). Available at www.ama-assn.org/ama/pub/category/2512.html. Accessed June 18, 2006.

19. *Nicomachean Ethics*, Bk I, Chp 2, 1103a17.

20. *Nicomachean Ethics*, Bk I, Chp 2, 1103a25.

21. The following material on honesty was inspired by R. Hursthouse, "Virtue Ethics," *Stanford Encyclopedia of Philosophy* (2003). Available at http://plato.stanford.edu/entries/ethics-virtue/. Accessed May 12, 2006. I have rewritten it to fit healthcare professionals from its original, more general appeal.

22. *Nicomachean Ethics*, Bk. 6, Ch. 13, 1145a2–3.

23. This seeking of self-perfection has a major influence in Western culture, extending from the Greeks into the Roman stoics and then into Christianity. In some interpretations, Islamic *jihad* means a similar struggle with the self, a striving for spiritual self-perfection. Muslims knew Aristotle's teachings far in advance of Christendom. After the decline of Rome, Aristotle's work was lost in the West. However, in the ninth century, Arab scholars introduced Aristotle to Islam, and Muslim theology, philosophy, and natural science all took on an Aristotelian cast. After the Crusades, Arab and Jewish scholars reintroduced Aristotelian thought in the West. The correct interpretation of *jihad* is a matter of considerable debate and not a topic here.

24. T. L. Beauchamp and J. F. Childress, *Principles of Biomedical Ethics*, 5th ed. (New York: Oxford University Press, 2001).

25. T. F. Hoad (Ed.), "Justice," in *The Concise Oxford Dictionary of English Etymology* (New York: Oxford University Press, 1996). Available at www.oxfordreference.com/views/ENTRY .html?subview=Main&entry=t27.e8229. Accessed June 19, 2006.

26. For example, a teacher might say, "your response did the subject justice," meaning it was right and it was a more than merely adequate response, it was good. Or, one might say, "The person showed the justice of their claim," meaning it was a proper and correct claim.

27. T. L. Beauchamp and J. F. Childress, *Principles of Biomedical Ethics*, 5th ed. (New York: Oxford University Press, 2001).

28. Aristotle thought slavery was okay, because some could comprehend the rational principle, but not possess it. They acted from instinct. *Politics*, Bk II, Chp. 5. Aristotle described barbarians as brutish, along with people of vice. *Nicomachean Ethics*, Bk VII, Chp 1, 1145a30 and Chp. 5, 1148a15–30. By nature, some people should rule and others be ruled. He thought Greeks should rule barbarians "for by nature what is barbarian and what is slave are the same." *Politics* Bk I, chp.2, 1252 b 8. Women were inferior by nature to men as well: "The relationship between the male and the female is by nature such that the male is higher, the female lower, that the male rules and the female is ruled." *Politics*, Bk I, Chp. 4, 1254 b 12–14. The hierarchy of being and value had significant importance politically for millennia and such views still do today. Obviously, metaphysics influences our lives. The common morality has changed relative to many of these views.

29. *Nicomachean Ethics*, Bk. X, Ch. 9, 1179b5–10.

30. *Nicomachean Ethics*, Bk. X, Ch. 9, 1179b18. The other sentiments are written directly preceding this line. A *tincture* of something seems to suggest that it is not quite the real thing, although it could do some good. So many various definitions of the term *tincture* exist that it is difficult to get a precise understanding of the meaning of the phrase.

31. See B. Justice, *Who Gets Sick: How Beliefs, Moods, and Thoughts Affect Your Health*, 2 ed. (Houston: Peak Press, 2000). This book reviews the scientific literature on the subject. Although dated, it still provides an excellent introduction to the field.

32. In the realm of healthcare management, providing cues to quality to assure the patients that the services are appropriate is part of the management of the dimensions of quality. See V. A. Zeithaml, M. J. Bitner, and D. D. Gremler, *Services Marketing*, 4th ed. (New York: McGraw Hill, 2006). See S. B. Frampton, L. Gilpin, and P. A. Charmel, *Putting Patients First: Designing and Practicing Patient-Centered Care* (San Francisco: Jossey-Bass, 2003).

33. Some of these issues are discussed in *Nicomachean Ethics*, Bk. VII, Chs. 1–10, 1145a15–1154b30.

34. T. A. Mappes and J. S. Zembaty, *Biomedical Ethics*, 2nd ed. (New York: McGraw Hill, 1981), 7. The brush seems much too wide that paints all ethical theories as either more or less consequentialist.

35. For an extremely informative philosophical overview of natural law theory in general and Aquinas' version of it in particular, including an excellent defense of how natural law does not neatly fall into either deontology or consequentialism, see M. Murphy, "The Natural Law Tradition in Ethics," *Stanford Encyclopedia of Philosophy*, Edward N. Zalta, Ed. (2002). Available at http://plato.stanford.edu/archives/win2002/entries/natural-law-ethics/. Accessed June 19, 2006.

36. On how the heavens have never changed in their orderly cycles, see *On the Heavens*, Bk. I, Ch. 3, 270b10–17.

37. See G. Kemerling, *Thomas Aquinas* (*PhilosophyPages.com*, 2002). Available at www.philosophypages.com/ph/aqui.htm. Accessed June 19, 2006. See also S. Richards, *Faithnet.org.uk* (2006). Available at www.faithnet.org.uk/Theology/aquinas.htm. Accessed June 19, 2006.

38. For more modern writers in the field of natural law see, in alphabetical order, T. D. J. Chappell, *Understanding Human Goods* (Edinburgh: Edinburgh University Press, 1995); J. Finnis, *Aquinas: Moral, Political, and Legal Theory* (Oxford: Oxford University Press, 1998); P. Foot, *Natural Goodness* (Oxford: Oxford University Press, 2000); J. E. Hare, *God's Call* (Grand Rapids: Eerdmans, 2001); M. Moore, "Good without God," in *Natural Law, Liberalism and Morality*, R. P. George, Ed. (Oxford: Oxford University Press, 1996); and M. C. Murphy, *Natural Law and Practical Rationality* (Cambridge: Cambridge University Press, 2001).

39. The entire work is available online. St. Thomas Aquinas. 1259. Benziger Bros. edition, 1947. *Summa Theologica*. Translated by Fathers of the English Dominican Province. Christian Classics Ethereal Library. The online index is available at www.ccel.org/a/aquinas/summa/home.html. Accessed June 20, 2006. Question 94 is found at www.ccel.org/a/aquinas/summa/FS/FS094.html#FSQ94OUTP1. The standard reference format for something in *Summa Theologica* is, for example, ST IaIIae 94, 4. This is interpreted to mean it is the *Summa Theologica*; it is the first part of the second part; it is question 94; and it is article four.

40. J. S. Rakish, B. B. Longest, Jr., and K. Darr, *Managing Health Service Organizations*, 3rd ed. (Baltimore: Health Professions Press, 1992), 103; K. Darr, *Ethics in Health Services Administration*, 2nd ed. (Baltimore: Health Professions Press, 1991), 18.

41. For a better account within the healthcare literature, see J. W. Carlson, "Natural Law Theory," in *Biomedical Ethics*, 2nd ed., T. A. Mappes, and J. S. Zembaty (Eds.) (New York: McGraw Hill, 1981), 37–43, and M. C. Brannigan and J. A. Boss, *Healthcare Ethics in a Diverse Society* (Mountain View: Mayfield Publishing, 2001), 23–25.

42. Debating how something can have partial perfection need not concern us here.

43. This also contradicts some commentators, who say that it assumes all rational beings will agree on the content of the natural law. For this error, see M. C. Brannigan and J. A. Boss, *Healthcare Ethics in a Diverse Society* (Mountain View: Mayfield Publishing, 2001), 24.

44. For an extensive discussion of this approach in the healthcare literature, see T. L. Beauchamp and J. F. Childress, *Principles of Biomedical Ethics*, 5th ed. (New York: Oxford University Press, 2001), 128–132.

45. To go further into such controversies, see, as examples, P. J. Cataldo, "The Principle of the Double Effect," *Ethics & Medics*, 20 (March 1995), 1-3; B. Ashley and K. O'Rourke, *Healthcare Ethics: A Theological Analysis*, 4th ed. (Washington, D.C.: Georgetown University Press, 1997), 191–195; and D. B. Marquis, "Four Versions of Double Effect," *Journal of Medicine and Philosophy* 16 (1991): 515–544.

46. A similar insight was noted by T. L. Beauchamp and J. F. Childress, *Principles of Biomedical Ethics*, 2nd ed. (New York: Oxford University Press, 1983), 115.

47. M. Murphy, "The Natural Law Tradition in Ethics," *Stanford Encyclopedia of Philosophy*, Edward N. Zalta (Ed.) (2002). Available at http://plato.stanford.edu/archives/win2002/entries/natural-law-ethics/. Accessed June 19, 2006.

48. V. Cathrein, "Ethics," *Catholic Encyclopedia Online*, K. Knight (Ed.) (2003). Available at www.newadvent.org/cathen/05556a.htm. Accessed June 20, 2006.

49. V. Cathrein, "Ethics," Catholic Encyclopedia Online, K. Knight (Ed.) (2003). Available at www.newadvent.org/cathen/05556a.htm. Accessed June 20, 2006.

50. This theory does not appear to protect nonhuman animals, plants, dammed rivers, strip-mined mountains, and the like. Given their lack of rationality, not being made in the image of God, their lower level in the hierarchy of being, being a means to our ends, their potential would matter less. In the Aristotelian scheme, only angels were between humans and the unmoved mover, or God. Later on, Descartes, although not favored by either Catholics or Protestants in his time, made a fundamental distinction between mind and matter. Only humans were believed endowed with mind capacity. Mind easily translated into concepts like soul. Thus, the rest of the natural world, being without mind or soul, did not require us to worry about whether its potential was going to be circumscribed by our actions upon it.

51. For persons not familiar with this Latin term, the exact translation is "without that nothing." The typical way to understand it is that whatever is referred to is the essential element.

52. For some classics in this field, see R. M. Veatch, *Death, Dying, and the Biological Revolution: Our Last Quest for Responsibility* (New Haven: Yale University Press, 1976); J. Rachels, "Euthanasia," in *Matters of Life and Death: New Introductory Essays in Moral Philosophy*, T. Regan (Ed.) (New York: Random House, 1980).

53. V. Cathrein, "Ethics," *Catholic Encyclopedia Online*, K. Knight (Ed.) (2003). Available at www.newadvent.org/cathen/05556a.htm. Accessed June 20, 2006.

54. Most of his works appear to be available free online at http://oll.libertyfund.org/Intros/Kant .php, along with works of many other authors. I do not know whether the translations are those most accepted by scholars.

55. Although in near complete disagreement about the substance of their respective views, John Rawls and Robert Nozick are considered deontologists. Their views are key to understanding current political debates.

56. I. Kant, *Critique of Pure Reason*, trans. N.K. Smith, (New York: St. Martin's Press, 1781 [1965 ed.]).

57. I. Kant, *The Moral Law*, trans. H. J. Patton, (London: Hutchinson University Press, 1785 [1948 ed.]).

58. I. Kant, *The Critique of Practical Reason*, translated by L. W. Beck, (Indianapolis: Bobbs-Merrill, 1788 [1956 ed.]).

59. I. Kant, *Critique of Pure Reason*, trans. N. K. Smith, (New York: St. Martin's Press, 1781 [1965 edition]), pp. 29. The "B xxix" refers to the standard paging of the work. The "B" indicates this passage is in the *Critique*'s second edition only.

60. There is vast literature on the issues involved in whether free will exists. Different flavors of determinism are discussed and different perspectives on what it means to say someone acts freely. Although these issues are important, they simply cannot be broached here. For a good overview of the issues and the approaches taken by various religions, as well as various

thinkers, see W. K. Frankena, *Ethics: Foundations of Philosophy Series* (Englewood Cliffs, NJ: Prentice Hall, 1963), 54–62, and T. O'Conner, "Free Will," *Stanford Encyclopedia of Philosophy*, Edward N. Zalta (Ed.) (2005). Available at http://plato.stanford.edu/entries/freewill/. Accessed September 17, 2006.

61. What the moral law is will be taken up with the discussion of the categorical imperative.

62. I. Kant, *Critique of Pure Reason*, trans. N. K. Smith, (New York: St. Martin's Press, 1781 [1965 ed.]), 26–29 (Bxxv–bxxx).

63. I. Kant, *Critique of Pure Reason*, trans. N. K. Smith, (New York: St. Martin's Press, 1781 [1965 ed.]), 29.

64. I. Kant, *Critique of Pure Reason*, trans. N. K. Smith, (New York: St. Martin's Press, 1781 [1965 ed.]), 28.

65. I. Kant, "Fundamental Principles of the Metaphysics of Morals," translated by T. K Abbott, *Basic Writings of Kant*, A. L. Wood, Ed. (New York: Modern Library, 1785 [2001 ed.]), 151.

66. *Eudaimonia* is often improperly translated as "happiness."

67. I. Kant, "Fundamental Principles of the Metaphysics of Morals," translated by T. K Abbott, *Basic Writings of Kant*, A. L. Wood, Ed. (New York: Modern Library, 1785 [2001 ed.]), 152.

68. I. Kant, "Fundamental Principles of the Metaphysics of Morals," translated by T. K Abbott, *Basic Writings of Kant*, A. L. Wood, Ed. (New York: Modern Library, 1785 [2001 ed.]), 154–155.

69. I. Kant, *Foundations of the Metaphysics of Morals*, translated by L. W. Black (Indianapolis, IN: Bobbs-Merrill, 1959). The "AK 20" is the conventional page numbering used in Kant scholarship, locating this quote within the 22 volumes in the Preussische Akademie edition. Different pagination is used when referring to the *Critique of Pure Reason*.

70. T. L. Beauchamp and J. F. Childress, *Principles of Biomedical Ethics*, 5th ed. (New York: Oxford University Press, 2001), 57–112, provides a good discussion of autonomy in the context of medical ethics. E. E. Morrison, *Ethics in Health Administration: A Practical Approach for Decision Makers* (Sudbury, MA: Jones and Bartlett, 2006), 25–44, provides a discussion tailored to health care managers.

71. *Eudaimonia* is often improperly translated as "happiness." For its full meaning, see the discussion in text.

72. R. Johnson, "Kant's Moral Philosophy," in *Stanford Encyclopedia of Philosophy*, E. N. Zalta (Ed.) (February 26, 2004). Available at http://plato.stanford.edu/archives/spr2004/entries/kant-moral/. Accessed June 22, 2006. Given this understanding, Rousseau's famous statement that if people do not value freedom they must be "forced to be free" makes somewhat more sense. Nonetheless, forcing people to manifest your ideas of their highest purpose is *prima facie* paternalism.

73. T. L. Beauchamp and J. F. Childress, *Principles of Biomedical Ethics*, 5th ed. (New York: Oxford University Press, 2001), 348–351, provide a useful summary of these issues.

74. Kant posits a third version of the categorical imperative, "The Idea of the Will of Every Rational Beings as a Universally Legislative Will." (AK 4:431). I. Kant, "Fundamental Principles of the Metaphysics of Morals," translated by T. K Abbott, *Basic Writings of Kant*, A. L. Wood (Ed.) (New York: Modern Library, 1785 [2001 ed.]), 188. However, since this seems to mostly restate the emphasis on autonomy found in the second version, I shall not take up analysis of it separately.

75. I. Kant, "Fundamental Principles of the Metaphysics of Morals," translated by T. K Abbott, *Basic Writings of Kant*, A. L. Wood (Ed.) (New York: Modern Library, 1785 [2001 ed.]), 178.

76. For a sampling of sources stating or suggesting Kant's categorical imperative is the Golden Rule, see J. S. Rakish, B. B. Longest, Jr., and K. Darr, *Managing Health Service Organizations*, 3rd ed. (Baltimore: Health Professions Press, 1992), 103; K. Darr, *Ethics in Health Services Administration*, 2nd ed. (Baltimore: Health Professions Press, 1991), 18; M. C. Brannigan and J. A. Boss, *Healthcare Ethics in a Diverse Society* (Mountain View: Mayfield Publishing, 2001), 29; J. O. Hertzler, "On Golden Rules," *International Journal of Ethics* 44, no. 4 (1934): 418–436; S. B. Thomas, "Jesus and Kant, a Problem in Reconciling Two Different Points of View," *Mind* 79, no. 314 (April 1970): 188–199; P. Weiss, "The Golden Rule," *Journal*

of Philosophy 38, no. 16 (July 31, 1941): 421–430; J. E. Walter, "Kant's Moral Theology," *Harvard Theological Review* 10, no. 3 (July 1917): 272–295, esp. 293. Those who write about ethics without having philosophical training are even more likely to make this mistake. A Web site on engineering ethics simply indicates that the categorical imperative is the Golden Rule; see www.engr.psu.edu/ethics/theories.asp. Accesed September 9. 2006. I have even made the error myself in discussing ethical theories in the healthcare literature. The following articles were part of a column on healthcare ethics. See J. Summers, "Managers Face Conflicting Values," *Journal of Health Care Material Management* 7, no. 5, (July 1989): 89–90; J. Summers, "Clinicians & Managers: Different Ethical Approaches to Honoring Commitments," *Journal of Health Care Material Management* 7, no. 4 (May–June 1989): 62–63; J. Summers, "Determining Your Duties," *Journal of Health Care Material Management* 7, no. 3 (April 1989): 80–81; J. Summers, "Duty and Moral Obligations," *Journal of Health Care Material Management* 7 no. 2 (February–March 1989): 80–83; J. Summers, "Ethical Theories: An Introduction," *Journal of Health Care Material Management* 7, no. 1, (January 1989): 56–57. The fact something looks like something else does make it that something else.

77. The disavowal occurs in a footnote in I. Kant, "Fundamental Principles of the Metaphysics of Morals," translated by T. K. Abbott, *Basic Writings of Kant*, A. L. Wood (Ed.) (New York: Modern Library, 1785 [2001 edition]), 187, note. 13. To the normal reader the footnote would not clearly indicate it references the Golden Rule since Kant cited it in Latin and none of the terms have any resemblance to the English version of the Golden Rule.

78. I. Kant, "Fundamental Principles of the Metaphysics of Morals," translated by T. K. Abbott, *Basic Writings of Kant*, A. L. Wood (Ed.) (New York: Modern Library, 1785 [2001 ed.]), 186.

79. I. Kant, "Fundamental Principles of the Metaphysics of Morals," translated by T. K. Abbott, *Basic Writings of Kant*, A. L. Wood (Ed.) (New York: Modern Library, 1785 [2001 ed.]), 190–191.

80. I. Kant, *Foundations of the Metaphysics of Morals*, translated by Lewis White Black (Indianapolis: Bobbs-Merrill, 1959), 31.

81. I. Kant, "Fundamental Principles of the Metaphysics of Morals," translated by T. K. Abbott, *Basic Writings of Kant*, A. L. Wood (Ed.) (New York: Modern Library, 1785 [2001 ed.]), 186.

82. I. Kant, "Fundamental Principles of the Metaphysics of Morals," translated by T. K. Abbott, *Basic Writings of Kant*, A. L. Wood (Ed.) (New York: Modern Library, 1785 [2001 ed.]), 186.

83. For a good history of the Golden Rule, including versions that precede the Christian formulation at Matthew 7:12, see J. O. Hertzler, "On Golden Rules," *International Journal of Ethics* 44, no. 4 (July 1934): 418–436.

84. I. Kant, "Fundamental Principles of the Metaphysics of Morals," translated by T. K. Abbott, *Basic Writings of Kant*, A. L. Wood (Ed.) (New York: Modern Library, 1785 [2001 ed.]), 187, no. 13.

85. I. Kant, "Fundamental Principles of the Metaphysics of Morals," translated by T. K. Abbott, *Basic Writings of Kant*, A. L. Wood (Ed.) (New York: Modern Library, 1785 [2001 ed.]), 156.

86. I. Kant, "Fundamental Principles of the Metaphysics of Morals," translated by T. K. Abbott, *Basic Writings of Kant*, A. L. Wood (Ed.) (New York: Modern Library, 1785 [2001 ed.]), 183.

87. Some of the ideas in this section were drawn from F. Feldman, "Kant's Ethical Theory", in *Biomedical Ethics*, T. A. Mappes and J. S. Zembaty (Eds.) (New York: McGraw-Hill, 1981), 26–37, esp. pp. 36–37.

88. Healthcare managers do have a fiduciary duty to the organization and its patients. Such duties are described as duties of care and loyalty created when a person undertakes to act for the benefit of another as to whom he has a relationship implying confidence and trust and creating the expectation that he will act with a high degree of good faith.

89. For a very good overview of these views and a critical review as well, see A. Gandjour and K.W. Lauterbach, "Utilitarian Theories Reconsidered: Common Misconceptions, More Recent Developments, and Health Policy Implications," *Health Care Analysis* 11, no. 3 (September 2003): 229–244. A different source lists ten versions of consequentialism, see W. Sinnott-Armstrong, "Consequentialism," *The Stanford Encyclopedia of Philosophy* (Winter 2003 ed.), Edward N. Zalta (Ed.). Available at http://plato.stanford.edu/entries/consequentialism/. Accessed September 14, 2006. At least three versions of rule consequentialism are described;

see B. Hooker, "Rule Consequentialism," *The Stanford Encyclopedia of Philosophy* (Winter 2003 ed.), Edward N. Zalta (Ed.). Available at http://plato.stanford.edu/entries/consequentialism-rule. Accessed May 12, 2006.

90. Deontology can also be divided into rule and act deontology, although I did not find the distinction useful here. See W. K. Frankena, *Ethics: Foundations of Philosophy Series*, (Englewood Cliffs: Prentice Hall, 1963), 21–25.

91. J. S. Mill, *Utilitarianism* (1863). Available at www.utilitarianism.com/mill1.htm, Chapter II, para. 2. Accessed September 10, 2006. Owing to the many printed versions, I am citing it by reference to chapter and paragraph.

92. J. S. Mill, *Utilitarianism* (1863). Available at www.utilitarianism.com/mill1.htm, Chapter II, para. 2. Accessed September 10, 2006. Owing to the many printed versions, I am citing it by reference to chapter and paragraph.

93. *Eudaimonia* was discussed previously and is human happiness that necessarily includes pursuit of the good for humans qua humans.

94. See D. Lyons, "Mill's Theory of Morality," *Nous* 10, no. 2 (April 1976): 101–120, esp. pp. 103–104. He draws this conclusion from Mill's discussion of duty and punishment in *Utilitarianism*, Chapter V, para. 14–15, where Mill finds that punishment is necessary for persons not fulfilling their duties, without regard to any specific calculation of consequences. The fact that this begins to sound like deontology we shall leave unchallenged.

95. For example, D. Lyons, "Mill's Theory of Morality," *Nous* 10, no. 2 (April 1976): 101–120, notes the considerable debate over whether Mill was an act utilitarian or a rule utilitarian and over whether considerations other than utility entered into the decision calculus. He cites considerable sources on both sides of the debate.

96. Discussed by S. Gosepath, "Equality," *The Stanford Encyclopedia of Philosophy* (Winter 2003 ed.), Edward N. Zalta (Ed.). Available at http://plato.stanford.edu/entries/equality/. Accessed September 10, 2006.

97. For an extremely well-written, even witty, analysis of this difficulty, see M. Sagoff, "Should Preferences Count?" *Land Economics* 70, no. 2. (May 1994): 127–144. For a very abstruse and technical paper reaching essentially similar conclusions, see D. M. Hausman, "The Impossibility of Interpersonal Utility Comparisons," *Mind* 104, no. 415 (July 1995): 473–490.

98. See J. Summers, "Managers Face Conflicting Values," *Journal of Health Care Material Management* 7, no. 5 (May–June 1989); J. Summers, "Clinicians & Managers: Different Ethical Approaches to Honoring Commitments," *Journal of Health Care Material Management* 7, no. 4 (May–June 1989): 62–63; J. Summers, "Determining Your Duties," *Journal of Health Care Material Management* 7, no. 3 (April 1989): 80–81; J. Summers, "Duty and Moral Obligations," *Journal of Health Care Material Management* 7, no. 2 (February–March 1989): 80–83.

99. One of the common texts used for teaching healthcare managers the principles of management includes a section on ethics. Although much of the section is on point and the overall text is excellent, the discussion of consequentialism does not even mention that the typical understanding is the "the greatest good for the greatest number," but instead simply says "a summary statement that describes utilitarian theory is 'the end justifies the means.'" See J. S. Rakish, B. B. Longest, Jr., and K. Darr, *Managing Health Service Organizations*, 3rd ed. (Baltimore: Health Professions Press, 1992), 102. The author of the statement, Kurt Darr, had previously written K. Darr, *Ethics in Health Services Administration*, 2nd ed. (Baltimore Health Professions Press, 1991). In that text he did mention the idea of "the greatest good for the greatest number" along with "the end justifying the means," but thought both attributable to utilitarians, although not to be "applied without qualification" (p. 16). Those qualifications were not discussed. Unfortunately, many healthcare managers who were only exposed to the more general management theory book never would know about the greatest good for the greatest number and would likely perceive consequentialism as inherently allowing an evil to seek a good. For one of many other examples of misunderstanding consequentialism, see K. Anderson, *Utilitarianism: The Greatest Good for the Greatest Number* (Probe Ministries, 2004). Available at www.probe.org/content/view/1379/130/. Accessed Sep-

tember 10, 2006. G. Koukl, "Means and Ends," *Stand To Reason* (1994). Available at www.str.org/site/News2?page=NewsArticle&id=5444. Accessed September 10, 2006. Many of the sites making the claim that utilitarianism means the end justifies the means were religious sites. For an example of a business misreading of Mill's consequentialism, see R. Scruton, "Thoroughly Modern Mill," *Wall Street Journal*, May 19, 2006, A10. Available at http://online.wsj.com/article_email/SB114800167750457376-lMyQjAxMDE2NDI4Mj AyMDIxWj.html. Accessed September 10, 2006. Scruton considers Lenin, Hitler, Mao, Stalin, and common criminals as "pious utilitarians." See also http://en.wikipedia.org/wiki/ The_ends _justify_the_means for how this publicly edited source ties consequentialism to the theory. To define a theory by one of its criticisms is exceedingly off base.

100. B. Hooker, "Rule Consequentialism," *The Stanford Encyclopedia of Philosophy*, (Winter 2003 ed.), Edward N. Zalta (Ed.). Available at http://plato.stanford.edu/entries/consequentialism-rule. Accessed May 12, 2006. Hooker provides the reasons for this rejection and cites a large body of scholarship to support his contention. See also E. Millgram, "What's the Use of Utility?" *Philosophy and Public Affairs* 29, no. 2 (Spring 2000): 113–136, esp. p. 126.

101. A criticism in the philosophical literature is that revision of the rule to deal with exceptions leads inevitably back to act consequentialism. See B. Hooker, "Rule Consequentialism," *The Stanford Encyclopedia of Philosophy*, (Winter 2003 ed.). Edward N. Zalta (Ed.). Available at http://plato.stanford.edu/entries/consequentialism-rule. Accessed May 12, 2006. Practical experience as a manager and an educator of managers suggests that any manager worth having learned long ago not to let this happen.

102. T. L. Beauchamp and J. F. Childress, *Principles of Biomedical Ethics*, 5th ed. (New York: Oxford University Press, 2001), 98–102, discuss the substituted judgment approach and find it lacking. They promote the phrase "pure autonomy standard" for what I understand as the substituted judgment approach. Their change in terminology has not been picked up in the healthcare literature as a replacement for substituted judgment.

103. See E. E. Morrison, *Ethics in Health Administration: A Practical Approach for Decision Makers* (Sudbury, MA: Jones and Bartlett, 2006), 28; and T. L. Beauchamp and J. F. Childress, *Principles of Biomedical Ethics*, 5th ed. (New York: Oxford University Press, 2001), 102–103.

104. In political decision making, we fall back on the idea of having an elected person who represents us. Those representatives collect information about what their constituents think in a number of ways. In the organizational setting, the entire discipline of market research can be brought to bear. However, these information-gathering methods are seldom quick or inexpensive.

105. For an extremely well-written, even witty, analysis of this difficulty, see M. Sagoff, "Should Preferences Count?" *Land Economics* 70, no. 2 (May 1994): 127–144. For a very abstruse and technical paper reaching essentially similar conclusions, see D. M. Hausman, "The Impossibility of Interpersonal Utility Comparisons," *Mind* 104, no. 415 (July 1995): 473–490.

106. J. S. Mill, "On Liberty." (1863). Chapter I, para. 13. Available at www.utilitarianism.com/ol/htm. Accessed September 10, 2006. Owing to the many printed versions, I am citing it by reference to chapter and paragraph.

107. I again refer the reader to P. Tillich, *The Courage to Be* (New Haven: Yale University Press, 1952) for helpful thoughts on coping with difficult quandaries about the meaning of life and difficult choices in life.

108. See J. S. Rakish, B. B. Longest, Jr., and K. Darr, *Managing Health Service Organizations*, 3rd ed. (Baltimore: Health Professions Press, 1992), 106. Authors stress the balancing and eclectic nature of the work of the manager in drawing on the ethical theories and principles. See also M. C. Brannigan and J. A. Boss, *Healthcare Ethics in a Diverse Society* (Mountain View: Mayfield Publishing, 2001), 28, for a similar view. See E. E. Morrison, *Ethics in Health Administration: A Practical Approach for Decision Makers* (Sudbury, MA: Jones and Bartlett, 2006), 20–22, for thoughts on what it means to healthcare managers to draw these ideas together into a personal ethic.

109. Whereas nurses can trace their origins to Florence Nightingale (1820–1910), the professional society of healthcare managers, the American College of Healthcare Executives,

traces its origins to 1933. The organization was founded for the purpose of developing a profession of healthcare managers. See www.ache.org/CARSVCS/wesbury_fellowship.cfm. Accessed September 16, 2006. Many other healthcare professions are even more recent in origin.

110. See J. Summers, "Doing Good and Doing Well: Ethics, Professionalism and Success," *Hospital and Health Services Administration* 29, no. 2 (March–April 1984): 84–100 for an early discussion in the healthcare literature about the integration of these values and approaches.

CHAPTER 2

Principles of Healthcare Ethics

Jim Summers

OVERVIEW

In this chapter, Summers presents another scholarly approach to the foundations of ethics. He discusses the principles derived from the theories of ethics that provide a practical basis for making practice decisions. These four principles are nonmaleficence, beneficence, autonomy, and justice, with justice being the most complex. In addition, the author presents a model to assist with making ethics-based decisions about current issues and those that may emerge in the future. Coupled with Chapter 1, this reading provides a firm foundation for discussing the issues that follow in this text.

INTRODUCTION

Chapter 1 presented the major ethical theories and their application in health care as part of a foundation for the study of ethics. This chapter extends that foundation by showing how those theories inform the principles used in health care and apply to the issues in that field. The principles commonly used in healthcare ethics—justice, autonomy, and beneficence—provide you with an additional foundation and tools to use in making ethics decisions. Each of these principles is reviewed in this chapter. Because the concept of justice is the most complex, it is presented last. In addition, this chapter presents a model for decision making that uses your knowledge of theory and principles of ethics.

NONMALEFICENCE

If we go back to the basic understanding of the Hippocratic ethical teaching, we arrive at the dictum of "first do no harm, benefit only." The principle of *nonmaleficence* relates to the first part of this teaching and means "to do no harm." In healthcare ethics, there is no debate over whether we want to avoid doing the bad or harm. However, the debate occurs when we consider the meaning of the word *harm*. The following ethical theories come into play here:

- A consequentialist would say that harm is that which prevents the good or leads to less good or utility than other choices.
- A natural law ethicist would say that harm is that which is opposed to our rational natures, that which circumscribes or limits our potential.
- A deontologist would say that harm is that which prevents us from carrying out our duty or that which is opposed to the formal conditions of the moral law.

- A virtue ethicist, a person seeking *eudaimonia*, a person of practical wisdom, would find that harm is that which is immoderate, that which leads us away from manifesting our proper ends as humans.
- An ethical egoist would find harm as that which was opposed to his or her self-interest.

What Is "Harm" in the Clinical Setting?

In the clinical setting, harm is that which causes harm to the patient. However, deciding what *harm* means is no simple matter. Much of health care involves pain, discomfort, inconvenience, expense, and perhaps even disfigurement and disability. Using the natural law theory of double effect, we justify harm because there is a greater good. A consequentialist would say that the greater good, the greater utility, occurs from accepting the pain or dismemberment as part of the cost to get the benefit the healthcare procedures promise. The due care standard to provide the most appropriate treatment with the least pain and suffering sounds almost like a deontological principle.[1]

Most healthcare workers consider harm to mean physical harm, because the long history of healing has focused primarily on overcoming bodily disorders. However, harm can occur in other ways. For example, healthcare managers can cause harm by failing to supervise effectively. The result may be inadequate staff or equipment that is not maintained or kept up-to-date. Either of these can lead to adverse patient outcomes. Harm also comes from strategic decisions that lead to major financial losses and jeopardize the ability of the organization to continue. For example, making the decision to dispose hazardous materials without taking proper precautions puts the community at risk. In another example, healthcare policymakers can cause harm by changing eligibility requirements that lead to patient populations being unable to afford or to access the care they need. The ways harm can occur are infinite.

Harm as Negligence

Given the vast number of ways that harm can occur, healthcare workers have developed numerous protocols to protect patients, families, the community, and themselves. Failure to engage in these protocols is then an act of omission, as opposed to directly doing harm, which is an act of commission. A substantial body of law and ethical understanding supports the view that such a failure is negligence (omission). The person has not exercised the due diligence expected of someone in his or her role.

Healthcare financial managers also face a number of laws to ensure that they are not engaging in fraud and abuse, which also cause harm. For example, failure to follow the expectations of good financial management is essentially malfeasance. This term is very close to *maleficence* and represents neglect of fiscal responsibility. Medical professionals find a similar term with *malpractice*. Part of the education of all healthcare professionals concerns what it takes to avoid doing harm; to ensure that due diligence is followed.

Part of the development of a healthcare professional is to create a person of integrity who would consider it a violation of self to put those who trust in him or her at risk. Persons who avoid this violation are the persons of practical wisdom. They have achieved *eudaimonia* in their professions and in their lives. They can sit down together and discuss what should be done in a complex ethical situation. In the healthcare community, we believe that persons working within the healthcare ethic share a common understanding of the mission, vision, and values of health care. They are able to reason together, even if they get to their conclusions by different ethical theories and principles. The shared values of 'first do no harm, benefit only' provide a foundation that is often lacking in ethical disputes outside of health care.

Harm as Violations of Autonomy

An exceedingly large number of issues come to the surface as soon as you begin to address the issue of what harm is in a thoughtful way. For example, quality of life issues come into play. If a person elects not to receive a treatment because of a loss of life quality, then many people believe that imposing the treatment on that person is wrong. This would violate the principle of autonomy and evidence paternalism. Using the principle of autonomy, persons own their lives.

However, if the person is incompetent, the ethical approach is to determine if the person's wishes are known, and, if known, to follow them. This is called *substituted judgment*. If the person's wishes are not known, then the usual approach is what is called the *best interests* or *reasonable person decision*. The assumption is that the reasonable person would choose what is in their best interest.

BENEFICENCE

The other part of the Hippocratic ethical dictum is "benefit only." This is covered by the principle of beneficence. The *bene* comes from the Latin term for "well" or "good."

Beneficence and a Higher Moral Burden

Beneficence implies more than just avoiding doing harm. It suggests a level of altruism that is absent from simply refraining from harm. The ethical principle of having to engage in altruistic or beneficent acts means that we are morally obligated to take positive and direct steps to help others. Relative to the ethical theories, the underlying principle of consequentialism, the greatest good for the greatest number, is itself a statement of beneficence.[2] Early writers in the consequentialist tradition argued for the theory because of their belief that human nature was benevolent.[3]

Because beneficence is a fundamental principle of healthcare ethics, ethical egoism (our primary obligation is to ourselves and selfishness becomes a virtue) disconnects from health care. This is true because most people enter health care as a profession because they want to help people. Health care also is different in terms of the common morality. In the larger society, we are not necessarily held as negligent or deficient for failure to perform beneficent acts. However, in health care the professional roles carry that expectation.

Healthcare Roles and the Expectation of Beneficence

Acts of kindness and courtesy that are not expected of typical strangers are expected of healthcare workers. Failure to open a door to help someone in a wheelchair may be discourteous in most settings or perhaps even rude. However, it is unprofessional if you are a healthcare worker. Beneficence is part of the common morality of health care.

Nonmaleficence and Beneficence Are Insufficient Principles

Historically, the main problem that has emerged from emphasis on non-maleficence and on beneficence is that in most healthcare situations the physician was the person who defined "harm" and "good." Historically, most people were ignorant of what the physician was doing or talking about or why certain treatments were prescribed. Thus, the physician defined the patient's self-interest and carried it out. When the person who is receiving benefit or avoiding harm has little or no say in it, that person is being treated paternalistically. The term *paternalism* comes from the Latin *pater* that means "father." Paternalism, by definition, means that a person is being treated as one would treat a child. However, one of the major developments in health care over the last several decades has been patients' assertion of their desire to make decisions for themselves. Thus, we have to move beyond nonmaleficence and beneficence to include the principle of autonomy.

AUTONOMY

If you make a decision for me from the "first do no harm, benefit only" perspective without involving me in the decision, then my autonomy has been violated. Even if your entire intent is to put my interests before your own, leaving me out of decisions about myself violates my "self." Your intention to execute an act of beneficence does not mean I experience it as such an act.

Autonomy and the Kantian Deontological Tradition

Autonomy as a concept means that the person is self-ruling. The term *auto* is from the Greek and means "self." The rest of the term comes from the Greek *nomos*, which means "rule" or "law." Terms such as *normative* are derived from it. Thus, autonomy can be understood as self-rule. Underlying the concept of autonomy is the idea that we are to respect others for who they are. This view is honored in the medical tradition as far back as the Hippocratic writings. Therefore, the duty of the physician is to treat people's illnesses, not to judge them for why they are ill. It might be necessary for the physician to try to get patients to change what they are doing or who they are, but that is a part of the treatment; not a character judgment.

Autonomy in Health Care

In the healthcare setting, the conditions for autonomy are often unclear concerning whether the patient possesses them or not. Two important conditions must be met for autonomy: Are patients competent to make decisions for themselves? Are patients free of coercion in making the decision? These questions reflect the idea that autonomy implies the freedom to choose. Typically, people have an understanding of what it means to be competent and be able to make choices on their own behalf. However, that is not all there is to competence and autonomy.

The competent person also needs to be free of coercion. Coercion could mean they are trying to please someone—their parents, their children, or the providers—and thus are hiding their "real" choices. Forms of coercion that might prevent free choice in health care are myriad. Providers often encounter patients whose choices are compromised or coerced. For example, an abused spouse may not feel free to discuss the causes of bruises. A raped daughter may avoid discussion of a sexually transmitted disease. Drug abusers may hide their condition for fear of job loss.

An interesting approach to competence is the idea of specific competence, as opposed to general competence.[4] *Competence* can be understood as the ability to complete a task. This may mean you are able to do and understand some things, but not others. For example, a person with a temporary ischemic attack might be unable to balance a checkbook. However, that same person might be able to understand the consequences of medical procedures and thus assent to them or not. This is an example of specific competence. A person may be intermittingly competent owing to their medical condition. Thus, the person is competent to assent to treatment right now, but was not two hours previously, and might be unable to do so two hours in the future.

At this point, we have seen the importance of nonmaleficence, beneficence, and autonomy as principles of healthcare ethics. Now we move to the last of the four principles of healthcare ethics: justice.

THEORIES OF JUSTICE

In general, to know something is unjust is to have a good reason to think it is morally wrong. We can ask, "What sorts of facts make an act unjust rather than simply wrong in general?" Several reasons are available.

The term *injustice* often is used to mean unfairness in treatment. Injustice in this sense occurs when similar cases are not treated in the same fashion. Following Aristotle, many believe that we are required, as a formal principle of justice, to treat similar cases alike except where there is some relevant or material difference. The equity requirement in this 2400-year-old principle is critical. Now I shall break down the concept of justice into its components.

The Formal Principle of Justice

Justice usually comes in two major categories: procedural and distributive. *Procedural justice* asks, "Were fair procedures in place and were those procedures followed?" *Distributive justice* is concerned with the allocation of resources. In some cases, both of these issues will be in play at the same time. Both justice principles start from the idea that in the distribution of burdens and benefits the allocation should be equal unless there is a material reason to discriminate.

Procedural Justice

Procedural justice can be defined as "due process." For example, in the legal system we speak of being equal before the law as a part of procedural justice. In the legal sense then, procedural justice or due process means that when you get your turn you are treated like everyone else. This concept can also be applied to health care. For example, if you are waiting to see your primary care physician, did others get to go ahead of you without any clear medical reason?

Procedural injustices occur, but they are more common when dealing with employees. For example, if a healthcare manager has to terminate employees due to economic considerations, are the procedures for determining who will go applied without bias? In such cases, the issue is not so much whether what happened was itself just or fair, but whether the method by which it was done followed the stated procedures. No one would claim that it is fair to terminate good employees with long careers of service who have done nothing wrong. However, if economic circumstances dictate that employees must be terminated, the procedural justice question emerges as to whether there were standards and procedures for making the selection and if they were followed.

Failures of due process can also occur in the health policy arena and are closely watched by those participating in policymaking. For example, at a public hearing the time limit for speaking is three minutes. You will not think justice is done if some are allowed to speak 10 minutes, whereas others are constrained to three, or perhaps told to sit down after only one. We now turn to a review of the principles of distributive justice.

Distributive Justice

The concept of distributive justice relates to determining what is fair when decision makers are determining how to divide up burdens and benefits.[5] Kaiser Family Foundation data suggest the extent of the resource allocation disparity in healthcare demand and spending.[6] One percent of the U.S. population consumes 23.7 percent of healthcare resources. Half the U.S. population consumes only 3.4 percent of healthcare resources. The other half consumes 96.6 percent of healthcare resources. This is an extraordinary mismatch in the use of healthcare resources. Is it fair?

When it comes to distributive justice, several questions can emerge. Why are so many using so little? Are they healthy or simply unable to access the system? Are we seeing an improvement in the lives of that one percent who are taking up nearly 25 percent of the spending, whether measured by the patients or by the medical community? Are there less expensive ways to achieve healthcare goals? Do the healthcare goals, whatever they are, make sense relative to the world in which we find ourselves? Such questions are debated endlessly; however, they will not sidetrack us here. The point is to see the difficulty of the task of distributing the burdens of healthcare costs while seeking the holy grail of access, availability, and quality all at the same time.

To understand distributive justice, you must first understand that resource allocation issues occur at all levels. For example, a physician has to decide how much time to spend with each patient. Busy nurses have to decide how quickly to respond to a call button relative to the task they are engaged in when it sounds. Nurse managers have to allocate too few nurses to too many patients. Healthcare managers hire employees and must decide which to fund out of numerous requests. If they are going to increase pay, they must decide what method to use. Should the increase be across the board or by merit or longevity? If by merit, who decides if it is deserved and is the method fair? The latter question is one of procedural justice. This is an example where the two types often occur together.

Organizational leaders have to decide whether to spend scarce money on capital improvements on buildings and equipment, new employees, more money for the current employees, new services, advertising, or save the money. In health care, allocation of scarce resources can be a matter of life and death. For example, in Texas, persons with AIDS and HIV pleaded for funding not to be cut at a Texas Department of Health public hearing. On the line was a drug-assistance program facing budget cuts. The drugs for this treatment cost $12,000 per year, and the state was considering only allowing coverage if income levels were not in excess of $12,400. If a person made $13,000 a year, he or she would have only $1,000 on which to live. Desperation prevailed, as people told the panel to look them in the eye so they would know whom they were killing. Attendees promised, "not to slip quietly into their graves."[7]

Regardless of the outcome of that policy decision, in the midst of such emotions the need for the reflective equilibrium (discussed later) is high. Decisions are difficult when you are facing people who claim they are in such a crisis. Many related issues can be explored to understand why decisions are made with regard to distributive justice.

Material Reasons to Discriminate

The basic principle of justice is that each person should get an equal share of the burdens and benefits unless there is a material reason to discriminate. What are the reasons to discriminate?[8] The multiple reasons to discriminate typically boil down to two different areas: that the person deserves it or the person needs it. Society believes that those who work hard and do well deserve their success. That is the common morality in the United States. In contrast, a person who breaks the law and hurts people deserves prison. Health care shares this common morality but also includes a more complex element—need. The following list includes the most common candidates for material reasons to discriminate, all of which are subsets of need or being deserving:

1. Being deserving or worthy of merit includes one's contribution or results and effort
2. It also includes the needs of individuals or groups, such as:
   * Circumstances characterized as misfortune
   * Disabilities of a physical or mental nature or, more generally, unequal natural endowments
   * A person's special talents or abilities
   * The opportunities a person might have or might lose
   * Past discrimination against a group that is perceived as having negative effects in the present or simply a person's special legal status
   * Structural social problems perceived as restricting opportunity or even motivation

In the larger society, there is also a need to discriminate based on material need. One of society's views of distributive justice is that you get what you deserve or merit. Your results or contribution is what counts the most in getting what you deserve. The most common form of getting what you deserve in the larger society comes from the market. Therefore, if you are good at what you do, the market rewards you. If you are not, the market does not reward you, or even punishes you. For example, the physician who sees the most patients is sometimes the one with the higher income. Healthcare managers who meet revenue or productivity goals should get higher pay than their peers who fail to do so.

In the larger society, effort matters, too. Many want rewards based on effort, and often this effort is what our culture and our institutions reward. In some cases, we cannot determine if the results that did or did not occur are within the person's control. However, we can observe their effort, and it translates as reward. Thus, the healthcare manager who supervises the more complex healthcare system is paid more than a department manager. Researchers in biomedicine might work long and hard without necessarily getting the results they seek, yet they are compensated for their expertise and their labor.

Many of us are willing to help a person who we perceive as putting forth effort and will give up on the one who is not. This applies to healthcare treatments as well. For example, patients who follow "doctor's orders" to the letter and are clearly working hard to solve their health problems will likely elicit more support and effort from the clinical team. These situations are common in the management of chronic diseases and in behavioral health. Now let us take up the reasons to discriminate based on need.

Discrimination Based on Need

It is exceedingly difficult to put an upper limit on the concept of need. For example, the World Health Organization (WHO) defines *health* as "a state of complete physical, mental and social well-being and not merely the absence of disease or infirmity."[9] However, this definition sets up a model of need that is theoretically impossible to meet. However, some approaches are more useful. These include the following:

Need Based on Misfortune. In health care, the common morality is to discriminate for or against patients based on their need for care. For example, persons with emergencies are treated first, no matter how long you have waited in line. Persons in accidents, regardless of whose fault it is, are seen as having experienced a misfortune. Victims of natural disasters generally are perceived the same way. However, many of the conditions we treat in healthcare organizations are not owing to an infection, a bad series of decisions, or a natural disaster. People may suffer from genetic defects that vastly restrict their functioning. Others have reduced abilities in physical or mental capacity. These conditions can be considered a form of misfortune.

Even in the healthy population, significant disparities exist between people as to physical and mental ability, including factors such as motivation. For example, one could consider a person's special talents or abilities as a potential area for discrimination. Although we normally do not think of discriminating in favor of someone owing to special talents or abilities, it does occur. In health care, the clinical team may make more efforts to help someone with a special talent. For example, during cancer treatment, Lance Armstrong, who later was a seven-time Tour de France bike race winner, was administered a different chemotherapy than the protocol to protect his aerobic capacity.[10] Although that may not sound significant, it is a special treatment.

Healthcare managers make hiring and promotion decisions on perceived ability, speculating that past performance will be a guide to future performance. In that sense, the criteria are a mix of something you have done and a gamble that you will continue to perform. Policy decisions sometime are made this way as well, such as when awarding a contract, a grant, or funding a program. It appears that those involved have the ability to accomplish the goals of the policy makers.

Children and the elderly also receive special consideration based on abilities or talents. For example, the argument for spending money on children's health care ties into the idea of their future abilities. In a sense, this echoes the natural law argument to maximize potential. Many clinical workers will go to great lengths to help a child become whole, because they have so much life yet to live. Advocates for the disabled and the elderly also are concerned with ability. They worry that the reduced potential and ability of the elderly can lead to discrimination and thus loss of opportunity.[11] Obviously, the needs of children fall into this category, too.

Need Based on Past Discrimination. Other forms of need might include redress of past injustices to social groups, which overlaps with the need to provide opportunity and prevent the loss of ability. Such thinking led to the Civil Rights Act of 1965 and affirmative action. It could also be argued that past discrimination means that the protected groups deserve special dispensations. Clearly, the opportunities of many persons in those groups were restricted. Many special talents went undeveloped.

In the United States, health care long ago gave up institutionalization of segregation by race or gender. Nonetheless, in health care we have seen the nation respond to special groups and their needs by development of entire healthcare systems for them. For example, the Veterans Administration system is the largest healthcare system in the world. In addition, the Indian Health Service is designed to provide care to a very limited and specific group.

For some disadvantaged groups, the effects of adverse discrimination have led to structural problems that prevent some of the members from taking advantage of available opportunities. These structural burdens, such as poverty, poor educational and housing systems, and even poor transportation systems, often are blamed for the difficulties experienced by some. Regardless of what led to the problems, structural burdens are well known to have adverse health consequences. Many people who claim to have a need also say they have a right to our services. Let us look at the concept of rights, because it is intertwined with the concept of justice.

Distributive Justice and Rights

In the United States, debate continues over whether access to health care is a right or a commodity that must be purchased. Much of the language is confusing, because there are many types of rights. One thing is clear: To make a claim of a right means that you believe there is some legal reason you are entitled to something or that there is at the least a moral claim that your right is supported by ethical principles and theories. Rights range from ideal rights to legal rights. When someone makes a claim that something is a right, the typical reaction of the other party is to consider the basis of the claim. Is it a legal one? Is it moral? Alternatively, is it simply a wish or a statement of a preference?

Ways of Categorizing Rights

The diagram in Figure 2–1 shows the types of rights and their relationships. All the rights are found within the circle of ideal rights, which are rights we wish we had. Rights that are within another circle are subsets of that right. Rights that are partially within one or more other circles are rights that share common characteristics with their shared circles. For example, natural rights include elements of substance rights and negative rights. Some of the substance rights and negative rights have become legal rights. A positive right is a certain type of thing or social good to which you have a legal right. All positive rights are a subset of legal rights.

The size of the circle also indicates their relative importance within the common morality of the United States. For example, in the United States our common morality puts more emphasis on the negative rights than on the substance rights. Some nations place a greater emphasis on the collective welfare as opposed to individual opportunity. In these cases, the substance rights category would be larger and more of it would fit inside the legal rights circle.

The list of rights here is by no means exhaustive. The following discussion of the types of rights in Figure 2–1 is meant to provide a synopsis of the issues involved. Major literature exists for the topic of rights and includes others that are not part of Figure 2–1.[12] Nonetheless, the list is sufficient for the purposes of reflective equilibrium in healthcare ethics. The best of all rights from the point of view of the claimant are enforceable and are legal rights.

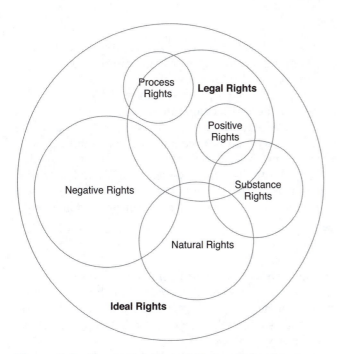

Figure 2–1   Types of rights and their relationships.

Legal and Positive Rights

Margaret Mahoney notes that positive rights used to be called "social goods," which society may or may not provide. The change to calling them "rights" was part of a rhetorical technique to give them a greater sense of legitimacy to the public.[13] A *legal right* means that someone has a legal obligation to fulfill your right, whatever it happens to be. A *positive right* is a narrow example of a legal right, because it is a specific social good. For this reason, it is shown in the diagram in Figure 2–1 as a circle completely within the set of legal rights. These rights are written into the law and are described as *entitlements*. However, a legal right can include more than simply entitlements. For example, the right to due process is legally protected, but it is not the provision of a good. The same could be said of the legal right to privacy under HIPAA laws. Thus, like due process, a right to privacy is not a positive right even though it is a legal right.

When rights are under pressure due to budget shortfalls, political pressure to cap government spending, or the like, the real meaning of a legal right is that you can go to court to get it enforced. Legal rights are not as strong as they were once thought to be in protecting the person with the right. For example, you may have a legal right to abortion or to Medicare and Medicaid, but if no one is providing it, your right has little value. Apparently, even the strongest version of a right does not mean that you will get whatever rights you have.

Substance Rights

Substance rights can be legal rights or not. They are rights to a particular thing, such as health care, housing, a minimum wage, welfare, food stamps, safe streets, a clean environment, and the like. In this sense, they are similar to positive rights, but not necessarily legal, as with an entitlement. This is somewhat of a nuanced difference, because a substance right might imply that it is a right to something basic needed to maintain life. Nations, such as those in Europe, can be more concerned with substance rights and attempt to guarantee an outcome or a basic minimum for their citizens. In those nations, the substance rights became legal rights. The positive legal rights noted earlier for health care also are substance rights, as would be the right in the United States to get treatment, or at least stabilized, at an emergency department regardless of ability to pay.

Negative Rights

In Figure 2–1, based on the common morality of the United States, the circle for negative rights is relatively large and extends into the legal rights domain. The terminology used for negative rights comes from the British tradition and essentially means that you have the right to be left alone. You have the right to do anything not strictly forbidden by the law.

Negative rights are clear and enshrine liberty. For example, the Bill of Rights is primarily a list of negative rights, such as speech and assembly will not be restricted. The Bill of Rights also includes the idea that a state will not enforce a religion. It also reinforces the negative right that people are allowed to have weapons because a well-regulated militia, being necessary to the security of a free state, means the right of the people to keep and bear arms shall not be infringed.

In the realm of health care, one major negative right is that we have the freedom to pursue our lives as we see fit. For example, motorcyclists claim they have a negative right to be free of having to wear protective helmets. Another negative right enshrined in law in some places is the right not to have smokers in your workplace, your eating area, or public areas generally. Smokers maintain this is a major affront to their freedom. One person's negative right to be free of smoke is the cancellation of another person's negative right to be free to smoke.

Other legal protections that assure you are left alone involve the protections against sexual harassment and hostile work environments. The privacy protections from HIPAA are yet one more legal negative right. Your medical information should be left alone unless you authorize it or it is for medically necessary reasons related to your care. Like the positive substance rights, the costs on the part of those who have to honor or take responsibility for assuring you are free of these hazards can be large.

Process Rights

Given the Bill of Rights, many laws relate to ensuring that due process is followed, at least for most people. As noted in the discussion of the layout of the diagram in Figure 2–1, process rights do overlap with natural rights. In the United States and in most developed nations, process rights also are going to be legal rights.

Natural Rights

Natural rights have a long history. The concept of a natural right means that we should respect attributes that humans have by nature.[14] For Aristotle and St. Thomas Aquinas, these features would be those that best support our achievement of our highest good. The most well-known appeals to natural rights within our common morality go back to the Founding Fathers. Drawing heavily on John Locke, Thomas Jefferson proclaimed in the Declaration of Independence that "We hold these truths to be self-evident, that all men are created equal, that they are endowed by their Creator with certain unalienable Rights, that among these are Life, Liberty, and the pursuit of Happiness."

One practical advantage of the natural rights approach to determining a person's rights is that people from very different perspectives use the same language. Thus, even if their views are philosophically inconsistent, they can agree that someone has a natural right. For example, many will say that there exists a natural right to that which is necessary to move toward one's full potential, and health is important to this. To the extent that health care is related to health, one should be able to sustain that morally one has a right to health care. Note that the philosophical reasons for why anyone should be able to develop his or her potential are manifold. However, people of differing religious and philosophic views could agree about having a natural right to develop potential without having to argue or even acknowledge their underlying philosophical differences. Thus, simply as a matter of rhetoric, the language of natural rights plays an important role in making right claims within our common morality.

Ideal Rights

An ideal right is a statement of a right that is meant to be motivational, a goal to seek. The WHO definition of health and its subsequent claim that everyone has a right to the highest attainable health care falls into this category.

Reflections on Rights

One element of the reflective equilibrium model (discussed later) that comes into play is the weighting of rights. Because we have a right seldom means that it trumps all other considerations. Consider the issue at the policymaking level. Assume there is a right to national security, education for the young, transportation, protection of property rights, and health care. Does one right trump the others at all times? Probably not, even though sometimes people think that their right claim should trump all the others. Even within health care, do the healthcare needs of the old trump those of the young?

What Does Having a Right Mean?

The U.S. Supreme Court has noted that you have no rights unless they are legal rights backed by statute. The fact that a strong moral case can be made is not sufficient. This applies directly to a healthcare case that can be used as an example. Recruiters for the military sold military service to World War II and Korean War veterans by stating that if they put in 20 years or more of service, they could obtain free medical care at VA hospitals. However, the Pentagon ended those benefits for veterans over age 65 in 1995 because they were eligible for Medicare. However, Medicare is not a complete healthcare system, and it is not free. Further, some veterans over age 65 say they cannot afford the premiums, deductibles, and co-payments of supplemental programs.

When the veterans filed suit to stay in the VA program, they learned that a promise by recruiters does not equal a law on the books. Thus, in one sense they had a right to something because they were promised it, but in the strictest sense of the word they had no rights if a law did not compel their treatment. A review of the laws dating from just after the Civil War found that the VA was treating people without statutory authorization. The Supreme Court ruled 5–4 that although the recruiters had made the promises in good faith, there was no contractual obligation. Thus, the federal government had no contractual obligation to the veterans.[15] This ruling is very significant, because it sanctifies that the only rights you have are strictly legal ones. As the nation and the world struggle increasingly with resource allocation issues, concerns about rights and distributive justice will become ever more common.

REFLECTIVE EQUILIBRIUM AS A DECISION-MAKING MODEL

The reflective equilibrium model is depicted in Figure 2–2. The middle of Figure 2–2 shows the basic facts of the situation, the healthcare issue where a decision is needed. In discussions of ethics, those making decisions about what to do use what are called *considered judgments* as decision-making guides.[16] Another term for such considered judgments is *ethical intuitions*, although the terms are not exactly the same.

A *considered judgment* implies that a degree of thinking and reasoning occurs before a decision is made. To many people, an intuition is simply a feeling, but to ethicists a moral intuition includes an element of reasoning. In moral reasoning, our considered judgments are tested against our feelings and back and forth. Clearly, the common morality will have a considerable influence on these judgments and intuitions as well.

Intuitions or considered judgments, as understood by ethicists, are essentially moral attitudes or judgments that we feel sure are correct.[17] These are of two types: (1) intuitions or considered judgments about particular cases (e.g., letting people stay in the Superdome during the Katrina incident without doing anything to supply or protect them adequately was not a good thing) or (2) regarding general moral rules (e.g., people whose lives or property are threatened by a natural disaster should be helped). Many such considered judgments exist in health care. For example, a person with a medical emergency should receive treatment regardless of his or her ability to pay.

Ethical theory comes into play in examining people's motivations. Some people may believe they should do something because they have a duty to help

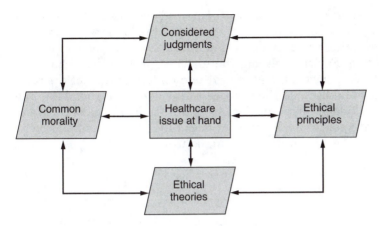

Figure 2–2 Reflective equilibrium at work.

others. Others may believe that assisting in a decrease of suffering is appropriate and the more people our decisions can help the better. Still others might appeal to our basic inclinations as humans to do the right thing or suggest that God or some deity or deities want us to fix the problem. When asked to justify their actions and decisions, these same persons might rely on these explanations or they might rely on ethical principles.

As discussed earlier, ethical principles include advancement of liberty, respect for autonomy, and acting out of beneficence to advance welfare. They also include ensuring that we do nothing to harm by following the principle of nonmaleficence and try to do this all fairly by upholding principles of justice. The typical portrayal of the healing ethic—first do no harm, benefit only—captures at least two of these principles: nonmaleficence and beneficence. The questions become just what to do. In the midst of all the decision making, the people involved are unlikely to consciously draw upon ethical theories or principles. They have internalized these foundations for making decisions and simply do so. This is what it means to be a person of practical wisdom, a person exhibiting the *eudaimonia* described in Chapter 1.

The term *reflective equilibrium* describes this back and forth process of coming to a coherent solution. John Rawls has described this method,[18] and its hallmark is its lack of dogmatism. The person involved in making the decision revises the decision as new information becomes available. The person may choose to draw upon one principle or ethical theory more heavily than he or she did previously.

Such movement back and forth among competing ethical theories and the quick reweighing of the importance of ethical theories and principles can sometimes look like incoherence or arbitrariness. However, people making healthcare decisions are not as troubled by the requirements of doctrinal purity as they are by the need to come to a decision. They need to have a sound ethical basis to explain that decision, get action on that decision, and get on to the next task. Ethical theories and ethical principles can help them to reach those decisions, explain them, and motivate others to act decisively, urgently, or passionately on them. With this foundation, the outcome is better, assuming the decision was sound. If not, the reflective equilibrium begins again. For this reason, the toolbox approach was chosen to better equip healthcare decision makers with an understanding of the principles and theories of ethics, so they can better decide, better explain, and better motivate. As Beauchamp and Childress put it, disunity, conflict, and moral ambiguity are pervasive features of moral life. Thus, it should be no surprise that untidiness, complexity, and conflict should be part of the process, too.[19]

SUMMARY

The principles of healthcare ethics complete the elements necessary for the reflective equilibrium. The primary principles of healthcare ethics are autonomy, beneficence, nonmaleficence, and justice. Justice is by far the most complex principle, because it includes the various conceptions of rights and there is greater dispute about what justice is and how to achieve it. Understanding the various nuances of rights and justice is of considerable importance in making resource allocations at the bedside, at the organizational level, or at the health policy level of government.

In using the reflective equilibrium model, a person will have to use reason to pick from among the principles, the theories, the common morality, and the considered judgments to apply them to the issue at hand. In health care, we have a great advantage over most organizational approaches to dealing with ethical issues. With the tradition of ethics committees and consults, a group of persons who are skilled and experienced in applying the reflective equilibrium is more likely to reach a decision that is reasonable than one made by a single person. This process will be messy; it will be error prone. That is the human condition and there seems to be no way around it.

Ethics is a complex field. Over thousands of years, humans have yet to develop an ethical theory that will satisfactorily handle all the issues. Nonetheless, some approaches have proven more satisfactory than others and have led to the development of principles. You might ask, "Now what?" Are there any final answers for healthcare issues now and in the future? The answer is "no." However, the important role of the study of ethics and ethics issues and the use of the reflective equilibrium model is to keep the inquiry going. The process matters as much, or even more, than the products. Although certain beliefs have been accepted for relatively long periods, the process eventually leads to a change. Let us hope the changes will result in improvement to our lives and an increase in the good. It is the job of each of us to keep the process going.

QUESTIONS FOR DISCUSSION

1. What do you think is the most important principle for clinical health-care professionals? Explain.

2. Why is beneficence a more complex principle than nonmaleficence?

3. Why is respecting autonomy so important to the future of health care?

4. Why is justice in health care more complicated than just doing what is fair?

5. How can the reflective equilibrium model assist you in making practical ethics decisions in the future?

NOTES

1. See E. E. Morrison, *Ethics in Health Administration* (Sudbury, MA: Jones and Bartlett, 2006), 46.

2. J. J. C. Smart, "Distributive Justice and Utilitarianism," in *Justice and Economic Distribution*, J. Arthur and W. Shaw (Eds.) (Englewood Cliffs, NJ: Prentice Hall, 1979), 103–115, esp. p. 103. In contrast, Richard Hare, also a consequentialist, specifically disavows that intuitions are sufficient upon which to base an ethical theory; R. M. Hare, "Justice and Equality," in *Justice and Economic Distribution*, J. Arthur and W. Shaw (Eds.) (Englewood Cliffs, NJ: Prentice Hall, 1979), 116–131, esp. p. 117.

3. D. Goleman, "The Roots of Compassion," *New York Times*, December 19, 2006. Available at http://happydays.blogs.nytimes.com/2006/12/19/the-roots-of-compassion/?8ty&emc=ty. Accessed December 20, 2006. *New York Times* surveys brain research and finds that humans may be hard wired to have empathy, compassion, and thus beneficence. T. L. Beauchamp and J. F. Childress, *Principles of Biomedical Ethics*, 5th ed. (New York: Oxford University Press, 2001) point out this early history on page 166.

4. This approach was pioneered by T. L. Beauchamp and J. F. Childress, *Principles of Biomedical Ethics*, 5th ed. (New York: Oxford University Press, 2001) who point out this history on pages 70–72.

5. Robert Nozick in *Anarchy, State, and Utopia* (New York: Basic Books 1974), 149–150, argues that the very language of "distribution" implies a central organization deciding who gets what and why. To him this improperly frames the discussion to imply a state and its attendant mechanisms when the problem is the state itself and its inevitable oppression.

6. Kaiser Family Foundation, "Illustrating the Potential Impacts of Adverse Selection on Health Insurance Costs in Consumer Choice Models," Kaiser Family Foundation, November 2006. Available at www.kff.org/insurance/snapshot/chcm111006oth2.cfm. Accessed November 24, 2006.

7. M. A. Roser, "Don't Cut State Drug Funds, AIDS, HIV Patients Plead," *Austin-American Statesman*, January 17, 2003, B1, B6.

8. J. Arthur and W. H. Shaw (Eds.), *Justice and Economic Distribution* (Englewood Cliffs, NJ: Prentice Hall, 1979), 1–11 was helpful here.

9. World Health Organization Constitution, "About WHO," World Health Organization. Available at www.who.int/about/en/index.html. Accessed November 24, 2006.

10. L. Armstrong, *It's Not About the Bike* (New York: G.P. Putnam's Sons, 2000), 108–109.

11. For a sampling of complaints, see K. Hausman, "Mentally Ill Workers Rarely Prevail in ADA Discrimination Claims, Survey Finds," *Psychiatric News* 37, no. 16 (2002): 6. Available at http://pn.psychiatryonline.org/cgi/content/full/37/16/6-a. Accessed November 24, 2006. See also M. Weiss, "Study Finds Discrimination against Disabled Patients," *ABC NewsHealth.com*. Available at http://abcnews.go.com/Health/story?id=2633167&page=1

&CMP=OTC-RSSFeeds0312. Accessed November 24, 2006. See also R. Longley, "Disabled Face Discrimination in Rental Attempts," *About.com*. Available at http://usgovinfo.about .com/od/rightsandfreedoms/a/disablerents.htm. Accessed November 24, 2006.

12. See L. Wenar, "Rights," *The Stanford Encyclopedia of Philosophy* (Fall 2006 Edition), Edward N. Zalta (Ed.). Available at http://plato.stanford.edu/entries/rights/. Accessed December 20, 2006.

13. M. E. Mahoney, "Medical Rights and the Public Welfare," *Proceedings of the American Philosophical Society* 135, no. 1 (1991): 22–29, especially p. 23.

14. L. Wenar, "Rights," *The Stanford Encyclopedia of Philosophy* (Fall 2006 Edition), Edward N. Zalta (Ed.) was helpful here. See especially section 6.1 on status rights. Available at http://plato.stanford.edu/archives/fall2006/entries/rights/. Accessed November 26, 2006.

15. Associated Press, "Veterans Lose Health Care Suit against Pentagon," Associated Press and *Washington Post*, November 20, 2002. Available at www.americasveterans.org/news/112002 .html. Accessed November 26, 2006. For a sample of unhappy commentary, see M. Marquez, "Government Must Honor Promises from the Past," *Austin-American Statesman*, January 21, 2003: A11.

16. J. Rawls, *A Theory of Justice* (Cambridge, MA: Harvard University Press, 1971), 47–48.

17. J. Arthur and W. Shaw (Eds.), *Justice and Economic Distribution* (Englewood Cliffs, NJ: Prentice Hall, 1979), 10.

18. J. Rawls, *A Theory of Justice* (Cambridge, MA: Harvard University Press, 1971), esp. 20–21, 48–51.

19. T. L. Beauchamp and J. F. Childress, *Principles of Biomedical Ethics*, 5th ed. (New York: Oxford University Press, 1971), Chapter 9, especially 389–390.

Critical Issues for Individuals

Part II of *Health Care Ethics: Critical Issues for the 21st Century* is concerned with issues that affect individuals. It is the largest section in the text, examining topics ranging from the moral status of gametes to end-of-life issues. The majority of the chapters focus on issues concerning the beginning of life and its end, because these stages bring with them many ethics concerns. The emphasis on this topic area makes sense given the complexity of its nature.

Chapters 3 through 6 are concerned with ethical dilemmas related to reproduction and prenatal care. Today and into the immediate future, this part of life will continue to present critical concerns for practitioners who wish to be ethical and honor patient needs and desires. Ethically thorny issues such as the use of assisted conception and abortion promise to be part of professional decision making in the future. In addition, advances in technology complicate decisions surrounding care during this stage of life because it offers more options than were previously available. For example, technology introduces the idea of cloning, which has previously been the purview of the science fiction writer.

Chapters 7 and 8 present issues related to the treatment of adults. The idea of competency is complex and promises to become more so as the population ages. Chapter 8 presents a discussion of the Patient Self-Determination Act, which has become an important part of clinical practice.

Chapters 9 and 10 examine some of the issues faced by adults as they age. The aging of the baby boomers means that issues of access to care and the autonomy of elders are certain to be a part of decision making for the twenty-first century. The authors of these chapters raise important ethical concerns for practitioners who will be part of the health care experience of this population group.

Finally, Chapters 11 through 13 present ethical concerns surrounding the process of death and dying. The topics discussed here have been the focus of recent media attention, which has added emphasis to their ethical concerns. Of course, as the bolus of boomers reach this stage of their lives; their sheer numbers will increase its ethical concerns. As we saw in earlier chapters, technology will also add to the decision to be made especially in the area of assisted death and withholding nutrition.

Part II of this text challenges your thinking about the ethical issues that you will face in providing health care in the twenty-first century. It also assists you in applying the theory and principles that you learned in Part I to future situations surrounding this care. Be prepared for some serious thought and lively discussions as you complete this section of the text.

CHAPTER 3

The Moral Status of Gametes and Embryos: Storage and Surrogacy

Glenn C. Graber

OVERVIEW

Graber presents the ethically challenging topic of the moral status of gametes and embryos by introducing us to "40 Ways to Make a Baby!" He uses the term moral community *to describe those deserving of our attention in ethical decisions. As you read his chapter, think about the contrast between deontology and teleological thinking in the area of value of persons. Graber uses animal rights and the rights of human children as examples to help you clarify your thinking about how we define rights of pre-embryos. He suggests that we need to expand our thought processes when analyzing the controversial issue of the rights of individuals prior to birth.*

INTRODUCTION

Technology complicates issues about human reproduction by increasing the number of choices available to us. The chart in Table 3–1, which I have whimsically entitled "40 Ways to Make a Baby" illustrates this.[1]

Technology has made possible a separation of the roles of the genetic mother (who contributes germ cells, perhaps for in vitro fertilization) from that of the gestational mother (in whose uterus the fetus develops). In addition, the social mother (who cares for the child after its birth through adoption or foster parenting) might be different from either of these. The roles of genetic and social father have always been separable. The ultimate possibility is expressed in line 32 of the chart where the baby has five parents—or perhaps six if you count the technician who delivers the sperm to the ovum as a sort-of father. In line 34 (male cloning), the source of the enucleated ovum might be different from the gestational mother, and the social mother might be still a different woman—or perhaps the genetic father might choose to raise the child in a life partnership with another male, giving the child two male and two female "parents."

Who among these four or five or six are *really* the parents of the resulting baby? Who should be given authority to make decisions about whether to continue the pregnancy if complications develop? Who should have a say in decisions about terminating treatment after birth if the newborn is severely compromised?

Not only are these relationships complex, but the decision points are multiplied greatly beyond the traditional possibilities. Until the advent of the birth control pill, no safe way was available to stop the process between fertilization and implantation, because these took place in the inaccessible regions of the

Table 3–1   40 ways to make a baby.

		Source of germ cells		Delivery of sperm	Site of fertilization	Site of gestation	Social parents		
		♂	♀				♂	♀	
1	Traditional	S♂	S♀	S♂	S♀	S♀	S♂	S♀	1
2	AIH	S♂	S♀	technician	S♀	S♀	S♂	S♀	2
3	IVF	S♂	S♀	⚲	in vitro	S♀	S♂	S♀	3
4	ICSI	S♂	S♀	Intra cytoplasmic Sperm Injection	in vitro	S♀	S♂	S♂	4
5	rent-a-womb	S♂	S♀	⚲	in vitro	surrogate	S♂	S♀	5
6	artificial womb	S♂	S♀	⚲	in vitro	artif. womb	S♂	S♀	6
7	adultery-a	G♂	S♀	G♂	S♀	S♀	?	S♀	7
8	AID	G♂	S♀	technician	S♀	S♀	S♂	S♀	8
9	AID + IVF	G♂	S♀	⚲	in vitro	S♀	S♂	S♀	9
10	AID + rent-a-womb	G♂	S♀	⚲	in vitro	surrogate	S♂	S♀	10
11	AID + artif. womb	G♂	S♀	⚲	in vitro	artif. womb	S♂	S♀	11
12	adultery-b	S♂	G♀	S♂	G♀	G♀	S♂	?	12
13	surrogate (AID)	S♂	G♀	technician	G♀	G♀	S♂	S♀	13
14	ovum donor	S♂	G♀	⚲	in vitro	S♀	S♂	S♀	14
15	surrogate (IVF)	S♂	G♀	⚲	in vitro	surrogate	S♂	S♀	15
16	#14 + artif. womb	S♂	G♀	⚲	in vitro	artif. womb	S♂	S♀	16
17	fornication	G♂	G♀	G♂	G♀	G♀	?	?	17
18	bachelor motherhood	G♂	S♀	G♂	S♀	S♀	—	S♀	18
19	#18 + AID	G♂	S♀	technician	S♀	S♀	—	S♀	19
20	#18 + IVF	G♂	S♀	⚲	in vitro	S♀	—	S♀	20
21	#19 + rent-a-womb	G♂	S♀	⚲	in vitro	surrogate	—	S♀	21
22	#19 + artif. womb	G♂	S♀	⚲	in vitro	artif. womb	—	S♀	22
23	bachelor fatherhood	S♂	G♀	S♂	G♀	G♀	S♂	—	23
24	#23 + AID	S♂	G♀	technician	G♀	G♀	S♂	—	24
25	#23 + IVF	S♂	G♀	⚲	in vitro	G♀	S♂	—	25
26	#24 + rent-a-womb	S♂	G♀	⚲	in vitro	surrogate	S♂	—	26
27	#24 + artif. womb	S♂	G♀	⚲	in vitro	artif. womb	S♂	—	27
28	adoption	G♂	G♀	G♂	G♀	G♀	S♂	S♀	28
29	#28 + AID	G♂	G♀	technician	G♀	G♀	S♂	S♀	29
30	#28 + IVF	G♂	G♀	⚲	in vitro	G♀	S♂	S♀	30
31	embryo adoption – IVF	G♂	G♀	⚲	in vitro	S♀	S♂	S♀	31
32	Five Parents (or is it 6?)	G♂	G♀	⚲	in vitro	surrogate	S♂	S♀	32
33	#29 + artif. womb	G♂	G♀	⚲	in vitro	artif. womb	S♂	S♀	33
34	clone—male E♀	S♂	—		in vitro	?	S♂	?	34
35	clone—female E♀	—	S♀		in vitro	?	?	S♀	35
36	twin fission (blastomere separation)	?	?	?	twin fission	?	?	?	36
37	ZIFT	G♂	G♀	G♂	embryo transfer	?	S♂	S♀	37
38	GIFT / DIPI	S♂	S♀	technician	S♀	S♀	S♂	S♀	38
39	cryopreservation	?	?	?	?	?	?	?	39
40	genetic therapy	?	?	?	gene therapy	?	?	?	40

KEY TO ABBREVIATIONS

S♂	=	social father
S♀	=	social mother
?	=	unknown—indicates multiple possibilities
AID	=	artificial insemination by donor
IVF	=	in vitro fertilization & embryo transfer
E♀	=	source of enucleated ovum [Germ Cell source contributes cell nucleus only. Mitochondrial genes NOT transferred.]
DIPI	=	direct intraperitoneal insemination
GIFT	=	gamete intrafallopian transfer

G♂	=	genetic father (merely)
G♀	=	genetic mother (merely)
—	=	none
AIH	=	artificial insemination by husband
ICSI	=	intracytoplasmic sperm injection
ZIFT	=	zygote intrafallopian transfer

woman's reproductive tract. Now many of the early steps in the reproductive process can be carried out in the laboratory, and we may have to decide at each stage whether to move forward to the next stage as well as with whom to consult about the decisions. One dramatic example of this is the practice of removing one cell from a pre-embryo created through in vitro fertilization to test for genetic anomalies that might help the parents decide which pre-embryo to implant.[2] Microinvasive surgical techniques allow physicians to manipulate ova within the fallopian tubes or the uterus, including assisting a sperm in penetrating the wall of the ovum.

These are possibilities with which we are not conceptually, emotionally, or ethically prepared to deal. We must sort out myriad questions about the status of the entity at each stage and the relationship of the other parties to this entity.

I am convinced that the thorny question of the moral status of the materials of human reproduction will be settled, if at all, by decision rather than by discovery. It is less an ontological question than a political one (in the broadest sense of the term *political*, referring to the conventions and agreements among the members of a community or a society). Information about the entities in question may, of course, be relevant to the outcome—but not in anything like the way that further analysis of the molecular structure of a soil sample retrieved from Mars may furnish evidence for or against the question of whether there is life on that planet.

The issue here is to establish the boundaries of the moral community—who counts, morally; who stands to us (i.e., to those of us in the acknowledged moral community) in a way that requires us to take them into account directly in our decisions and actions. These boundaries are ones that the community draws for itself, not lines that we discover embedded in the ontological landscape.

This issue transcends the usual divide in ethical theory between teleological and deontological theories. Before teleologists begin to calculate the consequences of their actions, they must determine *whose* welfare is to count; only then can they begin the process of calculating which action is optimal. I have elsewhere[3] distinguished between several characterizations of what I there called the "moral reference group" (Table 3–2).

Table 3–2   Moral reference groups.

Label	Scope
Personalism	Persons and only persons
Humanism	Humans and only humans
Vitalism	All and only living entities
Racism	All and only members of one race
Nationalism	All and only citizens of one nation
Sexism	All and only those of one gender
Universalism	All and only sentient creatures

Two teleologists with identical theories of value may come up with very different assessments of a given course of action if they approach their welfare calculations from the perspective of different moral reference groups. For example, a thoroughgoing sexist, who refuses to take into account the interests of one gender, would come to a very different conclusion about the optimal division of household tasks in a typical family than one who took the interests of all members of the household into account.

Determination of the moral reference group is also a meta-theoretical issue for deontologism. Kant's categorical imperative, for example, glosses together the moral reference group of personalism with that of humanism when it is phrased to read: "Act so that you treat humanity, whether in your own person or in that of another, always as an end and never as a means only."[4] It might be unclear whether this definition applies to persons only or to all humanity, but it is clear that it does not countenance sexism, racism, or nationalism and that it does not include the lower animals in the moral community. Kant was no animal-rights advocate.

The debate about animal rights can help to illuminate the issues here. Animal-rights advocates point out the features of (lower) animals that are similar to human attributes (especially the capacity to suffer pain). They accuse us of inconsistency if we uphold moral rules against certain sorts of treatment of humans at the same time that we allow similar treatment of animals. I contend that, even if successful, this argument is not enough to establish so-called rights in any full-blooded sense or to establish genuine moral standing for animals. Even if we are persuaded by these arguments that we have been needlessly cruel in our treatment of animals in food production, research, and other activities and resolve to treat them in less cruel and more humane ways in the future, we are still a long way from granting them genuine moral standing or membership in the moral community.

Moral standing involves going beyond describing actions as cruel or inhumane. For members of the moral community, another, more serious category of wrong is possible: the wrong of moral affront, indignity, or disrespect. One can show disrespect without being cruel (e.g., through diffidence), and one can cause pain (and perhaps even be cruel in a sense) without showing disrespect (as when a father refrains from rescuing his son from a painful experience in the interest of allowing him to experience the natural consequences of a mistake that he has made so that he will learn the wrongness of it). The common element in instances of disrespect or affronts to dignity has to do with the breakdown in an established system of cooperative mutual interaction. Instead of treating you as a peer engaged in a joint enterprise, I fail to acknowledge your interests or concerns and "use" you to further goals of my own. This notion of indignity or disrespect is the core notion in moral standing. If nothing we do to an individual qualifies as an indignity, they lack full moral standing.[5]

Individually, some of us may form such a bond with our pets that they are virtually admitted to our moral circle, and thus we regard a slight to them as an indignity. However, as a society we are a long way from having this sort of regard for lower animals generally. The day might come when we do, and we might then look back on our treatment of animals nowadays with the same disdain as we hold for the institution of slavery in our nation's past. But, unless and until we reach this sort of general understanding of their status, it cannot be said that animals are truly admitted into the moral community.

It is difficult to say precisely when (if ever) the status of moral standing will be established for animals. It is not enough for one or two visionaries to treat them in this way and to urge us to follow their example. At the other extreme, it is probably not necessary that each and every member of the moral community acknowledge their standing. Some (ill-defined) threshold of acceptance exists that would lead the moral anthropologist to say that this entity has become a full-fledged member of our moral community.

Questions can be raised, in this regard, as to whether children are fully established members of our moral community. Child abuse statutes are on the books throughout our society, but they are not always seriously enforced. Gross abuse of children by their parents is all too often condoned by the authorities as acceptable discipline or as within the domain of the privacy of the family and therefore none of the community's business. If we are still at this stage with regard to children well over a century after humane societies were established to campaign against cruelty to children and animals, it is not surprising that we are uncertain about the moral standing of reproductive materials or of the embryo at various stages of its development.

Technological developments in the reproductive area not only increase the points at which we may (and perhaps must) make decisions, but they also have an ambiguous impact on our attitude toward the developing embryo. On the one hand, the use of ultrasonography gives the expectant parent(s) prenatal contact and experience with the embryo. I have heard more than one couple describe the ultrasound images of their fetus in utero as "our first baby pictures." On the other hand, the greater awareness of the uncertainties of pregnancy that has come to our attention through our diagnostic technologies have led to what one commentator has called "the tentative pregnancy,"[6] in which women do not fully acknowledge that they are pregnant (especially to their friends but also attitudinally to themselves) until early ultrasounds and/or amniocentesis have established that the fetus is free from the sort of significant problems that might lead to miscarriage or to a decision to have an elective abortion.

How does the separation of roles within the reproductive process affect the stake of the various parties in the decisions to be made? It is far from clear. Parents I know who have both one or more children who are genetically theirs and one or more who are adopted uniformly insist that there is no fundamental difference in their commitment, emotional attachment, or sense of parenthood toward these children. Indeed, after a while, they may have to stop to remember which children are genetically theirs and which are not. Similarly, when the case was first in the news a few years ago about a child who had been switched at birth with another baby some dozen or so years earlier, I asked many of my friends who have children how they would feel if they were to learn after many years that the child they had been caring for was not genetically their child. I could not find anyone who would even begin to countenance the possibility of returning the child they now have to his or her genetic parents and taking on responsibility for the child who was genetically theirs. They uniformly and emphatically said that they considered the child now in their household as *their* child, and the other child, although having genetic links to them, would be a stranger to them.

Yet infertile couples expend enormous resources and effort in attempts to have a child who is genetically theirs, whereas many adoptable children languish in institutions or foster homes. To these people at this stage of the career of parenthood, genetics matters a great deal; to most people at a later stage of the career, it seems to matter a great deal less. The child who I have cared for and established a relationship with is clearly mine, no matter whether he or she is genetically mine; the child that I propose to care for is less obviously mine merely because I am entrusted with her or his care. I suggest that identification comes with extended contact with the child and getting to know that child as a person. Until that point has been reached, the child is, in a way, an abstraction—but the abstraction may be more nearly identified with me if I am aware of our genetic linkage. All this suggests that genetics, although not to be discounted entirely, is far from fundamental to the long-range bond between child and parent.

The interest of adopted children in learning about their genetic parents raises similar ambiguities. Most (but not all) adopted children report a strong interest in learning about their genetic parentage; but most also insist that this interest does not interfere with or diminish their emotional ties to the parents who cared for them since birth (what I call their "social parents").

One more complication has been introduced by new technologies. Even if the notion of the zygote and/or fetus as a *potential* person could be given sense in traditional reproduction—perhaps in terms of the course of development that would occur naturally if nature were left without interference to follow its course—this makes little or no sense nowadays. The natural course of events for a frozen pre-embryo[7] is inertial—it will remain in suspended animation until some intervention occurs to change its status. Little practical difference exists between the potential for personhood of a frozen pre-embryo and that for an individual germ cell that has not yet been joined with another. Only one additional laboratory step is required to move the individual sperm or ovum onto the path toward becoming a person (i.e., in vitro fertilization). Only one additional step is required to move the frozen pre-embryo onto the same path. Without technical intervention, the potential is nil in both cases.

These several ambiguities cannot help but be reflected in our valuation of the entity in question and our decision making about it. A pre-embryo is not the same as a child. In fact, a vast gap exists between the ways we experience and think of this stage of the reproductive process. The way we think about what constitutes a child also varies based on the time of gestation and the change in status from embryo to fetus.

It is argued by some that the pre-embryo is already genetically individuated and thus that it should be accorded the respect due to any human being; but this overlooks at least two respects in which a pre-embryo falls short of human status. For one, twinning could occur after this stage, so we may have here the proto stage of two persons (i.e., identical twins) instead of one individual. Second, the cells at this stage are not yet differentiated in terms of which cell will become one organ and which another—and, indeed, some of the cells that form part of the unified organism at this point of development will differentiate into placental material and thus will ultimately be discarded. Thus, it flies in the face of genetic fact to insist at this stage that the person who will (perhaps) come into being is present in some inchoate form. Furthermore, the probabilities of carrying the pre-embryo to term are only in the neighborhood of five percent even if it is implanted, so the odds are decisively against having a child develop from this clump of cells.

At what point in development shall we rule that a baby becomes a member of the moral community in her or his own right? Some key candidates for the transition point, together with the underlying philosophical rationale for each, are sketched in Table 3–2. Furthermore, it might not be the case that a bright line comes to be established; but rather an increasing value may be placed on the entity as it develops, culminating finally in a full-fledged sense of dignity or moral personhood.

These sorts of considerations led the Ethics Committee of the American Fertility Society to conclude the following:

> We find a widespread consensus that the pre-embryo is not a person but is to be treated with special respect because it is a genetically unique, living human entity that might become a person. In cases in which transfer to a uterus is possible, special respect is necessary to protect the welfare of the potential offspring. In that case, the pre-embryo deserves respect because it might come into existence as a person. This viewpoint imposes the traditional duty of reasonable prenatal care when actions risk harm to prospective offspring. Research on or intervention with a pre-embryo, followed by transfer, thus creates obligations not to hurt or injure the offspring who might be born after transfer.[8]

Applying this reasoning to the various decisions that might arise leads to a sensitive and morally serious approach.

All the parties affected by choices ought to have some significant voice in decisions, and all parties should take into account the special respect owed to these entities at every stage, as well as the special precautions to be taken if there is a possibility the entities are to be implanted and allowed to develop.

Surrogate contracts ought not to be regarded as indistinguishable from, for example, a contract that a woman might enter into to keep some piece of property in trust for a period of time. In addition to fiduciary duties to the contracting parties, the surrogate mother has special obligations of due care to protect the life that is hoped to result. However, if her life or health became threatened from continuing the pregnancy, it would be unreasonable to expect her to jeopardize her future in order to continue the process—thus she would retain her right to abortion. The legal right to elective abortion might remain even if her reasons for ending the pregnancy were less weighty (e.g., the notorious case of the threatened deposit on a scheduled cruise or pique over a late expense payment by the contracting parties), but ethically we would surely criticize her in these cases for failure to show the special respect that is due to the fetus.

Surrogacy arrangements ought to be developed with caution, recognizing that we are not dealing with a mere material possession, but rather with an entity that merits special respect and that may well generate intense emotions in the gestational mother, thus making it difficult for her to carry through agreements to give the child up and sever all ties once the child is born. Several notorious court cases have dealt with these matters; but even more common are hurt feelings by surrogate mothers who had expected to continue to be involved in the child's life after birth. All these issues should be discussed thoroughly throughout the gestational process, and clear-cut agreements specified in detail.

It may be too much to expect the law to be responsive to all these ambiguities, at least immediately, but our ethical thinking in this area needs to take them into account. We are dealing here with issues in which our thinking must be stretched to provide nuanced, sensitive ethical guidance. It would be too heavy-handed to prohibit development of this technology because we do not have a ready set of rules for dealing with its ethical dimensions. It is simplistic to thrust these decisions into the Procrustean bed of our moral rules for dealing with already-born children. Instead, we must undertake the task of sorting through the complexities and ambiguities of these unprecedented human dilemmas and attempt to come to consensus on the courses of action that maximize all the values involved. Casuistry (in the best sense) is called for, because we have a moral landscape before us that has been heretofore uncharted and must be filled in through the most careful and sensitive analysis of all its features.

SUMMARY

In this chapter, Graber discusses the many reproduction options that will be a part of the creation of human beings in the twenty-first century. While these options are a tribute to the progress of reproductive technology, they pose serious ethical issues in terms of the moral status of gametes and embryos and the need to identify the boundaries of the moral community. Ethics theories are used to show how the members of this community may be defined.

In addition to complicating the definition of a moral community, reproductive technology also creates ambiguity about how one sees the nature of an embryo. The chapter discusses these issues and presents information about parents' attitudes toward the personhood of children whether they are their genetic offspring or not. Finally, it points out the gap between the advances of reproductive technology and the moral decisions it will generate. The twenty-first century will require the courage to travel this moral landscape and map our course though ethical reasoning and discourse.

QUESTIONS FOR DISCUSSION

1. How important is the definition of *moral community* to defining the moral status of gametes and embryos?
2. What elements of deontology apply to making ethical decisions about this topic?
3. How can the teleological thinking apply when defining the moral status of the gametes and embryos?
4. Autonomy seems to be a theme in this chapter. What are the ethical issues relating to autonomy for the surrogate?
5. What ethical parallels can you draw between the rights of animals and the rights of children in the United States?

ADDITIONAL READING

American Society for Reproductive Medicine, *Ethical Considerations of Assisted Reproductive Technologies: ASRM Ethics Committee Reports and Statements*. Available at www.asrm.org/Media/Ethics/ethicsmain.html.

Genetics and Public Policy Center, Washington, D.C. (www.dnapolicy.org) reports on:
- *Public Awareness and Attitudes about Reproductive Genetic Technology* (2002)
- *Reproductive Genetic Testing: What America Thinks* (2004)
- *Reproductive Genetic Testing: Issues and Options for Policymakers* (2004)
- *Preimplantation Genetic Diagnosis: A Discussion of Challenges, Concerns, and Preliminary Policy Options Related to the Genetic Testing of Human Embryos* (2004)

Glover, J., *Ethics of New Reproductive Technologies: The Glover Report to the European Commission* (DeKalb, IL: Northern Illinois University Press, 1989).

Humber, J. M., and R. F. Almeder (Eds.), *Bioethics and the Fetus: Medical, Moral and Legal Issues* (Totowa, NJ: Humana Press, 1991).

Post, S. G. (Ed.), *Encyclopedia of Bioethics*, 3rd ed. (New York: Macmillan Reference USA, 2004). See especially the following articles:
- "Embryo and Fetus"
- "Fetal Research"
- "Genetic Testing and Screening"
- "Moral Status"
- "Reproductive Technologies"

Walters, W., and P. Singer, *Test-Tube Babies: A Guide to Moral Questions, Present Techniques, and Future Possibilities* (New York: Oxford University Press, 1982).

NOTES

1. For an earlier version of this chart, see G. C. Graber, "Ethics and Reproduction," in *Bioethics*, R. B. Edwards and G. C. Graber (Eds.) (New York: Harcourt, Brace, Jovanovich, 1988), 635.

2. See, for example, N. Fost, "Conception for Donation," *Journal of the American Medical Association* 291, no. 17 (May 5, 2004): 2125–2126.

3. G. C. Graber, A. D. Beasley, and J. A. Eaddy, *Ethical Analysis of Clinical Medicine: A Guide to Self-Evaluation* (Baltimore: Urban & Schwarzenberg, 1985), 256–258.

4. I. Kant, *Foundations of the Metaphysics of Morals*, translated by Lewis White Beck (Indianapolis, IN: Bobbs-Merrill, 1959), 47.

5. For a fuller account of this argument, see R. B. Edwards and G. C. Graber, *Bioethics* (New York: Harcourt, Brace, Jovanovich, 1988), 16–18.

6. B. Katz Rothman, *The Tentative Pregnancy: Prenatal Diagnosis and the Future of Motherhood* (New York: Viking/Penguin, 1986).

7. The term *pre-embryo* was introduced by the American Fertility Society to mark the stage of development when cells have begun to divide but have not yet begun to differentiate. See Ethics Committee of the American Fertility Society, "Ethical Considerations of the New Reproductive Technologies," *Fertility and Sterility*, Supplement 2, 53:6 (1990).

8. American Fertility Society, "Ethical Considerations of the New Reproductive Technologies," *Fertility and Sterility*, Supplement 1, 46:3 (1986), 35S.

CHAPTER 4

The Ethical Challenges of the New Reproductive Technologies

Sidney Callahan

OVERVIEW

When thinking about technology and ethics, it is often asked, "Just because we can do something, should we?" In this chapter, Callahan addresses this issue for the new technologies associated with procreation. With the expansion and profitability of these new technologies, the answer to this question is important now and will be for the rest of the twenty-first century. Notice how Callahan balances her arguments by discussing the impact of these approaches to having a child on the parents and the family in general. More importantly, she considers a person who seems to be forgotten in discussions of this matter—the child.

INTRODUCTION

How should we ethically evaluate the new reproductive technologies that treat human infertility? National debate over this issue continues as the incidence of infertility increases and new techniques are devised. Without a moral consensus over what is morally acceptable, a huge profitable "baby business" has grown and expanded.[1] At this point, legal lacunae and regulatory inconsistencies exist amidst contested ethical views.[2] One cause for the confusion arises from the rapidity of technological innovations and burgeoning marketing practices that serve the growing demand.

One obvious sign of society's conflicts over the morality of sex and reproduction can be found in the ongoing bitter debates over abortion, stem cell research, the status of embryos and, to a lesser extent, contraception and sex education in the schools. Lacking societal consensus on the morality of using medical technology to plan, limit, or interrupt pregnancies, we are unready to evaluate the newest assisted reproductive technologies aimed at producing births. To add to the uncertainty, the developed world is experiencing cultural changes in attitudes toward women, children, and the family. These interrelated social and technological changes have produced a pressing need to discuss and develop a new ethic of responsible reproduction.

My focus here is on some of the recent challenges. How should we ethically assess the innovative array of recent techniques developed to assist reproduction, such as in vitro fertilization, embryo transplants, egg and sperm donations, and surrogate mothers?

TWO INADEQUATE APPROACHES TO EVALUATING ALTERNATIVE REPRODUCTIVE TECHNOLOGY

Two inadequate approaches to the ethical assessment of the new alternative reproductive technologies are mirror images of each other in the narrowness of their focus. A conservative approach adopts as a moral requirement an "act analysis," in which the biological integrity of each marital sexual act must be preserved without artificial interference. With this view, a heterosexual married couple's act of sexual intercourse and union must always remain open to procreation.[3] Morally, "lovemaking and baby making" must not be separated. It is forbidden to separate sexual acts from procreative powers for contraceptive effect and artificial techniques that separate conceptions from marital intercourse are similarly wrong. Nor should third-party sperm and eggs be used for assisted reproduction. The fact that many alternative reproductive technologies do not protect embryonic life gives further cause for condemnation. Although the use of medical knowledge of fertility and interventions that increase the probabilities of conception are countenanced, achieving procreation through in vitro fertilization, artificial insemination, cloning, or third-party surrogacy is judged to be immoral.[4]

At the other end of the ideological spectrum, another form of act analysis focuses on the private exercise of reproductive acts as an instance of individual autonomy, procreative liberty, and the human right to reproduce. Competent adult persons must be free to exercise their reproductive rights without interference. As long as due process and informed consent by competent adults are safeguarded through appropriate contracts, adults should be entitled to engage in any alternative reproductive procedure or technology that can be procured from providers.[5] This permissive stance toward individual choice and the acceptance of market transactions is held to be morally justified on the basis of the individual's right to privacy and autonomy. Those who would attempt to limit acts of reproductive liberty should bear the burden of proof and be able to demonstrate concrete harm from some practice. Naturally, an unprecedented new technology can hardly be shown to have long-term negative consequences. Therefore, in effect, almost all alternative reproductive technologies should be able to proceed as ethically acceptable choices as contracted services.

The premature ethical foreclosures implied in the above narrow approaches to reproductive technologies are not adequate for the complexity of the moral challenges of technologically-assisted reproduction. Moral considerations should not be limited to upholding only one value or one good. A reproductive ethic based solely on preserving the natural biological integrity of each marital act of genital intercourse will not suffice, because the mastery of biological nature through technological intervention is completely natural to rational human beings—indeed, it is the glory of *Homo sapiens*. Yet, because we are rational, humans can also see that a completely permissive attitude of free choice in the use of new reproductive technologies can present serious problems. Risks taken in individual reproductive practices involve the lives of children as nonconsenting third parties—as well as affecting their families and the larger society. Humans are "the self-interpreting animals," and they live in sociocultural intergenerational groups shaped by symbolic meanings that have social consequences. Adopting particular reproductive technologies will have effects beyond fulfilling an individual's desire to be a parent.

That unrestricted uses of technologies have resulted in ecological and ethical disasters is an incontestable and inconvenient truth. Harmful outcomes have arisen that may have been unforeseen, accidental, or inadvertent. In more rare cases, fully intentional evil purposes have made use of technologies to destroy lives or facilitate genocide. Countless innovative technological interventions have produced harmful side effects that outweighed their immediate advantages. A grain of truth is found in the warning that control of nature by some people can end up producing oppression and increased control of other people with less power. Technology itself is never neutral or value free, and it has to be ethically assessed to be used in a responsible way.

Faced with new assisted reproductive technologies, the technological imperative (i.e., what can be done should be done) must not be allowed to govern individual and group practices or policies. Rational regulation and limitation might sometimes be necessary. Fulfilling individual human desires, even good desires, might become harmful to the future well-being of humankind. The question of whether certain reproductive practices are right, good, and conducive to human flourishing for everyone concerned must be addressed. Complex moral and social concerns have to be taken into account.

THE BASIS FOR DEVELOPING AN ETHICAL POSITION

In the case of reproductive technology, ethical positions should be grounded upon consideration of what furthers the good of potential children, their individual parents and families, and the moral health and common good of the larger society. Conflicts will surely arise. When there are conflicts of goods, priority should be given to the good of the child and potential child who is the most vulnerable party in the process. Children constitute the future of humankind and their protection, care, and education is a central moral obligation. The 1989 United Nations Convention on the Rights of the Child recognizes this moral and social truth. Human communities have a moral imperative to protect children and institute practices that will provide for their well-being. Moral standards that demand adult responsibility in the procreation and caretaking of the next generation enable culture and civilization to continue.

Prudent and rational persons must consider the safeguards, norms, and ideals that have been developed in the past before encouraging innovations with unknown consequences for children and their families. As in other forms of scientific and social innovation involving unknown risks to vulnerable lives without their informed consent, the burden of proof should be upon those who wish to innovate. When there is a difference in power between parties, even more precautions should be exercised in instituting a practice or a policy. Because a child or potential child cannot give informed consent and is completely helpless, the larger society must be vigilant on the child's behalf. Fulfilling adult human desires and intentions, or exercising individual liberty and autonomy, cannot suffice as a moral justification for the use of a reproductive technology. Do no harm is the primary ethical mandate, always and everywhere.

One ethical approach to new assisted reproductive technologies argues that they will do no harm and, indeed, should be permitted because they are analogous to and an extension of the socially beneficial practice of adoption. The practice of adoption is an ancient and widespread human practice that flourishes in modern societies. The evidence demonstrates that children can be incorporated successfully into families by legal adoption without ties of biological and genetic kinship. Moreover, other children adjust and cope successfully with single-parent families and families split by divorce, death, or desertion. In many other cases, "fictive kin" successfully step in to rear children. Therefore, why not allow innovative infertility treatments that employ nonmarital third parties, such as egg and sperm donors and surrogate mothers? The claim is that the psychological and social aspects of parenthood are its most important characteristics, thus through technological assistance infertile heterosexual couples, single parents, and homosexual couples can be enabled to have babies.

However, the adequacy of the analogy from adoption and "after the fact" crisis management can hardly justify planning beforehand to voluntarily replicate childrearing situations. Emergency solutions and adaptations make for poor operating norms with unforeseen consequences.[6] Even a child conceived through rape or incest might adapt well, but surely it would be wrong to plan such conceptions beforehand. A child, once born, might rather exist than not, but such conceptions could not be justified on the grounds that a sexual abuser had no other means to reproduce. In cases of adoption, a child already exists and is in need of care. For the most part, adoption rescues a child in an altruistic and legally committed action that can also give great satisfaction and happiness to an adoptive parent.[7] However, to initiate, fabricate, make to order, or even purchase a baby to satisfy individual desire is a different act.

More to the point, heretofore we have not ethically or legally countenanced the practice of deliberately conceiving a child in order to give it up or sell it to others for adoption. The still prevalent horror of selling children into prostitution and sexual slavery is considered a monstrous crime. Commercial sale of any human being has been legally and morally unacceptable since the outlawing of slavery. In the interests of human dignity and embodied integrity, Western society has forbidden the purchase of brides, sexual intercourse, or bodily organs. These existing norms have safeguarded certain cultural goods and values. Ethical guidelines for employing alternative reproductive technologies must also operate to strengthen, rather than threaten, basic cultural values. What ethical norms should be defended?

A PROPOSED ETHICAL STANDARD

It is ethically appropriate to use an alternative reproductive technology if, and only if, it makes it possible for a normal, socially adequate heterosexual married couple to have a child that they could expect to have but cannot have because of infertility. Infertility does not seem to be classifiable as a disease, and it is never life threatening. However, infertility for a married couple can be a dysfunction and an unfortunate handicap that can cause intense suffering. Medicine and medical technology is morally charged to relieve human suffering and correct dysfunctions or deformities that cause severe distress. Consequently, it can be wonderful, almost miraculous, that medical knowledge and technology now can often remedy a couple's infertility and restore a normally expected function for reproduction.

However, as in all the moral practice of medicine the techniques used must be ethically acceptable; they must correct and restore without doing harm to the infertile who suffer, the child, or other important values of the society. Ethically-acceptable techniques that meet these requirements would be artificial insemination by husband (AIH), in vitro fertilization (IVF), or tubal ovum transfer methods that neither use third-party donors nor deliberately destroy embryonic lives. It would seem morally contradictory to destroy human life to obtain a new life or to co-opt another person's reproductive and genetic powers for one's own genetic project.

A remedial standard based on evolved biological and sociocultural norms requires that the genetic parents, the gestational parent, and the rearing parents should be the same and adequately prepared to rear the child that results from medical intervention. To this end, potential parents who are to be medically assisted to reproduce should be presently alive and well, in an appropriate time in their lifecycle, and possess average psychological and social resources to care for a potential child.

Helping the severely retarded, the mentally ill, the genetically diseased, the destitute, the aged, or a widow with a dead spouse's sperm to have a child they otherwise could not have would be ethically unacceptable. It would also be unacceptable to alter average expectable reproductive conditions through direct efforts to produce the risks of multiple births or to use genetic screening to select and destroy embryos to obtain a desired gender. (The latter practices of sex selection and other forms of genetic screening and reductions produce a whole host of other ethical problems that cannot be dealt with here.)

However, it can be generally accepted that the power to intervene in such a crucial matter as the procreation of a new life makes the medical professionals or institutions involved morally responsible trustees of a potential child's future. As trustees, skilled professionals have an ethical duty neither to take serious risks on behalf of non-consenting others nor to select and destroy lives at the will of the potential parents.

Moral judgments by professional workers are unavoidable. All individual members of a social group, and particularly well-trained professionals, have moral obligations to their larger communities and to the common good as well as to individual clients. Moreover, the fact that expensive medical resources and professional skills are employed for remedial infertility treatments means that larger questions of distributive justice cannot be avoided. The huge profits that arise from marketing and providing infertility services raise other ethical and political concerns.[8]

Already, many lives are being affected in a variety of problematic ways without public knowledge or moral deliberations to arrive at political decisions about regulation. The claim that an individual's right to reproduce would be violated if infertility treatments are not freely made available to any individual who requests them seems wrongheaded. A negative right not to be interfered with (e.g., the right to marry, which itself is not absolute) does not entail a positive right (e.g., that society is obligated to provide a spouse).

Moreover, as a society, we have already decided that when child welfare is in the balance, social, legal, and professional interventions and curtailments of liberty are justified. Adoption procedures, custodial decisions, and child abuse cases require that professionals make judgments on the fitness of parental capacities. As the frequent cases of child abuse leading to murder attest, it is better to err on the side of safety than take risks with children's lives. Should not medical professionals be similarly responsible and morally cautious in carrying out the interventions that will in essence create a baby for a couple?

Employing third-party donors or the different forms of surrogate mothers is not, in my opinion, an ethically acceptable use of reproductive technologies. Procedures using surrogates or sperm and egg donors can variously combine different sources of sperm and eggs to produce embryos that gestate in a hired gestational womb apart from the rearing parents. Such separations and fragmentations pose social and psychological risks arising from the disjointed process. The commitment to care for a child might also become broken or defused. To understand the problems with third-party donors, we need to consider what values, goods, and safeguards have been inherent in the biological and cultural norm: of having two heterosexual parents who are the genetic, gestational, and rearing parents of their biological child whom they rear over their mutual life cycle.

Many proponents of third-party donors in alternative reproduction— whether for married heterosexuals, single men and women, or homosexual couples, ignore what happens *after* a baby is conceived, produced, or procured. Little account is taken of the fact that individuals live out their intergenerational life spans in families within complex ecological systems.[9] The assumption seems to be that why and how one gets a baby makes no difference in what happens in the years of childrearing and family life afterwards. This might be true of breeding dogs and horses, but it is hardly true of complex thinking, feeling, imaginative self-aware human beings interested in their origin and destiny in the world. Knowing your family forebearers can be important in constructing one's self-identity, especially in adolescence. The identity of fathers and mothers are crucial in understanding one's self.

When a young person becomes sexually mature and wishes to marry and procreate, thoughts often turn to one's own progenitors and birth. Legitimizing and morally sanctioning third-party or collaborative reproduction can contribute directly to the confusion and difficulties of young persons developing into adulthood. We put at risk the well-being of the family, the parents, the child, the donor(s), and the focus on moral responsibility for one's offspring.

THE FAMILY

The advantages and safeguards for children in having two married heterosexual parents who also are the genetic, gestational, and rearing parents are manifold and becoming more clear in new sociological research.[10] This form of family produces biological and cultural advantages for its members. From an evolutionary point of view, mammalian "in vivo" reproduction and primate parent-child bonding provide effective means for the protection, defense, and complex long-term socialization of offspring. They far outperform reproduction by species that lay eggs that are left floating unprotected in the sea or buried in the sand to take their chances with passing predators.[11] With the advent of long-living rational animals, such as human beings, the basic primate models are broadened and deepened to include family groups that include fathers and other kinship bonds, such as grandparents.[12] Two heterosexual parents supported by kin can engage in even more arduous parenting, including nurturing the young over an extended period of time. The nuclear family is founded on biology and has evolved as a cultural phenomenon that generates intense altruistic bonds and mutual caretaking.[13]

The Western cultural family ideal has gradually become less patriarchal as the equal moral worth of women and children has been recognized. Families have ensured far more than law, order, and social continuity. As the heterosexual members of a couple freely choose each other, they make a commitment to share the vicissitudes of life. Bonded in love and legal contract, a man and woman mutually exchange exclusive rights, giving each other emotional, sexual, and economic priority. Sexual mating results in children, who then have a claim to equal parental care from both their father and mother. In addition, the extended families of both parents are important as supplemental supports for the couple, especially in case of death or disaster.

No analysis of one procreative act or brief period in a marriage can do justice to the social fact that the reproductive couple exists as a unit within a nuclear and extended family of kin. Siblings, cousins, aunts, uncles, grandparents, and other relatives are important in family life for both pragmatic and psychological reasons. Individual identity is rooted in biologically-based descent and kinship within cooperating social groups. The family is the one remaining institution where status is given by birth; it is not earned or achieved. The irreversible bonds of genetic kinship extend over time and through space to produce a rooted sense of identity. Psychologically and socially the family provides emotional connection, social purpose, and meaning to ongoing life. Those individuals who do not marry or find families of their own are still strongly connected to others through their families of origin.[14] Each human being exists within a familial and social envelope, and must do so to flourish. But as a cultural invention, why must kinship and family be based upon biology? Cannot any persons who declare themselves to be a family be a family?

Although the internalized psychological image of a family and the intention to belong to a family, and act like a family, are the foundations of a family, the bond created by genetic kinship cannot be denied. Because we now understand the importance of cultural constructs, we must not underestimate the power of genetic ties.[15] Adoption, for instance, models kinship on the biological genetic ties of reproduction. One definition of the family is that a family consists of people who share genes. Sociobiologists and evolutionary psychologists emphasize the power of genetic relationships for altruism and human bonding.[16] In fact, the unwillingness of some infertile couples to adopt and their struggles to have their own biological baby is testimony to the existence of a strong innate urge to reproduce oneself genetically with a beloved mate.

This is understood as the fusion of two genetic heritages, with the child socially situated within two lineages. Members of both lineages may be supportive, or one set of kin may by choice or chance be more important, but having two sets provides important social resources. The child is heir to more than money or property when situated in a clear and rooted kinship community.

The search by adopted children for their biological parents and possible siblings reveals the psychological need of humans to be situated and to know their origins.[17] When there are one or more third-party donors—of sperm, eggs, or embryo—the child is distanced or cut off from either half or all of its genetic heritage. If deceptive secrecy is practiced concerning the child's origins, then both the child and his or her extended family will be wronged. Grandparents and half-siblings are deprived from knowing their close kin. Because family secrets are rarely kept completely, delayed revelations produce disillusionment and distrust among those deceived. Even when a child and relatives know the truth, the identity of the donor (or donors) becomes an issue for all concerned.

Parents and Spouses

Psychology has come to see genetic factors as being more and more important in mating, parent-child interactions, and childrearing outcomes.[18] When rearing parents and genetic parents differ and the donor is unknown, there is a provocative void. If the donor is known and is part of the rearing parents' family or social circle, other psychological problems and potential conflicts might emerge over whom the real parent is and who has primary rights and responsibilities. When the third-party donor is also the surrogate mother, combining genetic and gestational parenthood, the social and legal problems can be profound. The much discussed Whitehead-Stern court struggle indicates the divisive chaos, struggle, and suffering that is possible in third-party surrogate arrangements.

In the average expectable situation, two married parents possess equal genetic investment in the child and become unified by their mutual relationship to the child. They are irreversibly connected and made kin to each other through the child they have jointly procreated. Their love, commitment, and sexual bond have been made manifest in a new life. The development of the child that occurs during pregnancy also unites the couple and prepares them for the parental enterprise.[19]

The parent's genetic link with the child is shared with his or her own extended family. Common genetic inheritance produces a family likeness. Biological kinship often leads to empathy and ease of affective attunement for family members. The child's genetic link to one's spouse and to each marital partner's own kin strengthens the marital and family bonds. But the fact that the child is also a new and unique organism formed by a random combination of the couple's genetic heritage gives enough difference to allow the child to be seen as separate. The child possesses what has been called an "alien dignity" as a unique human being that must be recognized.[20] (Cloning one's self would be wrong for its egotistic intent and for its denial of a child's possession of a unique new identity.) Because we are embodied creatures, the psychological bonds of caring and empathy are built upon the firm foundation of biological ties and bodily self-identity.

When technological intervention assists reproduction within the marriage without donors, the arduous process can also contribute to the marital unity. When techniques such as AIH or IVF or tubal ovum transfer are used to correct infertility, the time and money spent, the shared stress and discomfort, and the cooperative efforts required can serve to strengthen the couple's unity and commitment. Seeking to bear their child can focus two persons upon their marital relationship and their mutual contribution to childbearing. The psychological bonding between them can grow and transcend the stress and the unpleasant and painful procedures and interventions in their sexual and social lives. Mutual sacrifices are necessary. When successful, the resulting baby will, as in a spontaneous pregnancy, be a new life in whom they are mutually invested, and to whom they are equally related. (In adoption also, both parents have an equal legal and social relationship to the child to whom they are jointly rescuing and committing themselves.) Given the equal investment in their child, both parents are equally responsible for childrearing and support.

Unfortunately, in assisted reproduction the success rates for the arduous and expensive treatments are low and often disappointing.[21] A couple has to be able to withstand frustration together, not become dangerously obsessed with the quest, and be able to turn to adoption or accept childlessness. The temptation to move to ethically problematic methods "on the market" can be strong.

When employing third-party genetic or gestational donors, however, the marital and biological unity is broken asunder. One parent will be related biologically to the child and the other parent will not. True, the nonrelated parent might give consent, but the consent, even if truly informed and free, can hardly equalize the imbalance. Although there is certainly no question of adultery in such a situation, nevertheless, the intrusion of a third-party donor can have a psychological effect on the couple's union. Even if there is no jealousy or envy, the reproductive inadequacy of one partner has been dramatically defined and reliance has been placed on an outsider's potency, genetic heritage, and superior reproductive capacity.[22]

Asymmetry of biological parental relationships within a family or household has always been problematic, from Cinderella to today's stepparents and reconstituted families. Children who are unrelated to one of their married parents have less positive social outcomes and are in greater danger of abuse.[23] The most frequently cited cause of divorce in second marriages is the difficulty of dealing with another person's children.[24] Empathy and identification within a sense of shared biological kinship seems to buttress parental authority and commitment. In disturbed families under stress, one finds more incest, child abuse, and scapegoating if biological kinship is asymmetrical.[25] Biological ties become psychologically potent, because people fantasize in subjective emotional interactions with one another as both children and adults.

Parents' fantasies about a child's past and future make a difference, as all students of child development or family dynamics will attest. Identical twins might even be treated very differently because parents project different fantasies upon them.[26] Third-party donors and surrogates cannot be counted on to disappear from family consciousness, even if legal contracts could control other ramifications or overt interventions.

The Child

The most serious ethical problems in using third-party donors in alternative reproduction concern the well-being of the potential child. A child conceived by new forms of collaborative reproduction is being made subject to a biosocial experiment without his or her consent. Although no child is conceived with his or her informed consent, a child not artificially produced is begotten and born in the same way as life was transmitted to his or her parents. Even if there is no danger of transmitting unknown genetic disease or causing physiological harm to the child, the psychological relationship of the child to his or her parents is endangered, whether or not there is deception or secrecy about the child's origins. It should be clear, as already mentioned, that being adopted and rescued after the fact has a different meaning for a child than having been a contractual product involving third parties.

An adopted child, although perhaps harboring resentment against his or her birth parents, probably views the rescuing adopters differently than a child would look at parents who have procured or fabricated the child to order using strangers. Treating a child like a commodity—something to be manufactured and procured for the satisfaction of the purchasing parents—infringes upon the child's dignity as a gift received from one's progenitors, from nature's creativity, and for the faithful, a gift from God.

As ideals of parenthood have developed, those who seek a child not as a gift received for its own sake, but because of the need to satisfy some personal need or desired extrinsic end, are judged ethically suspect. Unfortunately, we are still struggling to overcome residual beliefs that view children as a kind of personal property. Only gradually have we welcomed children as new lives given to their parents in trusteeship. Children can now be valued as equal in moral worth to adults despite their dependency and their powerlessness. Having a child solely for some selfish reason has now become as morally unacceptable as marrying solely for money or status. In the past, some people have wanted children to prove sexual prowess, to secure domestic labor, to procure a scapegoat, to increase social power, or to have someone of their own to possess. Parental motives for procreating influence the future relationship of the child with its parents, as does the means used to have a child.

A person or a couple obsessively driven to produce a child might not be prepared to rear the actual child once born. Being wanted and being well reared are not the same. Parental overinvestment in "gourmet children" can be psychologically burdensome for a child.[27] Adolescent problems of anorexia, depression, and suicide have been seen as related to the dynamics of parental control.[28] A young person must achieve a separate identity in order to relate adequately with others or to become autonomous-in-relationship.

The child who was desired for all the wrong reasons is pressured to live up to parental dreams of the optimal baby or perfect child. Outright rejection of imperfect or nonoptimal babies contracted for by alternative reproductive technology is possible and should be a matter of grave concern. There also seem to be some risks for IVF children, due to multiple births and prematurity, but when the parents are married and committed to their own irreversibly-related children, resources can be made available to care for needs that may arise.

A child with a "clouded genetic heritage," however, has a more tenuous access to resources as well as to the achievement of a secure personal identity. In the course of a child's development, psychologists note that thinking and fantasizing about one's origins seems to be inevitable in the search for self. In alternative reproduction, the question "Whose baby am I?" becomes inevitable.[29] "Why was my biological parent not more concerned with what would happen to the new life he or she helped to create?" The need to know about possible half-siblings and other kin might become urgent at some point in development. Those first infants conceived from sperm donors now are entering young adulthood, and they have started new support movements and Internet blogs. Other such young adults join in searches for their biological parents and relations. More transparency and openness is advocated. The problem of inadvertent incest is one concern, but the main focus is on issues of identity. The asymmetry of biological relationships in a family exacerbates the existence of complex fantasies and psychological currents within them. Having two married parents with whom one is equally biologically related has advantages. A young person can safely identify with parents; love, hate, or come to terms with them; and then safely separate from them on the path to maturity.

DONORS AND THE CULTURAL ETHOS

Procuring donors of sperm, eggs, embryos, or wombs is an essential component of collaborative reproduction. The market has grown as the baby business has grown. Although a "gauzy shroud of sentimentality," cloaks the language of fertility clinics, such as "donors," "surrogate mothers," "family building," or "forever families," a growing market and profitable businesses exist.[30] Infertile persons are choosing and shopping as market forces operate to set prices. Brokers search for donors and recruit them for a profit; potential clients shop for the eggs and sperms they want and that they can afford. Donors, too, shop for the best deal.[31] However, in this burgeoning enterprise little research has examined the effect of the baby business on these donors. Nor has there been much critical analysis of the morality of what a donor is doing. It is as though the market processes and the sellers are being assimilated into the model of blood donors who are paid for their blood.

When persons sell their eggs and sperm, they are selling their unique genetic identity that they inherited from their own parents and grandparents. This generative capacity is not like blood, a kidney, or any other organ, because it contains the information and generative potential that is basic to personal identity. When an individual treats this gift of identity and power as less than precious or contracts to sell it, he or she breaks an implicit compact with the human group to respect and practice "procreative stewardship."[32] So, too, a surrogate mother is selling her womb and reproductive capacities that she has inherited as a gift from her mother. Some donors and surrogates who do not receive money for their services might consider that participating in assisted reproduction is an act of altruism, but the altruism is being directed to fulfill the desires of adult(s), not of the child who will be born. When money is taken for such services, it is analogous to selling sex in prostitution.

Another serious problem in the practice of donation by third parties is that it counters a basic principle of morality—taking responsibility for the consequences of one's actions. Adult persons are held morally responsible for the effect of their words and deeds. In serious matters, such as sex and reproduction, which have irreversible lifetime consequences, we rightly hold competent persons to a high standard of moral and legal responsibility. To counter tendencies toward sexual irresponsibility and child neglect, Western culture has insisted that men and women be held accountable for those sexual acts that create new life.

Donors, whether male or female, who take part in collaborative reproduction do not assume personal responsibility for their momentous reproductive act that results in the birth of their biological child. In fact, in most cases the donor contracts to abdicate any present or future personal responsibility. The donor is specifically enjoined not to carry through on what he or she initiates or causes, but instead to hand over to physicians or others, usually unknown others, their potent generative power. By design and contract, persons attempt to abdicate all consequences or responsibility for their reproductive act. Yet parental responsibility is a basic form of the natural responsibility that human beings possess.[33] Taking part in the procreation that results in a new life has traditionally given rise to moral obligations and moral claims from the life engendered. It seems doubtful that a legal convention can completely undo the obligation.

Donors who abdicate parental responsibility also deprive their own parents of grandparenthood and other close family members from knowing their relatives. Future children of the donor, or other children of a surrogate mother, might never know their half-siblings. To disregard the biological reality of our relationships promotes a mistaken disembodied view of how human beings actually function—or should function. If we succeed in isolating sexual and reproductive acts from personal responsibility, this approval of moral abdication can only increase existing problems within the culture. Do we want to encourage women to be able to emotionally distance themselves from their potential offspring or, in the case of surrogates, from the child in their womb who will be turned over to those who pay? When eggs are commodities sold to the highest bidder, personal identity also is under threat of becoming another commodity.

Do we wish to sanction male abdication from responsibility for their biological offspring? Already epidemics of male sexual irresponsibility, unmarried conceptions, and father abandonment are straining the family bonds. Commitment to support and care for children is weakened when we legitimize the isolation of genetic, gestational, and social parentage. When reproduction becomes commercialized and governed by contract and purchase, our familial culture becomes even more fragmented and alienated.

One of the requirements for a responsible ethic of sexuality and reproduction is to acknowledge sexual acts as personal acts involving the whole person. Lust is wrong because it disregards the whole person in the pursuit of sensual gratification. A person is reduced to a means to fulfill selfish desire, and, if money is involved, exploitation of the poor will occur. So, too, it seems wrong to isolate and use a person's reproductive capacity apart from his or her whole person. When a woman donates her eggs and gestational capacity there is a grave danger of exploitation, as feminists have warned.[34] The physiological risks attending the drastic intervention in a woman's reproductive system needed for surrogacy or egg retrieval are considerable. If a great deal of money is offered for surrogacy or eggs, needy women will be tempted to sell their bodies and suffer the consequences. Feminists rightly protest that it is all too easy to reduce women to baby machines who are bought and sold by those rich enough to pay. What will such attitudes and practices do to other children in the society? Can children comprehend, without anxiety, the fact that mothers can make babies, but also give them away for money? The great primordial reality of maternal commitment, mutual dependency, and irreversibly bonded kinship is demeaned.

SUMMARY

Our society faces a challenge to its traditional ethics of reproduction and family norms. The cultural norm, based on biological predispositions unifies genetic, gestational, and rearing parents in a nuclear family supported by an extended kinship system. The family exists as a dynamic intergenerational institution that is interrelated to the larger society and shores it up. In Western societies, technological progress has forced new and refined understandings of morally responsible reproduction. The parental enterprise is rightly seen as basically an altruistic one—children should not be viewed as a form of personal property or as a means to satisfy adult desires or needs. When making individual reproductive decisions or public policy, the good of the potential child, along with the general cultural conditions that support childrearing and family life should be the primary considerations.

I have argued for an ethical standard that limits alternative reproductive techniques to those that remedy infertility of a marital committed couple in average expectable conditions. The genetic, gestational, and rearing parents should remain unified in human reproduction. Collaborative reproduction risks the good of the child, the good of families, and the need of the culture to uphold moral responsibility. Certain limits should be set on using certain technologies for assisted reproduction. As Ghandi said, "Means are ends in the making."[35]

QUESTIONS FOR DISCUSSION

1. According to Callahan's ethical reasoning, why would a business to create "gourmet children" be unethical when the potential parents are able to provide informed consent?

2. Why does Callahan include the application of certain reproductive technology procedures for married people and not for single, aging, or gay potential parents? What is her ethical argument?

3. What ethical principles would apply in a decision to limit the use of current and future reproductive technologies?

4. How is Callahan's position on reproductive technology different from Graber's view in Chapter 3?

5. What ethical theories support Callahan's position in this chapter?

NOTES

1. See D. L. Spar, *The Baby Business: How Money, Science, and Politics Drive the Commerce of Conception* (Cambridge MA: Harvard Business School Press, 2006); D. L. Spar, "The Business of Babies," *Science & Theology News* (July-August 2006): 43–46.; D. L. Spar, "Buying Our Children, Selling Our Souls? The Commodification of Children," *Conscience* 27 (2006): 14–16.

2. E. Marguardt, *The Revolution in Parenthood: The Emerging Global Clash between Adult Rights and Children's Needs* (New York: Institute for American Values, 2006).

3. Congregation for the Doctrine of Faith, *Instruction on Respect for Human Life in Its Origin and on the Dignity of Procreation* (Washington, D.C.: United States Catholic Conference, 1987).

4. A statement of these principles can be found in Roman Catholic Church teaching "Instruction on Respect for Human Life in Its Origin and on the Dignity of Procreation" by the Congregation for the Doctrine of Faith, *Origins* 16 (March 19, 1987) and P. Lauritzen, *Pursing Parenthood* (Bloomington, IN: Indiana University Press, 1993).

5. John A. Robertson, *Children of Choice: Freedom and the New Reproductive Technologies* (Princeton, NJ: Princeton University Press, 1994).

6. J. Wallerstein, J. Lewis, and S. Blakeslee, *The Unexpected Legacy of Divorce: A 25-Year Landmark Study* (New York: Hyperion, 2000).

7. M. Stewart Van Leeuwen and G. Miller Wrobel, "The Moral Psychology of Adoption and Family Ties," In *The Morality of Adoption: Social-Psychological, Theological, and Legal Perspectives*, T. P. Jackson (Ed.) (Grand Rapids, MI: William B. Erdmans, 2005), 3-31.

8. Spar, op. cit. and M. Ryan, *Ethics and Economics of Assisted Reproduction: The Cost of Longing* (Washington, D.C.: Georgetown University Press, 2003).

9. A classical statement of this process can be found in E. H Erickson, *Childhood and Society* (New York: Norton, 1950); also J. Heckhausen, "Psychological Approaches to Human Development," in *The Cambridge Handbook of Age and Ageing*, M. L. Johnson (Ed.) (Cambridge: Cambridge University Press, 2005), 181–189; R. Martinson and S. A. Martinson, "The Nature of Parenting," in *Work of Families: Roles of Families*, Chapter 5, *The Family Handbook*, H. Anderson, D. Browning, I. S. Evison, and M. Steward Van Leeuwen (Eds.) (Louisville KY: Westminster John Knox Press, 1998) 63–89.

10. Institute for American Values, *Why Marriage Matters: 26 Conclusions from the Social Sciences*, 2nd ed. (New York: Institute for American Values, 2005); E. Marguardt, op. cit.

11. See J. Altman, "Sociobiological Perspectives on Parenthood," in *Parenthood: A Psychodynamic Perspective* (New York: Guilford Press, 1984); E. O. Wilson, *Sociobiology* (Cambridge, MA.: Harvard University Press, 1975). See also M. Daly and M. Wilson, "Evolutionary Psychology and Marital Conflict: The Relevance of Stepchildren," in *Sex, Power, Conflict: Evolutionary and Feminist Perspectives*, D. M. Buss and N. M. Malamuth (Eds.) (Oxford: Oxford University Press, 1996), 9–28.

12. The role of the father has been seen as critically important in both the female and male child's intellectual development, moral development, sex role identity, and future parenting; for a summary of relevant research, see R. D. Parke, *Fathers* (Cambridge, MA: Harvard Uni-

versity Press, 1981) and S. M. H. Hanson and F. W. Bonett, *Dimensions of Fatherhood* (Beverly Hills, CA: Sage Publications, 1985).

13. See K. Gough, "The Origin of the Family," *Journal of Marriage and the Family* (November 1971): 760–768; P. J. Wilson, *Man the Promising Primate: The Conditions of Human Evolution* (New Haven, CT: Yale University Press, 1980); G. P. Murdock, "The University of the Nuclear Family," in *A Modern Introduction to the Family*, N. W. Bell and E. F. Vogel (Eds.) (New York: The Free Press, 1968); and M. J. Bane, *Here to Stay: American Families in the Twentieth Century* (New York: Basic Books, 1976).

14. S. P. Bank and M. D. Kahn, *The Sibling Bond* (New York: Basic Books, 1982); I. Arnet Connidis, "Sibling Ties Across Time: The Middle and Later Years," in *Cambridge Handbook of Age and Aging*, op. cit., 429–436.

15. Wilson, op. cit., and Daly and Wilson, op. cit.

16. D. S. Browning, "Adoption and the Moral Significance of Kin Altruism," in *The Morality of Adoption* (Grand Rapids, MI: Wm. B. Eerdmans Publishing), 52–77.

17. C. Nadelson, "The Absent Parent, Emotional Sequelae," in *Infertility: Medical, Emotional, and Social Considerations*, M. D. Mazor and H. F. Simons (Eds.) (New York: Human Sciences Press, 1984); M. Stewart Van Leeuwen and G. Miller Wrobel, op. cit.

18. Twin studies and the recognition of inherited temperamental traits have followed studies showing a genetic component to alcoholism, manic depression, schizophrenia, antisocial behavior, and I.Q. For a popular discussion of the findings in regard to schizophrenia and criminal behavior, see S. Mednick, "Crime in the Family Tree," *Psychology Today* 19 (March 1985): 58–61. For a more general discussion by an anthropologist, see M. Konner, *The Tangled Wing: Biological Constraints on the Human Spirit* (New York: Holt, Rinehart & Winston, 1982). See also Daly and Wilson, op. cit.

19. A. Macfarlane, *The Psychology of Childbirth* (Cambridge, MA: Harvard University Press, 1977); M. Greenberg, *The Birth of a Father* (New York: Continuum, 1985).

20. H. Thielcke, *The Ethics of Sex* (New York: Harper & Row, 1964), 32ff.; Early beginnings of a philosophical reassessment of the status of children in J. Blustein, *Parents & Children: The Ethics of the Family* (Oxford: Oxford University Press, 1982), and in O. O'Neill and W. Ruddick (Eds.), *Having Children: Philosophical and Legal Reflections on Parenthood* (New York: Oxford University Press, 1979); S. Callahan, "An Ethical Analysis of Responsible Parenthood," in *Genetic Counseling: Facts, Values, and Norms; Birth Defects: Original Article Series* 15, no. 22 (New York: Alan R. Liss, 1979).

21. Assisted Reproductive Technology Success Rates 2003 National Summary and Fertility Clinic Reports 2003. U.S. Department of Health and Human Services Centers for Disease Control and Prevention CDC Reproductive Health; Spar, *The Baby Business*.

22. Daly and Wilson, op. cit.

23. Institute for American Values, op. cit.

24. B. Maddox, *The Half Parent: Living with Other People's Children* (New York: M. Evans and Company, 1975); R. Espinoza and Y. Newman, *Stepparenting: With Annotated Bibliography* (Rockville, MD: National Institute of Mental Health, Center for Studies of Child and Family Mental Health, 1979).

25. See "Explaining the Differences Between Biological Father and Stepfather Incest," and "Social Factors in the Occurrence of Incestuous Abuse," in *The Secret Trauma: Incest in the Lives of Girls and Women*, D. E. H. Russell (Ed.) (New York: Basic Books, 1986).

26. D. N. Stern, *The Interpersonal World of the Infant: A View from Psychoanalysis and Developmental Psychology* (New York: Basic Books, 1985).

27. See "The Child as Surrogate Self" and "The Child as Status Symbol," in D. Elkind, *The Hurried Child* (Reading, MA: Addison-Wesley, 1981).

28. S. Minuchin, B. L. Rosman, and W. Baker, *Psychosomatic Families: Anorexia Nervosa in Context* (Cambridge, MA: Harvard University Press, 1978).

29. L. Andrews, "Yours, Mine, and Theirs," *Psychology Today*, 18 (December 1984): 20–29.; Marguardt, op. cit.

30. See Spar's descriptions.

31. Donor 15, "Ova Sale: The Art of the Deal in the Gray Market for Human Eggs," *Reason* (October 2006). Available at www.reason.com/news/show/36867.html.

32. B. Waters, "Adoption, Parentage, and Procreative Stewardship," in *The Morality of Adoption*, 32–51 (Grand Rapids, MI: Eerdman's Books for Young Readers, 2005).

33. H. Jonas, *The Imperative of Responsibility: In Search of an Ethics for the Technological Age* (Chicago: University of Chicago Press, 1984).

34. B. Rothman, *The Tentative Pregnancy* (New York: Viking Press, 1986); H. Holmes, B. Hoskins, and M. Gross, *The Custom-Made Child: Women-Centered Perspectives* (Clifton, NJ: Humana Press, 1981); A. M. Jagger (Ed.), *Living with Contradictions: Controversies in Feminist Social Ethics* (Boulder, CO: Westview Press, 1994).

35. M. Gandhi, *The Essential Gandhi: An Anthology of His Writings on His Life, Work and Ideas.* (New York: Random House, 1962).

CHAPTER 5

Abortion: The Unexplored Middle Ground

*Carol Petrozella**

OVERVIEW

This chapter is a revision of one written by R. A. McCormick in the first edition (see note). In order to clarify comments which are different from the current author, his name is placed in parentheses for clarification. Petrozella discusses the issue of abortion and how it continues to divide the country. Some despair that there may never be public resolution of these differences. However, the author posits that in a democracy, we must seek common ground. She presents areas where both sides of the debate might find the beginning of dialogue and where agreement might even be possible. For the healthcare professional, it is important to understand all the arguments in this issue and to be aware of laws and organizational policies that govern its practice.

INTRODUCTION

During the Republican National Convention in August 1988, I (McCormick) listened to an interview with fundamentalist minister Jerry Falwell and Faye Wattleton, president of Planned Parenthood, on the subject of abortion. Falwell kept insisting that unborn babies were the last disenfranchised minority—voiceless, voteless, and unprotected in the most basic of civil liberties. Wattleton's statements all returned to the concept of privacy and the woman's right to decide whether she would or would not bear a child. It was a tired old stalemate; nether party budged an inch. The moderators identified their only common ground as the statement: "This is a great country where people are free to disagree."

Unfortunately, the Falwell–Wattleton exchange is an example of the current discussion on abortion. Each side makes one point that is central and absolute. The discussion accomplishes nothing except perhaps to raise everyone's blood pressure. All remarks return to and are interpreted from this single absolute starting point. Thus, Falwell sees nonviolent demonstrations at abortion clinics as signs of hope for a transformation of consciousness and a growing rejection of abortion. Wattleton sees them as unconstitutional and violent disturbances of a woman's exercise of her prerogative to make her own choice.

**Revised from R. A. McCormick, "Abortion: The Unexplored Middle Ground," in *Health Care Ethics: Critical Issues for the 21st Century*. Original ed., 1998, edited by John. F. Monagle and David C. Thomasma. (Sudbury, MA: Jones and Bartlett, 2005).*

Are we doomed forever to this kind of dialogue of the deaf? Perhaps, especially if the central principles identified by both sides are indeed central. However, one should note an important difference in these "central issues." Falwell and those who share his view are speaking primarily of the morality of abortion and only secondarily about public policy or the civil rights of the unborn. Wattleton says little about morality (though she implies much), but puts all her emphasis on what is now constitutional public policy. On his level, I (McCormick) believe Falwell is right. On her level, Wattleton is right (in the sense that *Roe v. Wade* does give women a constitutional right). The discussants are like two planes passing in the night at different altitudes.

In such heated standoffs, the idea of what public policy ought to be, especially in light of which morality, is rarely discussed. The linkage of these two in a consistent, rationally defensible, humanly sensitive way usually becomes victim to gavel pounding. Unless this linkage is made more satisfactorily in the public consciousness than it has been thus far, any public policy on abortion will lack supportive consensus and continue to be seriously disruptive to social life. The terms *pro-choice* and *pro-life* will continue to mislead, label, and divide our citizenry.

Can the public conversation be enlarged so that a minimally acceptable consensus might have the chance to develop? I (McCormick) am probably naive to think so. However, I (McCormick) have seen more unexpected and startling things happen—Vatican II, for example. Even Falwell and Wattleton could agree on a few things beyond their edifying puff that this is a great country because people are free to disagree. I call my proposed area of conversation "the unexplored middle ground."

If the public talked more about this middle ground, we could perhaps establish a public conversational atmosphere with a better chance at achieving a peaceable public policy. Before listing possible elements for this unexplored middle ground, I want to make three introductory points. First, diverting attention to the middle ground is not an invitation to compromise. To attempt to discover what we might agree on is not to forfeit our disagreements. It is only to shift the conversational focus. It is to discuss one's convictions with a different purpose, with different people, in a different way.

Second, my own moral position (McCormick) is abundantly clear from previous writings.[1] Therefore it is my conviction that the policy set in *Roe v. Wade* does not adequately reflect the position of a majority of Americans. Although that conviction should not hinder the search for a middle ground, it does warn the reader that the "middle ground" I propose is influenced by these postures. The consensus I would like to see develop and be reflected in policy is related to my own beliefs and will, undoubtedly, shape my identification and wording of the "unexplored middle ground." Indeed, some—from both sides—will see my middle ground as a poorly disguised presentation of only one point of view, hardly in the middle. I acknowledge the possibility in advance, but forge ahead nonetheless.

Third, when I speak of a common ground I do not mean that all or many now agree on these points. Nevertheless, I believe there is solid hope that they can begin to agree.

ELEMENTS OF A MIDDLE GROUND

1. ***There is a presumption against the moral permissibility of taking human life.*** This means that any individual or society sanctioning this or that act of intentional killing bears the burden of proof. Life, as the condition of all other experiences and achievements, is a basic good, indeed the most basic of all goods. If it may be taken without public accountability, we have returned to moral savagery. For this reason, all civilized societies have rules about homicide, though we might disagree with their particulars.

I (McCormick) take the presumption stated above to be the substance of the Christian tradition. The strength of this presumption varies with times and cultures. Cardinal Joseph Bernardin noted that the presumption is strengthened in our time.[2] By that he means that in the past capital punishment was viewed as a legitimate act of public protection. Furthermore, in war, killing was foreseen and was justified on three grounds: national self-defense, the recovery of property, and the redressing of injury. Now, however, many people (including several recent popes) reject capital punishment and view only national self-defense as justifying violent resistance. Although such applications remain controversial, they are not the point here. The key principle is the presumption against taking human life.

2. ***Abortion is a killing act.*** So many discussions of abortion gloss over the intervention as "the procedure" or "emptying the uterus" or "terminating the pregnancy." In saying that abortion is a killing act, I (McCormick) do not mean to imply that it cannot be justified at times; the statement does not raise that issue. I (McCormick) mean only that the one certain and unavoidable outcome of the intervention is the death of the fetus. That is true of any abortion, whether it is descriptively and intentionally direct or indirect. If the death of the fetus is not the ineluctable result, we should speak of premature delivery. To fudge on this issue is to shade our imagination from the shape of our conduct and amounts to an anesthetizing self-deception. All of us should be able to agree on this description, whether we consider this or that abortion justified or not.

A key issue is not addressed here, but there is no intention of ignoring it. At what point does interruption of the reproductive process merit the name abortion? That is a legitimate question. Plausible reasons exist for saying that only interruption of an implanted, fertilized ovum deserves this name. Here, however, I (McCormick) wish not to distract from the main assertion—one that applies to the 1.3 million abortions done per year in this country.

3. ***Abortion to save the life of the mother is morally acceptable.*** Readers may wonder why I (McCormick) bother to mention this point. I do so because those who are morally opposed to abortion frequently see their position caricatured into unrecognizability. Such a caricature only intensifies opposition and polarization.

However, recently passed laws in the United States and other countries are counter to this premise. For example, abortion has been illegal in Nicaragua for over 100 years. The exception to this law could be made if the women's life was threatened, but her condition needed certification by three doctors. A new law enacted in November 2006 no longer allows this exception. Women convicted of abortions in Nicaragua can be sentenced to six years in jail. (See www.nytimes.com/2006/11/20/world/americas/20nicaragua.html.) Latin American laws on abortion are among the most restrictive in the world. For example, El Salvador's abortion law, passed in 1998, does not include exceptions and abortions are punishable by up to 50 years imprisonment. Cuba is the only country in Latin America that does not bar abortion. (See www.philly.com/mld/inquirer/news/nation/16126957.htm?source=rss&channel=inquirer_nation.)

Recently, in the United States, South Dakota legislators passed a law banning all abortions except those that threatened the life of the mother. However, in the November 2006 elections, South Dakotans rejected the "Abortion Ban." (See www.nytimes.com/2006/11/08/us/ politcs/08issues.html.)

Even this issue remains controversial and does not achieve universal agreement. Often a distorted interpretation of a "fundamental individual right to life" exists that comes close to editorial hucksterism. Those who formulate their convictions in terms of a "fundamental right to life" by no stretch of the imagination deny a similar right to the mother. Nor does such a general statement about fetal rights even address situations of conflict. In thinking about common ground, it would be useful to recall the statement of J. Stimpfle, bishop of Augsburg: "He who performs abortion, except to save the life of the mother, sins gravely and burdens his conscience with the killing of human life."[3] The Belgian bishops made a similar statement.[4] Agreement on this point may seem a marginal gain at best. However, in the abortion discussion, any agreement can be regarded as a gain, especially when it puts caricatures to rest.

4. *Judgment about the morality of abortion is not simply a matter of a woman's determination and choice.* Pro-choice advocates often present their position as though the woman's choice were the sole criterion in the judgment of abortion. I (McCormick) believe that very few if any really mean this, at least in its full implications. It is simplistic and unsustainable. Taken literally, it means that any abortion, at any time, for any reason, even the most frivolous, is morally justified if the woman freely chooses it. That is incompatible even with the admittedly minimal restrictions of *Roe v. Wade*. No official church body and no reputable philosopher or theologian would endorse the sprawling and totally unlimited acceptance of abortion implied in that criterion. It straightforwardly forfeits all moral presumptions protective of the unborn. In this formulation, the fetus becomes a mere blob of matter.

Conversation about the fourth point will not bring overall agreement on the abortion issue. However, it might lead to a more nuanced formulation on the part of those identified with the pro-choice position. It might also lead to a greater sensitivity on the part of some pro-life advocates to the substantial feminist concerns struggling for expression and attention in the pro-choice perspective.

5. *Abortion for mere convenience is morally wrong.* This only makes explicit the above point. Once again, agreement on this point might seem to represent precious little gain. Agreement might even be fugitive because of the problem in defining the phrase "mere convenience." One person's inconvenience is another's tragedy. Yet for those not hopelessly imprisoned in their abso-lutisms, I think agreement is possible if discussion is restrained. Such discus-sion could be remarkably fruitful. Those who agree with the statement eventually would have to say why such abortion is morally wrong. Such a dis-cussion could go in one direction only: straight to the whys and wherefores of the claims of nascent life upon us.

6. *The conditions that lead to abortion should be abolished insofar as is possible.* In the above statement, the abolished conditions could include poverty, lack of education, and lack of recreational alternatives to sexual promiscuity among teenagers. Nearly everyone agrees with these prescrip-tions, but they are not addressed. In other words, we have tended to approach abortion too exclusively as a problem of individual choice rather than a social problem. Left at that, it tends to divide people. Were it also approached as a social problem, it could easily bring together those in opposition and move the issues beyond the level of individual choice.

7. *Abortion is a tragic experience to be avoided if at all possible.* Regardless of one's moral assessment of abortion, most people could agree that it is not a desirable experience. It can be dangerous, psychologically trau-matic, generative of guilt feelings, and divisive for families. Of course, it is invariably lethal to fetuses. No amount of verbal redescription or soothing and consoling counseling can disguise the fact that people would prefer to achieve their purposes without going through the abortion procedure. It is and always will be tragic.

8. *There should be alternatives to abortion.* This is a corollary to the preceding point. Its urgency is in direct proportion to the depth of our percep-tion of abortion as a tragic experience. It would seem likely that the need for alternatives should appeal above all to those who base their approach on a woman's freedom of choice. If reproductive choice is truly to be free, then alter-natives to abortion should be available. Alternatives include all the supports—social, psychological, medical, financial, and religious—that would allow a woman to carry her pregnancy to full term should she choose to do so. Expand-ing the options is expanding freedom.

Bishop Skylstad's letter to the Secretary General, International Secre-tariat Amnesty International dated September 12, 2006, supports this state-ment. Bishop Skylstad, President of the U.S. Conference of Catholic Bishops (USCCB), stated, "a far more compassionate response [abortion] is to provide support and services for pregnant women and to advance their educational and economic standing in society. The Catholic Church provides these ser-vices to many women around the world and commits itself to continuing to do so. The Catholic Church will also continue to advocate greater attention to these needs in all relevant international assemblies." This letter was in response to a proposal by Amnesty International to support as he stated an "assertive policy of advocating abortion on demand as a 'human right.'" The bishop urged Amnesty International to maintain its neutral stance on abor-tion and to ". . . not dilute or divert its mission by adopting a position that many see as fundamentally incompatible with a full commitment to human rights and that will deeply divide those working to defend human rights." (See www.usccb.org/comm/archives/w006/06-a74.shtml.)

9. *Abortion is not a purely private affair.* *Roe v. Wade* appealed to the so-called right of privacy to justify its invalidation of restrictive state abortion laws. In public debate, assertions about a woman's "control over her own body" often surface. Such appeals either create or reinforce the idea that abortion is a purely private affair. It is not; at least not in the sense that it has no impact on people other than the woman involved. It affects husbands, families, nurses, physicians, politicians, and society in general. We ought to be able to agree on these documented facts. I (McCormick) am proposing that the term *privacy* is a misleading term used to underline the primacy of the woman's interest in abortion decisions. Communal admission of this point, which is scarcely controversial, would clear the air a bit and purify the public conversation.

10. Roe v. Wade *offends many people.* So did previous prohibitive laws. On these matters, those who acknowledge facts must agree. However, to place these facts together invites people out of their defensive trenches. In other words, it compels them to examine perspectives foreign to their own.

11. *Unenforceable laws are bad laws.* Unenforceability may stem from any number of factors. For instance, a public willingness to enforce the law may be lacking. Alternatively, the prohibited activity may be such that proof of violation will always be insufficient. On the other hand, attempts to enforce might infringe other dearly treasured values. Whatever the source of the unenforceability, most people agree that unenforceable laws undermine the integrity of the legal system and the fabric of social life.

Our own American experience with Prohibition should provide sufficient historical education on this point. Its unenforceability stemmed from all the factors mentioned above and more and it spawned social evils of all kinds. In this respect, Democratic Senator Patrick J. Leahy of Vermont once remarked that amendments should be used not to create a consensus but to enshrine one that exists. He added:

> The amendments that have embodied a consensus have endured and are a living part of the Constitution. But where we amended the Constitution without a national meeting of minds, we were forced to retract the amendment, and only after devastating effects on the society.[5]

12. *An "absolutely prohibitive" law on abortion is not enforceable.* By "absolutely prohibitive," I (McCormick) mean two things. First, such a law would prohibit all abortions, even in cases of rape and incest and in cases where the life of the mother is at stake. Second, "abortion" would mean the destruction of the human being from the moment of conception. The latter was the intent of the Human Life Statute (S.158) introduced by Jesse Helms on January 19, 1981. It sought by a simple majority of both houses to declare the fetus a human being from the moment of conception. Thus, in effect it sought to redefine the terms *person* and *life* to bring them under the protective clauses of the Fourteenth Amendment.

I say that such an absolutely prohibitive law is unenforceable. First, it has no consensus of support, as poll after poll over the years has established. Even religious groups with strong convictions against abortion have noted its unenforceability. For example, the Conference of German Bishops (Catholic) and the Council of the Evangelical Church (Protestant) issued a remarkable joint statement on abortion some years ago.[6] After rejecting simple legalization of first-trimester abortions (*fristenregelung*), they stated that the task of the law-maker is to identify those conflict situations in which interruption of preg-nancy will not be punished (*straflos lassen*). I mention the German example because of the apparently ineradicable American tendency to identify moral conviction with public policy (i.e., "There oughta be a law!"). This penchant is visible in the refusal of some pro-life advocates to admit any toleration into public policy.

The second reason an "absolutely prohibitive" law would not work concerns specification of legal protection from the moment of conception. If this were enshrined in the penal code and attempts made to enforce it, we would be embroiled in conspiracy law (the intent to abort). Why? This is because in the pre-implantation period, there is no evidence of pregnancy. Lacking such evi-dence, one could not prosecute another for having performed an abortion, but only for having intended to do so. That is just not feasible.

13. *There should be some public policy restrictions on abortion.* This point may seem to lack bite: after all, those most polarized could agree on this "middle ground," and even *Roe v. Wade* admitted "some" control. This tiny island of agreement is not important in itself. By focusing on it, discussants must face these two questions: "What kind of control?" and "Why?" Discussing these questions could take us right back to square one, but it could also lead to a more nuanced and sophisticated notion of public policy in a pluralistic society.

14. *Witness is the most effective leaven and the most persuasive edu-cator concerning abortion.* I do not mean to discredit the place of rational discourse. We abandon such discourse at our own risk, and often the result is war. I (McCormick) mean only that genuine education is eye-opening. The most effective way of opening eyes is often the practical way of witness. We come to understand and appreciate heroism much more by seeing heroic activ-ity than by hearing or reading a lecture on it. Are we more selfless when sur-rounded by people who are concerned for others? Are we more fearlessly honest when friends we deeply admire exhibit such honesty?

Those with deep convictions about freedom of choice for women or about the sanctity of fetal life would be considerably more persuasive if they emphasized what they support rather than what they oppose and did so in action. Pro-life advocates (whether individuals, organizations, or institutions, such as dioceses) should put resources into preventing problem pregnancies and when those pregnancies occur they should support them in every way. Paradoxically, the same is true of those who assert the primacy of free choice. For if the choice is to be truly free, genuine alternatives must exist. In summary, "putting one's money where one's mouth is" is an effective alternative to other means such as bombing and picketing.

15. *Abortion is frequently a subtly coerced decision.* As ethicist, Daniel Callahan pointed out 15 years ago, "a change in abortion laws, from restrictive to permissive, appears—from all data and in every country—to bring forward a whole class of women who would otherwise not have wanted an abortion or felt the need for one."[7] The most plausible interpretation of this phenomenon, according to Callahan, is that the "free" abortion choice is a myth. He stated,

> A poor or disturbed pregnant woman whose only choice is an abortion under permissive laws is hardly making a "free" choice, which implies the possibility of choosing among equally viable alternatives, one of which is to have the child. She is being offered an out and a help. Nor can a woman be called free where the local mores dictate abortion as the conventional wisdom in cases of unmarried pregnancies, thwarted plans, and psychological fears.[8]

Interestingly, agreement that many abortion decisions are coerced might result in cooperation between pro-choice and pro-life advocates. The concern of pro-choicers for true freedom would lead them to attempt to reduce or abolish coercive forces by offering genuine alternatives. The pro-life faction should rejoice at this provision of alternate options because it would reduce the felt need for abortion and thus the number of abortions.

16. *The availability of contraception does not reduce the number of abortions.* I include this element because of exposure to discussions of abortion soured by the introduction of statements like the following: "The Catholic Church, being so staunchly opposed to abortion, should be in the forefront of those backing contraception to prevent it. By condemning contraception the church adds to the number of abortions." Someone making such a remark supposes that support for contraception will reduce the number of abortions performed.

One of a group of "minor" truths listed by Daniel Callahan in 1973 was the following: "There is no evidence yet from any country that, with enough time and [the] availability of effective contraceptives, the number of abortions declines."[9] Clearly the availability of effective means of contraception is one thing; official approval of their use is quite another. As witnessed by the number of Catholics who depart from official church teaching on contraception, official disapproval does not seem to make much difference. Callahan's assertion should therefore serve as a rebuttal to the above statement about Catholic inconsistency. I do not attach much conciliatory significance to this rebuttal except that it clears the air of distracting and one-sided statements.

Current findings also support the decline in abortions and relate this fact to improved family planning services. Henshaw (1998), cited in *Healthy People 2010*, stated, "Unintended pregnancy rates in the United States show a decline, probably as a result of higher contraceptive use and use of more effective contraceptive methods." *Healthy People 2010* also stated, "Induced abortion is another consequence of unintended pregnancy." The same source cites Forrest and Samara's (1996) data, stating,

> . . . approximately one abortion occurs for every three lives births annually in the United States, a ratio two to four times higher than in many other Western democracies. Just as unintended pregnancy occurs across the spectrum of age and socioeconomic status, women of all reproductive ages, married or unmarried, and in all income categories obtain abortions. Abortion results when women have unin-

tended pregnancies. Each year, publicly subsidized family planning services prevent an estimated 1.3 million unintended pregnancies.[10]

Healthy People 2010 reflects the government's concern about unwanted pregnancies and the decisions to have an abortion as the remedy. The U.S. Department of Health and Human Services' *Healthy People 2010*, has identified this concern. In fact, one of their leading key indicators is "Responsible Sexual Behavior" which has a goal of improving reproductive health and family planning. The document states that unintended pregnancies represent half of all U.S. pregnancies, and a large proportion of those are among teenage girls. Almost half of these unintended pregnancies result in abortions. *Healthy People 2010* also recommended increased use of condoms and abstinence as indicators of responsible sexual behavior. The document stated, "research has shown clearly that the most effective school-based programs are comprehensive ones that include a focus on abstinence and condom use."[11]

17. *Permissive laws forfeit the notion of "sanctity of life" for the unborn.* This is a hard saying, but that does not make it less true. Here Daniel Callahan is at his best—and most tortured. He grants a woman the right not to have a child she does not want. However, he is unflinchingly honest about what this means. "Under permissive laws," he notes, "any talk whatsoever of the 'sanctity of life' of the unborn becomes a legal fiction. By giving women the full and total right to determine whether such a sanctity exists, the fetus is, in fact, given no legal or socially established standing whatsoever."[12] Callahan does not like being backed into this corner. However, he is utterly honest. His legal position does not allow for any pious double-think. The law "forces a nasty either-or choice, devoid of saving ethical ambiguity."

18. *Hospitals that do abortions but have no policy on them should develop one.* I (McCormick) introduce this as a contribution to the unexplored middle ground because non-Catholic healthcare facilities have approached the problem almost exclusively in terms of patient autonomy. Some hospitals have grown nervous about this posture because it amounts to simple capitulation to patient preferences. They have begun to see that theirs is not a carefully reasoned moral stance on abortion, but an abdication of the responsibility to develop one. The counsel to develop a policy is relatively non-threatening because it does not dictate what that policy ought to be. It is promising because it suggests that ethical complexity and ambiguity might become more explicit, which would represent an advance in the dialogue.

19. *The "consistent ethic of life" should be taken seriously.* I (McCormick) happily borrow the term *consistent ethic of life* from Cardinal Joseph Bernardin. Many have observed that the most vociferous about fetal rights are among our most hawkish fellow citizens. Something is amiss here. Abortion must be considered within the larger context of other life-and-death issues, such as capital punishment and war making.

20. *Whenever a discussion becomes heated, it should cease.* This is the final proposed piece of middle ground. I am not suggesting that abortion is so trivial a concern that heat is inappropriate. Rather, I (McCormick) know from long experience that shouting sessions on abortion only alienate and divide the shouters. Nothing is illumined, not because the offerings are not illuminating, but because nobody is either listening or being heard.

The idea of an unexplored middle ground and the invitation to explore it will please few. Yet the abortion problem is so serious that we must grasp at any straw. A nation that prides itself on its tradition of dignity and equality for all and the civil rights to protect that equality cannot tolerate a situation denying 1.3 million human fetuses this equality and these rights. We must at least continue to discuss the problem openly. Quite simply, the soul of the nation is at stake. Abortion's pervasiveness represents a horrendous racism of the adult world. When it is justified in terms of rights, all of our rights are endangered because their foundations have been eroded by arbitrary and capricious application.

For this and many other reasons, it is important that abortion continue to occupy a prime place in public consciousness and conversation. If we settle for the status quo, we may be presiding unwittingly at the obsequies of some of our own most basic, most treasured freedoms. That possibility means that any strategy—even the modest one of keeping a genuine conversation alive by suggesting a middle ground as its subject—has something to recommend it.

Indeed abortion issues continue to be in the forefront of public consciousness and conversation. According to the editorial in the *New York Times* dated November 11, 2006, "The Court and Abortion," the U.S. Supreme Court will be hearing arguments again on the Partial Birth Abortion Ban Act of 2003. An important issue is the contention by Congress that a ban of this nature will not pose a risk to women's health. (See www.nytimes.com/2006/11/11/opinion/11sat1.html.) Justice Kennedy, it is considered, is the justice whose vote will determine the outcome of this case.

Linda Greenhouse, in her article "Justices Hear Arguments on Late-Term Abortion," stated that Justice Kennedy's comments "reflected arguments that the doctors challenging the law have made." They say that "partial-birth abortion—known medically as both "intact dilation and evacuation and D and X for dilation and extraction—is often safer because removal of an intact fetus avoids injury to the uterus. The more common method of second-trimester abortion, in which the fetus is dismembered, can leave behind bone fragments."[13]

Another issue garnering public attention is the recent approval and signing by President Bush of a law that makes the morning-after pill accessible to women over 18 without a prescription (Plan B). Garner Harris, in the *New York Times* article published August 25, 2006, states that "abortion rights advocates argue that the wide availability of Plan B may reduce abortions: abortion opponents assert that Plan B will cause them." Harris quoted Kirsten Moore, president of the Reproductive Technologies Project in Washington, D.C. She stated, "We are pleased that a common sense, common ground agenda for reducing unintended pregnancy and the need for abortion finally won out."[14]

The Pontifical Academy for Life Statement on the So-Called "Morning-After Pill" stated that the morning-after pill is used "within and no later than 72 hours after a presumably fertile act of sexual intercourse, has a predominantly 'anti-implantation' function, i.e., it prevents a possible fertilized ovum (which is a human embryo), by now in the blastocyst state of its development (fifth to sixth day after fertilization), from being implanted in the uterine wall by a process of altering the wall itself. The final result will thus be the expulsion and loss of this embryo."[15]

Other issues for consideration in abortion discussions and in finding the common ground include the wide availability of family preferred planning methods and the reimbursement of insurance companies for these services. Other areas of discussion might address questions like "Should churches that oppose contraceptive use be required to include these services in their employee health plan benefits?" Finally, questions like "What about politicians whose religious beliefs are in conflict with their public duty as they see it?" and "Should they be sanctioned by their religions if their vote conflicts with their religious teachings?" may have to be including in the discussion for common ground. Certainly, the issue of abortion and abortion policy will still be an area for discussion in health care into the twenty-first century.

SUMMARY

This chapter begins with a presentation of the two current and very divergent positions on abortion. Using McCormick's ideas as a starting point, Petrozella then describes the need to expand public conversation to include points of consensus or middle ground on this difficult issue. She presents twenty elements that should be considered in establishing this middle ground. Each of the elements is supported by examples and ethical reasoning. Finally, Petrozella presents additional areas for consideration in finding a common ground and makes the point the ethical issues around abortion will continue to be significant in the twenty-first century.

QUESTIONS FOR DISCUSSION

1. According to the author, why is even a dialogue about abortion difficult?
2. What are at least five common areas where both sides could find sufficient agreement for the beginning of dialogue toward a middle ground on this issue?
3. What is the role of the healthcare professional in relation to abortion?
4. How can the principles of ethics (autonomy, beneficence, nonmaleficence, and justice) assist in finding a middle ground on abortion?
5. How does your personal view affect your care for patients in this area?

NOTES

1. See, for example, R. A. McCormick, "Public Policy on Abortion," in *How Brave a New World?* (Washington, D.C.: Georgetown University Press, 1981).
2. J. Bernardin, *Origins* 13 (1983–1984): 491–95; Origins 14 (1984–1985): 707–709.
3. F. Scholz, "Durch ethische Grenzsituationen aufgeworfene Normen probleme," *Theologish-praktische Quartalschrift* 123 (1975): 342.

4. Les évêques belges, "Déclaration des évêques belges sur l'avortement," *Documentation Catholique* 70 (1973): 432–438.

5. Cited in M. C. Segers, "Can Congress Settle the Abortion Issue?" *Hastings Center Report* 12 (June 1982): 20–28.

6. Conference of German Bishops and the Council of the Evangelical Church, "Fristenregelung" entschieden abgelehnt, Ruhrwort, December 8, 1973, 6.

7. D. Callahan, "Abortion: Thinking and Experiencing," *Christianity and Crisis*, January 8, 1973, 296.

8. Ibid.

9. Ibid., 297.

10. See *Healthy People 2010*. Available online at http://opa.osophs.dhhs.gov/pubs/hp2010/hp2010_rh.pdf.

11. Ibid.

12. D. Callahan, "Abortion: Thinking and Experiencing," *Christianity and Crisis*, January 8, 1973, 296.

13. See Greenhouse article in the *New York Times*. Available at www.nytimes.com/2006/11//09/washington/09scotus.html. Accessed November 13, 2006.

14. See Gardner article in the *New York Times*. Available at www.nytimes.com/2006/08/25/halth/25fda.html. Accessed November 13, 2006.

15. See The Pontifical Academy for Life Statement on the So-Called "Morning-After Pill" Statement. Available at www.vatican.va/roman_curia/pontifical_academies/acdlife/documents/rc_pa_acdlife_doc_20001031_pillola-giorno-dopo_en.html. Accessed December 4, 2005.

CHAPTER 6

Proposals for Human Cloning: A Review and Ethical Evaluation

Kevin T. Fitzgerald

OVERVIEW

In this chapter, Fitzgerald presents an update on the current scientific and ethical status of human cloning. He clarifies the often-confused issues relating to cloning and stem cell research. He also discusses the rational given for the merits of cloning research. His ethical arguments include consideration of the need for cloning and its effects on individuals and society.

INTRODUCTION

In August of 1975, Dr. John Gurdon, a British scientist, reported the first successful cloning of frogs using nuclei from adult frogs transplanted into enucleated eggs.[1] This success generated great enthusiasm among scientists for developing techniques for cloning animals. Over the next two decades, the initial enthusiasm greatly declined, because not only did the cloned frogs never develop into adult frogs, but further experiments seemed to indicate that cloning a mammal from either adult or fetal tissue might never be possible. As scientific interest in cloning waned, so, too, did the apparent need for extensive ethical discussion concerning the possibilities of human cloning. At times, it seemed as though only Hollywood was still interested in human cloning, with movies such as *The Boys from Brazil* and *Multiplicity*.

On February 22, 1997, Dr. Ian Wilmut and his team of researchers from the Roslin Institute in Scotland regenerated scientific enthusiasm for animal cloning with their announcement of the successful cloning of a sheep. Speculation about human cloning and its moral implications was reignited in the media. In the wake of this renewed interest came various proposals concerning what could, might, and should be done with regard to applying this new cloning technique to human beings. It is the intent of this chapter to review some of these proposals and to evaluate them as to their scientific probability and ethical justification. Before evaluating these proposals, the wise course is to clarify the facts about human cloning—at least inasmuch as they are currently known.

The remarkable scientific article published by Wilmut et al., in the February 27 issue of the journal *Nature* demonstrated that it was now possible to use cells from the differentiated tissue of an adult mammal to produce a clone of apparently normal characteristics.[2] Differentiated tissue is primarily composed of cells that have taken on specialized functions, such as those performed by liver and muscle cells, and, consequently, have turned off all the other genes not needed to perform these specialized functions. Many researchers had feared that it would never be possible to turn these genes back on so that specialized cells from an adult mammal, or even a fetal mammal, might be used to produce a viable clone. However, using a kind of nuclear transfer (NT) similar to that used by Dr. Gurdon, the researchers in Scotland were able to create a mammalian clone.

The idea of what constitutes a viable clone can be divided into two categories: reproductive clones and research clones. If one is cloning for reproductive purposes, then the concept of a viable clone is the generation of an infant animal that is not burdened by significant health problems so that it might live a relatively normal life. Currently, only a few researchers or ethicists are arguing for reproductive human cloning.[3] The vast majority of experts and biomedical societies are against attempting reproductive human cloning at this time.[4] Research cloning is currently the most intense focus of debate. This process is designed to create cloned human embryos that will then be destroyed in order to study the embryonic stem cells that can be isolated from these cloned embryos. In either case, research or reproductive cloning, the cloned human embryos are created in the same fundamental manner as was Dolly the sheep.

Though the cloning of Dolly has been rightly heralded as a major breakthrough in science, many obstacles remain to the application of this technology in humans. In fact, the research done in South Korea and published in the journal *Science*, which was internationally touted as the big breakthrough in human cloning, turned out instead to be a complete hoax.[5] In fact, as of March 2007 no research group has presented verifiable evidence of the creation of any embryonic stem cell line that has been derived from a cloned human embryo.

In light of the lack of success in achieving human cloning, why then is there this renewed excitement about it? The reasons for pursuing human cloning have been enumerated in a variety of recent articles and reports. As mentioned earlier, these reasons currently focus primarily on the benefits that might be achieved in research on cloned embryos. These benefits include (1) creating tissues, organs, or other treatments that can be matched to individual patients or diseases; (2) creating cloned embryonic stem cell models for research on specific human diseases and how they arise during development, and (3) using cloned embryonic stem cells for research on human reproduction and development in general.

These proposals for the pursuit of human cloning for research will be reviewed first because they are currently of greatest relevance to the public discussion and debate. Reproductive human cloning will be reviewed second because the likelihood of pursuing reproductive cloning will depend on the success, or lack of success, researchers have with their attempts to clone human embryos for research cloning.

HUMAN CLONING FOR RESEARCH PURPOSES

The process of research cloning is currently focused on the creation of embryonic stem cell lines from cloned human embryos. The goal of the cloning procedure is to create human embryos that will develop to the blastocyst stage. At this stage of development, usually around 5 to 7 days after fertilization has occurred, the embryo is a small, hollow sphere with some cells in its interior, called the inner cell mass. The entire embryo may be about 200 cells at this point of development. The cells of the inner cell mass are the cells that are of interest to the researchers, because they will become the embryonic stem cell lines. These cells must be separated from the rest of the embryo in order to become a cell line.

Currently, embryos must be destroyed in order to create embryonic cell lines. This destruction of human embryos is one of the main points of contention in the public debate concerning human cloning for research. This issue will be examined in more detail in the upcoming ethics section of this chapter.

What do researchers propose to do with the cloned human embryonic stem cell lines they wish to create? As mentioned previously, several things. First, the primary advantage researchers think these cell lines will have is that they can come from an individual with a specific disease or condition. The idea then is that the underlying genetic or biochemical cause of the disease might be investigated more precisely by using the cloned embryonic stem cell line to produce the different types of cells affected by the disease and to observe how their proper functioning is disrupted by the disease during the process of differentiation and afterwards.

Using this information, the researchers might then be able to attempt with this cell line different types of interventions aimed at preventing, reversing, or compensating for the disease condition. If an intervention is found to be efficacious, then the cell line might even be manipulated to create cells, tissues, or even organs that no longer have the disease. If a given manipulation is demonstrated to be successful and safe, then the tissues or organs created might be useful for transplantation back into the person whose adult cell was used to create the cloned embryo that was the source of the embryonic stem cell line.

Though the creation of transplantable tissues and organs might be the ultimate goal, researchers could also claim that, even if they do not get to that goal, they might still learn some very important basic biology of disease processes from this research such that it will help treat diseases in some other way. Hence, the fundamental emphasis put forth to try to justify human research cloning is the widely-accepted idea that research is done primarily to benefit people. In other words, if the research will benefit people, we should do it. Whether this justification of human research cloning is legitimate will be analyzed in the upcoming section of the chapter on the ethical issues. However, currently much of the purported benefits of research cloning are still speculative, because no cloned human embryonic stem cell lines have been created. Next, we will look at reproductive cloning.

HUMAN CLONING FOR REPRODUCTIVE PURPOSES

In order to address the issue of reproductive cloning, one must first acknowledge the significantly higher level of control over the cloning process that will be required for reproductive cloning relative to that required for the research cloning process. The reason for this difference is basically safety. Proponents of research cloning are much less concerned about the loss of embryos or the creation of useless embryos than proponents of reproductive cloning can be regarding the creation of cloned children. Proponents of research cloning might well be satisfied with the creation of one useful cloned cell line out of several or many attempts, whereas those who desire to pursue reproductive cloning would likely be dissatisfied with the creation of one healthy child out of several or many that are born, or even carried in pregnancy. This safety issue is one that leads many research cloning proponents to back away from supporting reproductive cloning at this time.

If these safety issues could be adequately addressed, what reasons are then given for the pursuit of reproductive cloning? Can it be used for parents who face both genetic and reproductive obstacles to having their own children? Some have proposed that human cloning could be another alternative in the array of assisted reproductive technologies (ART) offered to such couples. One could propose the possibility that no other alternatives are available to the couple except attempting to clone one of them. Of course, the question arises at this point: What do we mean by having one's "own" child? A cloned child would actually be biologically more like the much-delayed identical twin of whichever parent is cloned. Because one's biological children are actually only half related to each parent, one could argue biologically that a cloned child is no more naturally related to either parent than an adopted child. After all, all humans share over 99 percent of their DNA. What sort of relatedness makes a child one's own?

When pushed to an extreme, it becomes evident that a genetic reductionism underlies this reproductive cloning perspective. Are genes the only possible basis for the parent-child relationship? Are human identity and personality merely genetic? What of adopted children who call their parents "Mom and Dad," or those who look to teachers or mentors as the ones who have been most instrumental in forming their identities? A consistent response from scientists during this furor about the possibility of human cloning has been to remind people that we are more than our genes, even on a physiological level. One's environment plays a significant role in shaping one's identity and characteristics. Examining still another proposed use for reproductive human cloning will help elucidate this point.

It has been proposed that human cloning might be employed so that a couple could "replace" a dying child or a person could replace a dying spouse. As in the previous case, there is a dangerous biological reductionism inherent in this proposal. No human being is replaceable—not even physiologically. We are all unique, including identical twins. The desire to clone a loved child or spouse to "replace" the lost loved one may well indicate a retreat to a biological solution from the age-old problem of dealing with the grief and trauma of death. Even if the psychological struggle with the loss of a loved one were eventually dealt with successfully, the cloned child or spouse would always have to live with the reality of having been cloned to replace another.

From this brief overview, one can see that even if the immense safety issues could be surmounted with regard to reproductive cloning, many other significant issues remain concerning what exactly the purpose would be in pursuing human reproductive cloning. In addition, there are ethical issues, which will be addressed in the following section.

ETHICAL ISSUES IN HUMAN CLONING

Before the ethical issues surrounding human cloning can be addressed, it will be necessary to clarify some details about the issue that are often confused in the mass media and the public debate. Evidence of this confusion can be seen in the differences that are obtained when people are polled about whether they agree with human cloning. Depending on how one phrases the questions asked, one can reliably get the majority of respondents to be either in favor of human cloning or against it. Comparing two past polls will help demonstrate this point.

On March 25, 2005, the results of a poll done by the Opinion Research Corporation, and commissioned by the Coalition for the Advancement of Medical Research (CAMR), indicated that "a strong majority of Americans solidly support embryonic stem cell and therapeutic cloning research."[6] As stated on the CAMR Web site:

> Of the 1,045 people responding, the specific breakdown of responses was as follows: 59% said they favored medical research that uses stem cells from human embryos, (30% strongly favor, 29% somewhat favor); 33% are opposed, (13% somewhat oppose and 20% strongly oppose), and 8% of respondents answered they did not know. Once a description of embryonic stem cell research was read, 68% said they favored it, (39% strongly favor, and 29% somewhat favor), only 28% opposed the research (11% somewhat oppose, and 16% strongly oppose), and 4% responded they did not know. For therapeutic cloning, 60% of Americans approved the research, (27% strongly approved, 33% somewhat approved), whereas 35% disapproved (12% somewhat, and 23% strongly), and 5% of respondents answered they did not know. Once a description of therapeutic cloning research was read, 72% favored it (30% strongly, 42% somewhat), and roughly 23% opposed the research (11% somewhat, 11% strongly), and 6% of respondents answered they did not know.[7]

Interestingly, a different poll focusing on the same issues, done by International Communications Research and commissioned by the United States Conference of Catholic Bishops (USCCB), was released on May 31, 2006, with the results stating that "48% of Americans oppose federal funding of stem cell research that requires destroying human embryos, while only 39% support such funding."[8] In addition, the USCCB Web site states:

> When survey respondents were informed that scientists disagree on whether stem cells from embryos, or from adult tissues and other alternative sources, may end up being most successful in treating diseases, 57% favored funding only the research avenues that do not harm the donor; only 24% favored funding all stem cell research, including the type that involves destroying embryos. . . . The new poll also shows overwhelming opposition to human cloning, whether to provide children for infertile couples (83% against) or to produce embryos that would be destroyed in medical research (81% against).[9]

Because these two polls were done a year apart, one might conclude that the public's attitudes had changed during that year. However, the USCCB Web site cites earlier polls done during the previous two years by the same company that showed similar negative responses to human embryonic stem cell research and cloning research.[10] How then can two presumably accurate polls reach opposite conclusions? The answer, in part at least, can be found in the contradictory descriptions and evaluations of the human embryo.

The current debates surrounding cloning often revolve around the biological and moral realities of human embryos. What was once a seemingly clear concept—a sperm fertilizes an egg and creates an embryo—has now become a convoluted intersection of cutting-edge biological research, ethical reflection, and religious perspective. For instance, some proponents of research cloning will argue that no human embryos are created or destroyed in the process of creating cloned stem cells. This argument is based on the fact that no sperm are used in the cloning procedure, only eggs. Because they define embryos as the union of sperm and egg, cloning cannot produce an embryo.

However, the cloning procedure created Dolly the sheep. No one argues that Dolly was not a sheep. If Dolly was a sheep, then she must have been a lamb at some point. If Dolly was a lamb, then she must have been a fetal sheep before she was born as a lamb. If Dolly was a fetal sheep, then what was she before she was a fetus? In mammalian developmental biology, Dolly must have been an embryo. Hence, cloning produces embryos, and does so without sperm.

Unfortunately, things are even more convoluted regarding the embryo definition problem than this issue of whether cloning produces embryos. For example, it is known in biology that the process of fertilization can create abnormal growths, some of which are cancerous, rather than generating developing organisms. One such growth is called the hydatidiform mole.[11] No one argues that a complete hydatidiform mole is an organism or a human being, yet it can arise from the union of sperm and egg. Hence, whereas the processes of fertilization and cloning can both create embryos (i.e., organisms in the earliest stage of development), they can also both create nonorganismal growths that are not embryos. Considering the apparent contradictory results of the two polls just cited, clarification of exactly what one means by the term *embryo* would be crucial when one is arguing for or against the destruction of human embryos in research.

This clarification is crucial, because it extends beyond the complexities described previously. Some proponents of cloning research will acknowledge that they accept the creation and destruction of full-fledged human embryos in research because currently the best chance for getting good stem cells comes from creating the best embryos one can. However, these embryos are not considered by these proponents to be of the same moral importance or standing as a human fetus, because they are created and developed outside the human body in a Petri dish. As long as the embryos are not transferred to a woman's body, they cannot ultimately develop to a stage equivalent to birth. Therefore, they argue, embryos created by the cloning process which are intended only for research purposes are not ethically the same as embryos that are developing within a women's body.

This argument also raises some contentious issues. Presume that two cloned embryos are created that are equally functional, developing, human organisms. This argument asserts that the embryo intended to be destroyed for research is somehow of less value or important than the embryo that is intended to be transplanted for reproductive purposes. What happens if the two embryos get mixed up in the lab and the one intended for research is transferred to a woman's uterus while the other is destroyed? Has some significant wrong occurred that would not have occurred if there had been no mixup? What if no one ever finds out about the mistake? Did no wrong occur because people think that their intentions were carried out properly? Can some human organisms be treated as disposable because some people decide that they should be treated as disposable?

Fundamentally, this argument of intentionality can be interpreted as treating embryos similar to property. One can treat one's possessions as preciously or not as one intends. The question is then: Are embryos to be treated the same as property, or does the fact that they are human organisms preclude such treatment?

Some opponents of cloning research argue that embryos must be treated the same as other human beings, at least to the extent that they should not be created and destroyed for research purposes. However, they recognize the potential usefulness that might come from research done on stem cells that have specific disease characteristics. Their proposal is to attempt to create stem cells with such disease characteristics, and which act like embryonic stem cells for research, but do not come from embryos. One way to do this creation of these embryonic-like stem cells would be to employ an altered nuclear transfer (ANT) technique. This ANT technique could be done several different ways.[12] The key point to all the ANT approaches is not to include the destruction of a human embryo in the process of generating the stem cell lines desired for research.

These ANT proposals can be placed alongside other proposals opponents of human cloning recommend researchers should pursue to gain the benefits of stem cell research, while avoiding the destruction of human embryos. Often all these antihuman-cloning proposals are lumped together in the adult stem cell research versus embryonic stem cell research choice. This designation of the adult versus embryonic is not completely accurate. If the goal of research is to gain understanding of disease and develop better treatments, then opponents of research that destroys human embryos can actually point to all the biomedical research being done on diseases and treatments that does not destroy human embryos. Considering that most biomedical research is not specifically stem cell research (either adult or embryonic), it is scientifically quite a stretch to claim that only human cloning research will provide an answer or treatment to a given disease.

Of course, it is part of the nature of scientific research not to be able to predict where and when the breakthroughs will come. Hence, proponents of human cloning research often respond that we need to do all the research we can in order to provide the best chance that answers or treatments will be found as soon as possible. In fact, more recently some proponents have even begun to claim that pursuing human cloning research is a moral obligation because it might help us achieve treatments for those suffering from terrible diseases earlier than we might otherwise.

Though these arguments might appear compelling at first glance, they rest on false assumptions. First, there is already a great deal of human research that could be done which might readily result in more rapid discoveries and treatments. This research is not done because it would harm human beings in the process. Due to many past tragedies involving biomedical research that unjustifiably harmed human beings, our society has decided to place limits on human research regardless of how useful the research might be. Hence, what is good for research is not always what is good for society. The key issue here regarding human cloning research is whether to create and destroy human embryos in research—not whether the research might lead us to treatments sooner.

The second false assumption presented is that we must do human cloning research because it might lead to earlier treatments for those suffering from terrible diseases. This claim assumes that the key aspect of disease treatment is research. In actuality, our world is replete with examples of cures and treatments that exist but are not getting to the people who are in desperate need of them. Hence, if everyone responded fully to the logic of the claim that we need to do all we can to treat those who are suffering from tragic diseases, then most, if not all, research would have to be stopped.

If the goal to provide treatment for those suffering from terrible diseases trumps all other concerns, then most of our resources would need to be shifted to healthcare delivery and preventive medicine. After all, what good is a treatment if those who need it cannot get it? In addition, would it not be better to avoid the disease altogether rather than having to treat it once some people get it? Because we are already faced with serious problems in preventing disease and getting the treatments we already have to those who need them, the logical response to the above moral claim about needing to treat people would be to reduce research and do better with the treatments and preventive strategies we already have.

In order to avoid confusion, the critique just presented will be clarified. The critique is not against biomedical research. Biomedical research can be a great good in a society. The critique is against those who would claim that a given type of research is morally obliged based on it possibly resulting in treatments for those suffering from terrible diseases. All health care is oriented toward the prevention and alleviation of suffering, if possible. Decisions regarding what elements of health care should get priority over others depend on many factors. The fact that a particular line of research might bring about good treatments is certainly not by itself a sufficient justification for that research to be done, especially when contentious ethical issues of human subject research are involved.

Contentious ethical issues are certainly involved in human cloning research, as has already been demonstrated. However, the ethical issues are not limited to those already described. Another issue that is only recently receiving adequate attention involves the acquisition of human eggs for cloning research.

Currently, animal cloning is a very inefficient process. In addition, as cited previously, no one has provided verifiable evidence of the creation of cloned human embryonic stem cell lines. Combine these two facts and one is faced with the daunting probability that it will require an enormous number of human eggs to achieve human cloning, even of embryos, on a scale that will be adequate for the number and kinds of cloning research programs envisioned by proponents of this research.[13] This probability is daunting because the process of procuring eggs for research involves the hyperstimulation of a woman's ovaries and this process involves risks to the woman's health. These risks are of such significance that people from many different perspectives—pro-life and pro-choice, Democrat and Republican, feminist, Green, and social conservatives—have joined in calling for a moratorium on the use of human eggs for cloning research.[14]

Again, society is faced with the challenge of protecting human beings from harm (i.e., the many young women who will be needed as egg donors) in the face of interest in pursuing research that is seen as desirable to many. Considering the fact that there are many alternative avenues of research that can be pursued without putting women or embryos at risk, the burden of proof should be on those who argue this research is not only good for science but also for society.

When arguing for human cloning research as a good for society, the argument often arises that if our society decides for whatever reason not to pursue this research we will put ourselves at a disadvantage because other societies or nations will do it. They then will get the benefits and we will lose out. Again, though this argument might seem compelling at first, closer examination reveals that it, too, is flawed. Many historical examples are available to remind us of the harms that may befall a society that too eagerly pursues technological advance at the cost of other societal values and goods. The past catastrophes of eugenic policies pursued both in the United States and Germany should be reminder enough of the harms that can occur in the name of medical advancement.

If research cloning can be questioned on the grounds of its potential harm to individuals and society, then reproductive cloning can also be questioned on these grounds. Even if cloning is the only reproductive option an individual or couple might have, should it be pursued? Proposing human cloning to solve reproduction problems depends heavily on the argument that people have the right to have genetically related offspring. When discussing such rights, it is important to distinguish between negative (liberty) rights and positive (welfare) rights.

In 1994, the Ethics Committee of the American Fertility Society (now the American Society of Reproductive Medicine) stated that in the context of procreation, "A liberty right would encompass the moral freedom to reproduce or to assist others in reproducing without violating any countervailing moral obligations. A welfare right to reproduce would morally entitle one to be assisted by another party (or other parties) in achieving the goal of reproduction."[15]

If society is troubled by the ethical problems associated with reproductive cloning, one can certainly argue that society is not obliged to support it as a welfare right. Additionally, if society concludes that the rights or dignity of the child to be born are violated by reproductive cloning (e.g., to be made as a copy of someone else), then society can also deny even a liberty right to clone one-self because of the countervailing moral obligation to protect the cloned child from harm.

SUMMARY

We have considered several proposals regarding the possibility of human cloning. These range from possible medical interventions for directly treating disease to meeting perceived reproductive needs. In the final analysis, considering the possibility of alternatives both in research and in reproduction, as well as the multitude of ethical problems still plaguing the cloning issue, the burden of proof regarding whether we should pursue human cloning should be on those who desire to clone human embryos—for research or reproduction. Currently, the arguments employed by human cloning proponents do not provide enough justifiable reason to apply the recent advances in cloning techniques to human beings.

QUESTIONS FOR DISCUSSION

1. Why do you think there is a renewed interest in human cloning? Does the media attention increase this interest?
2. Do you think science has an ethical obligation to present the public with both the benefits and burdens of cloning research?
3. What is the role of autonomy in cloning research? Whose autonomy should be considered?
4. What would be the deontologist's position on cloning?
5. The healthcare community also is concerned about the business aspects of cloning. Do you think cloning will become a good business opportunity?

NOTES

1. J. B. Gurdon, R. A. Laskey, and O. R. Reeves, "The Developmental Capacity of Nuclei Transplanted from Keratinized Skin Cells of Adult Frogs," *Journal of Embryology and Experimental Morphology* 34 (1975): 93–112.
2. I. Wilmut, A. E. Schnieke, J. McWhir, A. J. Kind, and K. H. S. Campbell, "Viable Offspring Derived from Fetal and Adult Mammalian Cells," *Nature* 385 (1997): 810–813.
3. For example, see: Gregory Pence, *Who's Afraid of Human Cloning?*
4. This perspective against reproductive cloning includes organizations that have taken positions in support of research cloning, such as the National Academies and the National Research Council. For example see their report, "2007 Amendments to the National Academies' Guidelines for Human Embryonic Stem Cell Research," at http://books.nap.edu.
5. D. Normile, G. Vogel, and J. Couzin, "CLONING: South Korean Team's Remaining Human Stem Cell Claim Demolished," *Science*, January 13, 2006, 311: 156–157.
6. Available at www.camradvocacy.org/press_releases_archive_details.aspx?rid=news_1326.

7. Ibid.

8. Available at www.usccb.org/comm/archives/commarc.shtml.

9. Ibid.

10. Ibid.

11. R. Slim and A. Mehio, "The Genetics of Hydatidiform Moles: New Lights on an Ancient Disease," *Clinical Genetics* 71, no. 1 (2007): 25–34.

12. For a good introduction to ANT, see the President's Council on Bioethics report, *Alternative Sources of Human Pluripotent Stem Cells*, May 2005. Available at www.bioethics.gov.

13. The number of eggs required can only be guessed at currently, because no one has yet succeeded in creating a cloned human embryonic stem cell line. However, considering that hundreds, if not thousands, of eggs have already been used in human cloning research, the number of eggs needed to create the disease-specific cell lines desired by researchers would easily be in the tens of thousands, and possibly into the millions.

14. One example of such a group can be found at www.handsoffourovaries.com.

15. The Ethics Committee of the American Fertility Society, *Fertility & Sterility* 62(1994): Supp.1, 18S.

CHAPTER 7

Competency: What It Is, What It Isn't, and Why It Matters

Byron Chell

OVERVIEW

As Chell points out, the issue of determining patient competence for medical decision making is often difficult because no absolute definition exists. Hopefully, the need to make decisions for the patient is rare, but circumstances requiring this practice may increase in the twenty-first century. To assist in this process, the author presents information about parameters for making these decisions and provides useful guidelines for practitioners and administrators.

INTRODUCTION

A competent adult has the absolute right to refuse medical treatment—even lifesaving medical treatment! Can there be any doubt that this is a correct statement of principle, medical ethics, and law?[1] In spite of this clear and seemingly straightforward declaration, however, when a patient refuses to accept needed medical care, we yet find much concern and confusion. This is especially true when the treatment is lifesaving.

The rule that a competent adult has the right to refuse any and all medical treatment emphasizes the importance of the concept of competency. In fact, if we are uneasy about a decision to refuse treatment, we immediately retreat to the thicket of competency.[2] Such a retreat is appropriate, however, because when confronted with a refusal of needed medical care the first and key question we should ask is whether the patient is competent to make the required decision.

Yet difficulties regarding competency remain, because the concept is confusing. What is a competent adult? What is the definition of competency? Are those who refuse lifesaving treatment on religious grounds really competent? How do we find the proper answers to these questions when evaluating patients? Anyone involved in bioethics and medical decision making regularly confronts such questions.

This chapter discusses what competency is and what it is not. It also discusses what we should and should not be doing in making determinations of competency for deciding whether to allow a patient to refuse medical treatment. If we have a clear understanding of what competency is, why we seek it, and why it matters, we will know how to approach and complete the task of determining competency without unnecessary anxiety and confusion.

WHAT COMPETENCY IS AND WHAT IT IS NOT

Competency is not a thing or a fact. It is not something we can look for and find if only we know how. Determinations of competency are not medical judgments. Clinical training is not required. Being competent does not necessarily mean being rational. We find many persons competent to make medical care decisions even though their refusal of treatment is based on irrational beliefs. When we make determinations of competency, we are not seeking truth or facts. We are not assessing the patient in light of a clear and neutral standard upon which we can make a definitive finding. It is not that easy.

Competent is simply a label we apply to persons after we examine various aspects of their physical and mental condition. Decisions relating to competency are legal and social decisions. They are legal decisions in that they are determinations of an individual's legal capacity to exercise the right to self-determination. No legal education is required, however. They are social decisions in that the statutory definitions we apply in the search are societal decisions. Additionally, when we make determinations of competency we are doing so with imprecise criteria, vague notions, and personal beliefs and prejudices, all of which affect the outcome.

Considering the importance of the concept of competency in making determinations relating to, respecting, or overriding the patient's refusal, it at first appears necessary that we fix upon a definition of the term *competency*. However, despite our attempt as a society to define it, we have failed to find an adequate definition.

THE SEARCH FOR THE DEFINITION OF COMPETENCY

We do not need to find the definition of competency to fulfill our task. This is fortunate, because there is no pre-existing single definition of the term. We can only create a definition—or various definitions. No standard definition of competency is to be found. No statutory consistency or line of cases can be uncovered that would allow the simple discovery of the meaning of the terms *competent* or *incompetent*. Definitions of competency can be found in a number of different and specific situations where society and the law have always had to deal with the concept. We generally recognize that people can be competent to do one thing and not another or can be competent to some extent and not another. For example, we have laws regulating a person's competency to make a will, to enter into contracts, or to stand trial.

Definitions of *incompetency* have generally fallen into two categories: definitions that emphasize end results and definitions that emphasize thought processes. Both types of definitions, however, are intimately and necessarily related in light of what we actually do in making determinations of competency.

Definitions in terms of end results essentially ask us to look at how persons live. What is their condition? What are the consequences or the end results of their thinking? For example, a former definition of the term *incompetent* for mental health commitment purposes is as follows:

> As used in this chapter the word incompetent shall . . . be construed to mean or refer to any adult person who . . . is unable properly to provide for his own personal needs for physical health, food, clothing or shelter, (or who) is substantially unable to manage, his own financial resources.[3]

A definition emphasizing end results tells us to look at what is happening to persons because of their thinking. We must examine the physical consequences that follow from their mental status. An incompetent person is one whose mental processes lead to bad or serious consequences. A competent person simply would not live like that or be in that situation.

Although such definitions are adequate in the context of mental health civil commitment proceedings, they are not very helpful in many cases of refusals of medical care. We question the competency of many persons who refuse medical treatment even though they are quite capable of providing for their own food, clothing, and shelter and can manage their daily affairs very well.

Because definitions in terms of living conditions or end results are not always adequate to the task, we also use definitions of competency that emphasize thought processes. A definition of incompetency in terms of thought processes involves determining if someone is competent by looking at how he or she relates to and decides things. One essentially tests the person's comprehension of reality, understanding, and ability to make rational judgments. One example of this type of incompetency definition is as follows:

> Several tests of competency might be applied, e.g., patients may be considered competent if (1) they evidence a choice concerning treatment, (2) this choice is "reasonable," (3) this choice is based on "rational" reasons, (4) the patient has a generalized ability to understand, or (5) the patient actually understands the information that has been disclosed. . . . [T]he courts have not settled on any single test of competency; in practice, doctors seem to apply an amalgam of some or all of these tests.[4]

A definition emphasizing thought processes involves listening to the patient and judging whether what is said "makes sense." Is the patient rational? The point is not to examine the physical consequences that follow from the patient's mental state, but rather to examine the mental state itself.

There are currently many competing definitions of competency, and this is simply a reflection of the fact that competency can be properly defined in many different ways.

The search for a single test of competency is a search for the Holy Grail. Unless it is recognized that there is not a magical definition of competency to make decisions about treatment, the search for an acceptable test will never end. "Getting the words just right" is only part of the problem. In practice, judgments of competency go beyond semantics or straightforward applications of legal rules; such judgments reflect social considerations and societal biases as much as they reflect matters of law and medicine.[5]

Competency is, of course, whatever we define it to be. The trick is to define it so that it best helps us to do the job that needs to be done. The job in this context is to make decisions involving decision making. We must decide whether we will allow the patient to decide. Thus, what are the proper considerations we must keep in mind in making our decisions? What is the essence of competency? What criteria should be reflected in a proper definition?

THE ESSENCE OF COMPETENCY

Competency is essentially the ability to make a decision. Regardless of the particular definition used, determining competency in a given situation involves answering one question: Should we allow this person to make this decision under these circumstances? Generally, but not always, the answer to this question is yes, and a person is labeled competent if (1) he or she has an understanding of the situation and the consequences of the decision and (2) the decision is based on rational reasons.

Determining whether the person does or does not understand his or her condition is usually not the troublesome part. Sometimes it is difficult to determine the seriousness of the patient's condition and sometimes physicians will disagree. However, if the medical conclusion is that intervention is required to prevent death or serious harm, it is normally not too difficult to determine whether the patient understands what the doctors are saying and whether the patient appreciates the consequences of his or her choice. This aspect of determining competency does not create philosophical and conceptual confusion. It can do so, however, in some cases of religious refusals.

Determining whether the patient's decision to refuse treatment is based on rational reasons can cause us much concern. Although the word *rational* might appear redundant, its meaning in this context is "sensible," "sound," "reasonable," or "lucid." The term *reasons* is used in the sense of "reasons why," "motive," or "explanation." Thus, the reason why or the explanation of the decision to refuse treatment is to be considered rational if it is sensible or sound, lucid and not deranged, and it conforms to reason. In other words—it makes sense! In lieu of rational reasons, we might require sound explanations, sensible motives, or even reasonable reasons why.

It is not possible to define specifically terms such as *rational reasons*, *sound explanations*, or *sensible motives* or to measure definitively what is rational or reasonable. These determinations will necessarily vary from person to person. We can set out cases where most persons would conclude that the reasons for the refusal are rational or sensible under the circumstances, and such examples can be instructive.

Suppose, for example, that an older patient is informed that her leg is gangrenous and that an amputation is necessary to save her life. Understanding the situation, she replies, "I refuse the amputation. I am not afraid of death. It is the natural end to life. I am 86. and I have lived a good and full life. I do not want a further operation, nor do I want to live legless. I understand that the consequence of refusing the amputation is death, and I accept that consequence."

This woman understands both her situation and the consequences of her choice. Additionally, her decision is understandable. It is based on facts and logic. Although we might wish her to choose otherwise (or we might choose otherwise), her reasons and reasoning are sane, sound, and sensible. She is competent.[6]

If she were to say, however, "I understand the consequences but I refuse the operation because the moon is full," it is not likely she would be considered competent. Although she understands her situation and chooses death to medical treatment, her decision is not understandable. Her decision does not rationally or reasonably follow from her premise. Her explanation does not make sense. She would be labeled incompetent.[7]

A thousand reasons for refusing treatment could be set out. Regarding each, we could ask the question, "Is this a rational or sensible reason?" On some, we might all agree. On others, there would be great disagreement. It is simply important to recognize that it can be no other way. Understanding this fact relieves the anxiety that accompanies the attempt to find out what competency is or to apply the proper definition of competency or rationality.

The fact that there can be neither a "true" finding of reasonableness nor a single test that will lead to uniform results should not, however, lead us to abandon our responsibility to make these judgments. Yet, when we weigh the reasons for the patient's choice, we many times discard the requirement of reasonableness and label persons competent even though their refusal is founded on irrational beliefs. Patients who refuse necessary medical care based on religious beliefs often are labeled competent even though their beliefs might be quite "irrational."

COMPETENCY IS COMPATIBLE WITH "IRRATIONALITY"— RELIGIOUS REFUSALS

We face many difficult questions when we confront a person who is refusing lifesaving medical care based on religious belief.[8] If the patient is going to die because he or she is refusing a readily-available medical procedure, we are puzzled, and we necessarily question the patient's competency. We find it difficult to accept that a rational and competent person would die when a simple act would save his or her life.

In considering competency and making judgments regarding those who refuse necessary medical treatment based on religious belief, we can apply the general definition of competency with a slight modification. In cases of religious refusals, a person is competent if (1) he or she has a proper understanding of the situation and the consequences of the decision and (2) the decision is based on religious beliefs ("irrational" beliefs) that are within our common religious experience or common notions of religion and do not appear to us "crazy" or "nonreligious." If this definition seems vague, it is because it is vague.

To demonstrate how to apply this definition of competency, consider the following four examples of religious refusals. In each of these cases, suppose that the patient is refusing a lifesaving blood transfusion. Suppose also that each patient expresses sincerely held beliefs.[9]

Patient A states, "I refuse the blood transfusion because I am a Jehovah's Witness and I believe it is a violation of God's law to accept such blood. I understand that the consequence of my refusal is my death and I accept that result." Patient B states, "I refuse the blood transfusion because I am one of Yoda's Children and, based upon Luke Skywalker's teachings, I believe the acceptance of blood is a violation of Yoda's law and the work of the Dark Side of the Force. I understand that the consequence of my refusal is my death and

I accept that result." Because we must make a determination relating to competency in these cases to decide whether we are going to respect or override the patient's refusal, what will be the likely result?

The first patient will be judged competent, and he will be allowed to refuse treatment and die. The second patient, although a more troubling case, will be labeled incompetent, and some other person will be allowed to give substituted consent to the treatment necessary to prevent his death.

Now, why is this the case? If we ask, "What is the difference between the statement of patient A as opposed to the statement of patient B?" the answer must be "none." Both are identical as statements of "irrational" religious belief or faith.

Belief and faith are irrational in at least one sense. In the context of this discussion, the term *irrational* means not derived logically from facts, data, or circumstances—that is, it is outside the scope of reason. Faith is essentially belief based on that which is incapable of proof. It does not involve logic, facts, or proof; it is trust and belief in a matter empirically unknowable. If it were knowable through facts or proof, we would speak in terms of knowledge and truth and not faith and belief. Theologians should know this.

A discussion that would attempt to label patient A's belief in Jehovah a religious belief and patient B's belief in Yoda a religious delusion would go nowhere. A conclusion in this situation that A's faith is based on a belief as opposed to a delusion would depend entirely on the beliefs, experiences, and prejudices of the person drawing that conclusion. In these cases, the label applied to the belief and the determination of competency depend on the novelty of the belief and on whether we want to give priority to the individual's continued life or to respecting the individual's choice. If the former, we would conclude that the decision is "crazy" and label the individual incompetent. If the latter, we would conclude that his belief is "religious" and label him competent.

In these two cases, the only difference is that patient A has voiced a religious belief held by organized and recognized groups within our society whereas patient B has voiced a belief totally outside our common religious experience. The Jehovah's Witness's belief relating to the refusal of blood is now well within our society's general "religious belief experience." Because of our concurrent societal belief in the free exercise of religion, we "respect" the Jehovah's Witness's belief even though it is irrational.[10] We recognize the belief as religious, and we label patient A competent. As far as patient B is concerned, sincere or not, religious or not, we conclude that his belief is too "crazy" to determine a life and death decision, and we label him incompetent.

However, what about the protections afforded by the First Amendment? If we do not accept patient B's belief, are we unlawfully discriminating against this Yoda's Child and denying him his right to the free exercise of religion? Although it is true that the U.S. Constitution guarantees certain rights relating to the free exercise of religion, it is emphasized that only "religious beliefs" are protected.[11] In addition, although it is often asserted that the courts will not assess or inquire into the truth or validity of individual religious beliefs,[12] the courts most certainly do decide what constitutes a "religion"[13] and what amounts to a "religious belief."[14] In making such decisions, the courts also apply imprecise criteria and vague notions.

In determining whether a belief is a religious belief entitled to protection, the courts have at various times required that the belief be "truly held"[15] or that it be "sincere and meaningful,"[16] and judges have often emphasized the helpful test of orthodoxy.[17] The courts have also noted that some beliefs may simply be "too crazy" to qualify for protection.[18] In sum, the courts do judge the validity of religious beliefs, and they do it in a manner similar to the method of determining competency described earlier. That is, if a belief is "too crazy," there is sufficient room within our law to conclude that the belief is "nonreligious," not "sincere and meaningful," not "truly held," or not sufficiently similar to orthodox religious beliefs. This is the conclusion that ought to be reached about patient B's belief in Yoda.[19] Because his belief is too crazy, we would label him incompetent, and the courts would label his belief as one not entitled to First Amendment protection. In doing so, both the courts and we would be acting properly.[20]

Some might object to making such judgments, but despite objections and difficulties, we ought and will continue to do so.[21] The only alternative to making such distinctions is to accept any statement of belief as consistent with competence and sufficient to support a life-and-death decision regardless of its apparent "craziness." Few would feel comfortable with such a rule.

Next, consider the following patients, who express slightly different reasons for refusing the lifesaving medical care. Patient C states, "I refuse the blood transfusion because the full moon, properly understood, is the source of the human spirit and the key to human happiness and cures all disease. When the moon rises in full next week you shall see that it will cure me without the need of your medical procedure."

This is the easiest case. As with patient B, patient C has based her choice on a belief quite outside our common religious experience. Additionally, she clearly does not appreciate either the nature of the situation or the consequence of her decision. She does not understand that her death is imminent. She fails both tests and is clearly incompetent. Is there any doubt that this patient's refusal would be overridden and action taken to provide the lifesaving care?

Patient D states, "I refuse the blood transfusion because I am a Jehovah's Witness and I believe it is a violation of God's law to accept such blood. God will heal me without the need of your medical procedures." This is a more difficult case. Would you allow this patient to refuse the lifesaving care?

This Jehovah's Witness has based her refusal on a belief within our common religious experience. However, it is also evident that she does not appreciate either the nature of her situation or the consequences of her decision. She does not understand that without the blood transfusion her death is imminent. Although we may accept this patient's belief relating to the prohibition of blood, her religious beliefs go too far. Her belief in a cure without medical intervention in this situation does amount to a religious delusion.

Patient D is similar to the patient in a recent Ohio case where treatment was allowed in spite of the patient's "religious refusal." The patient refused to consent to treatment because she believed that she was the wife of an evangelist who would arrive to heal her. The court noted the rule that a patient's honestly-held religious belief must be respected, but it decided that when those beliefs amount to a religious delusion, they may be disregarded.[22]

This might appear at first to be a subtle distinction, but it is a very important one. Carefully consider the difference between patient A and patient D. Patient A states, "I believe accepting blood is against God's will, and I will not accept blood even though I will die because of my belief." Patient D states, "I believe accepting blood is against God's will, and I will not accept blood. I also believe God will cure me and I will not die."

In failing to understand and recognize the consequences of her decision, patient D is not making the life-and-death decision required here. She is not deciding between the two, because she does not recognize one as being a consequence of her decision. The decision here is not simply to either accept blood or refuse blood. The decision that needs to be made involves the choice of either accepting blood and living or refusing blood and dying. In patient D's mind, she is simply choosing between life with treatment as opposed to life without treatment. One cannot freely decide between two choices if one does not understand what the choices actually are. If one cannot freely decide, one is not competent to decide.[23]

Because patient D is in fact not making the required decision between the two alternatives of life and death, in failing to respect her "nonchoice" we are denying neither the principle of personal autonomy nor freedom of religious expression. We are obligated only to respect a decision. In refusing treatment, patient D is not making the required decision based up a religious belief. Rather, her religious belief prevents her from understanding that her death is imminent and the decision that we require her to make. Her belief in this situation is a delusion—religious or not—in that it has adversely affected her ability to understand.

In summary, in religious refusal cases and following the general definition of competency just set out, we ought only label a patient competent and respect a refusal of medical treatment when the patient is not deluded and he or she understands the situation and appreciates the consequences of the decision. To respect the refusal the patient's refusal must also be founded on a religious belief that is within our common religious experience or our common notions of religion. It should not be perceived as extremely unreasonable, crazy, or nonreligious.

Some concepts involved in the issue of competency, the manner in which we should evaluate competency, and the conclusions that should be reached concerning patients A–D can be set out as shown in Table 7–1.

CONCLUSIONS RELATING TO COMPETENCY

The above view of how to determine competency in cases involving understanding, appreciation, rationality, and religious belief can be summarized in

Table 7–1   Competency decisions for patients A–D.

	Proper understanding[1]	Accepted belief[2]	Competent[3]
Patient A (Jehovah's Witness)	Yes	Yes	Yes
Patient B (Yoda's Child)	Yes	Yes	No
Patient C (Moon Child)	No	No	No
Patient D (Jehovah's Witness)	No	Yes	No

[1]*Proper understanding:* The patient understands his or her condition and the consequences of the decision. In these cases, the patient understands he or she is going to die without medical intervention. The patient's understanding is not "deluded" by religious belief.

[2]*Acceptable belief:* The person's decision is based on a belief that is within our common religious experience. It is a belief that has been held by a sufficient period of time or is sufficiently similar to other orthodox beliefs so that we label it a religious belief and not nonreligious, unsound, or insane.

[3]*Competent:* The label we apply in the various situations.

another fashion. As with the cards used by police officers to assist in giving *Miranda* warnings, a medical decision-making card might state the following:

Process for Determining Competency of Patients Who Refuse Medical Treatment

Answer the following questions concerning the patient:

1. Does the patient understand his or her medical condition?
2. Does the patient understand the options and the consequences of his or her decision?
3. Is the patient's refusal based on rational reasons?
4. If the refusal is based on religious beliefs, are the religious beliefs acceptable and entitled to First Amendment protection, i.e., beliefs held by a sufficient number of persons for a sufficient period of time or sufficiently similar to other orthodox beliefs such that we do not label the beliefs crazy or nonreligious?

If the answers to 1, 2, 3, and 4 are all yes, then the patient's refusal will be respected. He or she should be labeled competent. If the answer to either 1, 2, 3, or 4 is no, then the patient's refusal should not be respected and action should be taken to obtain substitute consent. He or she is incompetent.

Using this procedure, one will reach a proper result in all cases, no matter who makes the determination, physician, or judge, or what the particular statutory definition might be. If the answer to all four questions is yes, any proper statutory definition of competency will be fulfilled. If the answer to any of the four is no, any proper definition of incompetency will be met.[24] This is not to say that in any given case there is a proper conclusion or that different persons asking these same questions will not reach different conclusions. This is also not to say that such questions can be easily answered in all cases. Sometimes it is easy to answer these questions and we feel quite confident in our conclusions. Sometimes it is terribly difficult. Nevertheless, following this type of procedure will give a proper result simply because these questions are based on the essence of the concept of competency. They contain the necessary considerations, vague and slippery as they may be, to make the required decision. Such a procedure simply allows us to reach a conclusion in a straightforward manner, and this is all we can hope to do.

WHY IT MATTERS

It is always important to emphasize the significant ethical and moral issues involved in labeling a person incompetent. Such emphasis underscores our need to work hard at making proper determinations. Consider just what it is we are saying when we exercise the power of the state to override a patient's specific refusal of medical care because the patient is incompetent. We are, most assuredly, judging the validity of the patient's reasoning and the truth of the patient's beliefs. We do so without precise criteria or objective standards. We decide which reasons expressed by the patient are acceptable and which are proper religious beliefs entitled to protection.

As a society, we simply think that some persons, for one reason or another, should not be allowed to make certain decisions. We reach this conclusion for the same reason that we think certain defendants should not be held responsible for otherwise criminal actions. Based on our experience, some persons just do not appear to be rational, responsible, or competent human beings.

In medical decision making, we must distinguish between rational and irrational reasons and between acceptable religious beliefs and craziness (or whatever one wishes to call it). If we do not make such distinctions, then we must allow the refusal of any patient no matter what the basis, even though the patient's beliefs are such that they delude the patient's understanding of the situation and prevent him or her from making the required decision. What if the patient's beliefs seem clearly senseless and unacceptable, as nonsensical as the beliefs of an acutely psychotic person who chooses death based on "commands" from the television set?

As a further matter, consider this aspect of judging a person incompetent. In spite of the person's stated choice, we make a different choice and force our choice upon the person. We do so claiming that we have the right (and the duty) to force our decision on the person; it is for his or her "own good." We do so because, in spite of the person's choice (an incompetent choice), the person has a right to the benefits of our decision (a competent choice). We reason the person has a right to the benefits of the choice that he or she would have made if competent. If the person were competent to decide and had reached a different conclusion, he or she would be, in effect, a different person. When you change a person's understanding, beliefs, thoughts, conclusions, and choices, you have changed the person. In forcing our choice upon the patient, we are claiming that the patient has a right to the benefits of being a different person. Indeed, we are insisting that he or she be a different person. It is not difficult to understand and appreciate the ethical and moral problems involved in negating personal autonomy under such circumstances and in using power and force, if necessary, to insist that a person be another person.

Of course, most persons are aware that good intentions and the exercise of power for another person's own good can bring about horrendous results. Controversial decisions and disagreements have always and will always result from determinations of competency. Such is our condition, however, the nature and consequences of these decisions simply underscore the weight of our obligations.

SUMMARY

Although more needs to be said, this discussion has attempted to explain what competency is and to set out a straightforward process for making determinations of competency. The patient's competency is the first and foremost question that must be resolved in deciding whether we will respect or override the patient's refusal. There is no single definition of *competency*, and there are many different ways of stating the concepts involved in that term.

The term *competent* is nothing more than a label we place on a person when we conclude that we should allow him or her to make the decision at issue. Generally, we apply the label to the person who understands his or her condition and the consequences of the choices and whose reasons make sense to us. Sometimes, however, especially in cases of religious refusals and First Amendment considerations, we apply the term *competent* to persons who base their refusal on irrational beliefs as long as those beliefs are within our common religious experience and do not seem too strange.

In making determinations of competency and in forcing treatment on others, we are engaging in serious matters. These are decisions that should not be avoided, however. We must use our experience of the human condition and our best judgment in the attempt to make proper decisions. As long as they are made with proper motives and a proper understanding of the task, they are properly made. Although these decisions might be difficult in individual cases, they should be made without unnecessary concern or doubt because in doing so we are doing all that can properly be done. We are, after all, simply human beings attempting to make very difficult decisions relating to other human beings.

QUESTIONS FOR DISCUSSION

1. What demographic changes or healthcare practices might increase the need to determine patient competence in the future?

2. How do the principles of patient autonomy and beneficence conflict when making healthcare decisions that run counter to the patient's choice?

3. Why is it important for a healthcare professional to have a guideline for deciding patient competence?

4. In competency cases, how important is it to listen to the patient and clarify his or her wishes? Would you want more than one person to interview the patient?

5. What ethical theories support making a treatment decision for a patient even when he or she does not want treatment?

NOTES

1. Judge Cardoza stated it this way: "Every human being of adult years and sound mind has a right to determine what shall be done with his own body. . . ." *Schloendorff v. Society of New York Hospital* (1914) 105 N.E. 92,93. See also *Matter of Spring* (1980) 405 N.E.2d 115; *Superintendent of Belchertown v. Saikewicz* (1977) 370 N.E.2d 417; *Bartling v. Superior Court* (1984) 163 Cal.App.3d 186; *Barber v. Superior Court* (1983) 147 Cal.App.3d 1006.

2. "On balance, the right to self-determination ordinarily outweighs any countervailing state interests and competent persons generally are permitted to refuse medical treatment, even at the risk of death. Most of the cases that have held otherwise . . . have concerned the patient's competency to make a rational and considered choice of treatment." *Matter of Conroy* (1985) 486 A.2d 1209,1225.

3. California Welfare and Institutions Code Sec. 1435.2 (repealed Jan. 1, 1981).

4. R. Meisel and L. Meisel, "Toward a Model of the Legal Doctrine of Informed Consent," *American Journal of Psychiatry* 134 (March 1977): 285, 287.

5. R. Meisel and L. Meisel, "Tests of Competency to Consent to Treatment," *American Journal of Psychiatry* 134 (March 1977): 279, 283.

6. See *Lane v. Candura* (1978) 376 N.E.2d 1232 for a decision respecting a patient's refusal of an amputation under similar circumstances.

7. *Matter of Schiller* (1977) 372A.2d 360 is another case where the court struggled with the refusal of an amputation. In the *Matter of Schiller*, the patient was found incompetent and a guardian was appointed primarily because Mr. Schiller failed to properly evidence an understanding of his medical condition and the reality of death, the more likely situation in such cases.

8. Our additional concern is occasioned, of course, by the First Amendment to the Constitution of the United States. "Congress shall make no law respecting an establishment of religion, or prohibiting the free exercise thereof. . . ."

9. Of course, in making determinations of competency one would always want to know more and would question the patient carefully and thoroughly.

10. It should be emphasized that the beliefs of Jehovah's Witnesses are not used to single out those beliefs as being less rational than or deserving of less respect than any other religious beliefs. The Jehovah's Witness examples are used solely because the beliefs of Jehovah's Witnesses form the most widely-known religious basis for the refusal of medical care in this country.

11. "Only beliefs rooted in religion are protected by the Free Exercise Clause, which, by its terms, gives special protection to the exercise of religion." *Thomas v. Review Board* (1981) 450 U.S. 707,715.

12. "Men may believe what they cannot prove. They may not be put to the proof of their religious doctrines or beliefs. Religious experiences which are as real as life to some may be incomprehensible to others." *United States v. Ballard* (1944) 322 U.S. 78,86. "[R]eligious beliefs need not be acceptable, logical, consistent, or comprehensible to others in order to merit First Amendment protection." *Thomas v. Review Board* (1981) 450 U.S. 707,714.

13. See *Engel v. Vitale* (1962) 370 U.S. 421 (school prayer); *Loney v. Scurr* (1979) 474 F.Supp. 1186,1194. "[T]he Church of the New Song qualifies as a 'religion.'" *Theriault v. Silber* (1978) 453 F.Supp. 254,260. "The Church of the New Song appears not to be a religion." *Malnik v. Yogi* (1977) 440 F. Supp. 1284 (transcendental meditation).

14. See *Wisconsin v. Yoder* (1972) 406 U.S. 205, which contrasted the "religious beliefs" of the Amish with the "philosophical and personal" beliefs of Thoreau; also, *United States v. Seeger* (1965) 380 U.S. 163, which determined whether or not the beliefs of a conscientious objector qualified as "religious beliefs" to allow an exemption.

15. "[W]hile the 'truth' of a belief is not open to question, there remains the significant question whether it is 'truly held.'" *United States v. Seeger* (1965) 380 U.S. 163,185.

16. "We believe that . . . the test of belief 'in a relation to a supreme being' is whether a given belief that is sincere and meaningful occupies a place in the life of its possessor parallel to that filled by the orthodox belief in God of one who clearly qualifies for the exemption." *United States v. Seeger* (1965) 380 U.S. 163,166.

17. "[D]oes the claimed belief occupy the same place in the life of the objector as an orthodox belief in God holds in the life of one clearly qualified for exemption?" *Seeger* supra at 184. "[I]t is at least clear that if a group (or an individual) professes beliefs which are similar to and function like the beliefs of those groups which by societal consensus are recognized as a religion, the First Amendment guarantee of freedom of religion applies." *Loney v. Scurr* (1979) 474 F.Supp. 1186,1193 citing *Welsh v. United States* (1970) 398 U.S. 333,340. "While recently acquired religious views are worthy of protection, the history of a religious belief and the length of time it has been held are factors to be utilized in assessing the sincerity with which it is held." In re *Marriage of Gove* (1977) 572 P.2d 458,461, citing *Wisconsin v. Yoder*.

18. "One can, of course, imagine an asserted claim so bizarre, so clearly nonreligious in motivation, as not to be entitled to protection under the Free Exercise Clause . . ." *Thomas v. Review Board* (1981) 450 U.S. 707,715.

19. If a professed belief in Star Wars characters and making a life and death decision based on faith in Yoda and Luke Skywalker is not sufficiently "crazy" for you, create your own patient. Consider, for example, a refusal by the patient who tells you he is "Serumzat, believer in the teachings of the Prince of Liquids and Tabletops; I believe that accepting blood is wrong and will prevent my passage to the afterlife, which I am destined to rule."

20. As a further example of how courts make these decisions, see *Powell v. Columbian Presbyterian Medical Center* (1966) 267 N.Y.S.2d 450. The facts presented the classic case of the Jehovah's Witness who did not want to die but who refused a lifesaving blood transfusion. In a most candid decision that demonstrated the reality of the difficulty, vagueness, and room for legal discretion involved in these matters, the court stated in part: "This matter generated a barrage of legal niceties, misinformation and emotional feelings on the part of all concerned—including the Court personnel. . . . Never before had my judicial robe weighed so heavily on my shoulders. . . . I, almost by reflex action subjected the papers to the test of justiciability, jurisdiction and legality. . . . Yet, ultimately, my decision to act to save this woman's life was rooted in more fundamental precepts. . . . I was reminded of 'The Fall' by Camus, and I knew that no release— no legalistic absolution—would absolve me or the Court from responsibility if I, speaking for the Court, answered 'No' to the question 'Am I my brother's keeper?' This woman wanted to live. I could not let her die!" 267 N.Y.S.2d at 451,452.

21. It should be noted that in all cases of refusals of medical care, religious or not, as our certainty in the prognosis decreases, our willingness to allow the refusal increases. See, for example, *Petition of Nemser* (1966) 273 N.Y.S.2d 624, which contains an interesting discussion of these issues, although in some areas the court's analysis is incomplete or incorrect.

22. In re *Milton*, 505 N.E. 2d 255 (Ohio 1987). What would we do if this patient was Mrs. Oral Roberts?

23. Consider how terribly subtle these distinctions can be, however. Does it make a difference if the patient says "I leave my fate to Jehovah," as opposed to "I believe Jehovah will cure me"? Or if the patient states "God will save me" as opposed to "God may save me"? Again, we would explore this patient's understanding and beliefs carefully.

24. It should also be remembered that if the answer to any of these questions is no, the patient also is unable to consent to treatment.

CHAPTER 8

The Patient Self-Determination Act

David B. Clarke

OVERVIEW

In this chapter, Clarke provides a comprehensive overview of the Patient Self-Determination Act (PSDA) and its impact on healthcare practice. Although the PSDA became effective in 1991, it is still a major player in healthcare practice, particularly where the ethical challenges at end-of-life are concerned. Clarke traces the effects of the law as enacted and describes its influence on current healthcare practice. A serious reading of this chapter will provide you not only with information on the PSDA, but also a deeper understanding of the issues surrounding it and its future influence in healthcare practice.

INTRODUCTION

The Federal Patient Self-Determination Act (PSDA) became effective on December 1, 1991—more than 15 years after California passed its Natural Death Act. This enactment was also more than 22 years after Louis Kutner coined the term "living will" in a law journal proposal.[1] Planning for and implementation of the PSDA began in 1990, shortly after the law was passed as part of the Omnibus Budget Reconciliation Act (OBRA) and continued throughout 1991. By now, it is assumed that state agencies and healthcare providers affected by the legislation will have initiated programs and protocols designed to meet its basic requirements.

It also is presumed that programs initiated to meet PSDA requirements, either by states or institutions, will not be static. The PSDA instituted a dynamic process intended to foster communication between healthcare providers and consumers and between persons and their chosen healthcare decision-making surrogates. Although the core requirements of the PSDA can be implemented at a superficial level, the long-term benefits will only be realized through significant and fundamental changes in institutional policy, public and professional education, and social awareness.

The PSDA requires the following of Medicare and Medicaid institutional providers:

1. Provide written information to inpatients upon admission (or upon enrollment or initial entry into service) about:
   a. The person's rights under law to make healthcare decisions, including the right to accept or refuse treatment and the right to complete state-allowed advance directives.
   b. The provider's written policies concerning implementation of those rights.

2. Document in the person's medical record whether the person has completed an advance directive.

3. Not discriminate or condition care based on whether the person has completed an advance directive.

4. Ensure compliance with state laws concerning advance directives.

5. Provide education for staff and the community on issues concerning advance directives.

In addition, each state (acting through a state agency, association, or other private nonprofit entity) must develop a written description of the law of the state—whether in statute or case law—concerning advance directives and distribute the document to local healthcare providers (see 1a above).

The PSDA, then, is a call to states and healthcare providers to educate professionals and the public about local laws concerning healthcare decision-making rights and advance directives. As such, it is a federal law necessitating broad agreement among legal and healthcare professionals on current rights and obligations in the healthcare arena and resulting in massive and persistent education efforts directed at medical professionals, administrators, social service providers, and the lay public.

The PSDA does not provide for a universally-accepted advance directive, although many would argue that that would certainly facilitate the process of public information and awareness. It does not force healthcare professionals to talk more candidly with patients, nor does it prompt consumers to initiate discussions with their providers. The PSDA will not resolve the issues arising from the provision of care to persons who have neither completed an advance directive nor expressed to others their wishes about treatment preferences or desired quality of life.[2] Nor does the PSDA deal directly with the developing issues of physician-assisted suicide and euthanasia. However, both supporters and critics of the PSDA believe that the new law will raise public awareness of these and related issues as healthcare decision making generally becomes more focused.

Because the PSDA relies on state law for the content of implementation efforts, the process of satisfying the PSDA will inevitably change in the months and years ahead. Legislation and court decisions at state and national levels will prompt states to revise and redistribute the "statement of state law" on healthcare decision-making rights and advance directives. As laws and institutional policies change, healthcare facilities will modify and reprint materials included in pre-admission packets and provide them to patients upon admission. In addition, professionals charged with patient and community education might develop effective teaching skills they never dreamed of using. This chapter will address each of the major sections of the PSDA in light of the aforementioned comments. Attention will also be given to issues that have already arisen during this initial implementation period and to problems that are only tangentially related to the PSDA and its implementation.

BACKGROUND

In order to fully understand the impact of the PSDA, some background information is needed. The next section explains the types and uses of advanced directives and some of the concerns about these documents. It is followed by a section on the history of the enactment of the PSDA.

Advance Directives

All states now have at least one kind of advance directive.[3] *Advance directive* is the general term for a variety of documents designed to enable competent adults to make healthcare decision-making plans in advance of future incapacity, including terminal illness. At present, advance directives are prescribed exclusively by individual state law. Federal law does not provide for a uniform directive to be honored in all states, and states are not required to honor directives signed in other states. Efforts are under way, however, on both of these fronts.[4]

Advance directives are generally of two types: instructional and proxy. An *instructional directive* (most often called a *living will* or *terminal care document*) allows a competent adult to specify treatment wishes in advance of a terminal illness or condition during which the person is not capable of making sound healthcare decisions. Most living will laws specify a written form patterned loosely on the original document circulated widely by what is now the New York-based organization Choice in Dying. Whether called a *natural death act*, a *right of the terminally ill declaration*, or a *declaration of a desire for a natural death*, most instructional directives share common features. They are written statements, to be signed by a competent adult, witnessed and perhaps notarized, that affirm that in the event of terminal illness, the person wishes to forgo treatments that would serve only to prolong the dying process and would not effect a cure or recovery.

A *proxy directive* is very different. Patterned after a well-established legal document called a *durable power of attorney*, a healthcare proxy (or durable power of attorney for health care) allows a competent adult to choose another person to make healthcare decisions for him or her, according to his or her wishes, if—at any time and for any reason—the person becomes unable to make his or her own healthcare decisions. The chosen healthcare agent (or attorney-in-fact, in the case of a healthcare power of attorney) can make any healthcare decision that the person could him- or herself, except where the law or the person sets limits on the agent's authority to make certain kinds of decisions.

Some states have both directives, and, in fact, both might be needed in certain states to ensure that certain treatments are selected or avoided. No two states have the same laws, and no one form is accepted in each of the 50 states. The PSDA simply requires states and providers to give information about what is legally permitted in that state.

Researchers continue to express concern about the efficacy of advance directives, both instructional and proxy ones.[5] Typical was a letter to the *New England Journal of Medicine* in December 1991 signed by 16 physicians, nurses, lawyers, and ethicists.[6] The authors listed reservations about both forms of directive, including assertions that patients prefer to avoid discussions of future incapacity and death, that patients cannot predict accurately their future preferences, that patients might change their minds, that an appointed agent might turn out to be a poor choice as a surrogate decision maker, and that the documents or agents might specify treatments that the provider has sincere conscientious objections to using.

In many states, implementation of the PSDA has followed close on the heels of new or recently-modified advance directive legislation. It is understandable that both providers and consumers will have to "feel their way" for the foreseeable future in assessing the value of both the PSDA and any state-specific advance directive legislation. Perhaps more than with other kinds of legislation, the development of advance directives has been characterized by a high degree of modification and compromise. Concerted efforts of interest groups, such as the professional medical community, institutional and agency providers, senior advocates, and religious associations, have combined to produce legislation that might be virtually immune from legislative modification, at least in the near term. Those who favor extended trial implementation periods often get their wish, and more. Those who favor legislative "fine-tuning" of the law may have to be unusually patient. Answers to some questions will neither come quickly, nor will they come as succinctly as advocates and critics might hope.

Almost everything known about the effect of advance directives—on professional practice, public opinion, patient preferences, courts, and consumer tendencies—is based on studies done prior to the PSDA. Advance directives have been in legal use since 1977. However, the PSDA has given the concept a "bump start" by requiring facilities to provide education to staff, patients, and the community. The professional literature has been disappointingly slow to indicate whether research studies were conducted before or after the wave of public and professional education on advance directives and the PSDA during 1991 and early 1992. It was encouraging in early 1993 to see articles emphasizing the need for empirical research in this complex field.[7]

Patient Self-Determination Act

The PSDA was introduced in the U.S. Senate by John C. Danforth (R–Missouri) and Daniel Patrick Moynihan (D–New York) in October 1989, shortly before the case of Nancy Cruzan was first heard in a Missouri district probate court. Six months later, Representative Sander M. Levin (D–Michigan) sponsored a significantly revised version of the bill in the U.S. House of Representatives. Many of the original provisions proposed by Danforth, Moynihan, and Levin were ultimately deleted from the "ambitious" legislation, including requirements that:

- States have advance directive legislation (at the time, six did not).
- Agencies "document the treatment wishes of such patient, and periodically review such wishes with the patient."[8]
- Agencies "implement an institutional ethics committee which would initiate educational programs for staff, patients, residents and the community on ethical issues in health care, advise on particular cases, and serve as a forum on such issues."[9]

The PSDA was signed by President H. W. Bush in December 1990 as part of OBRA, and it became effective December 1, 1991. In retrospect, political caution and expediency prevailed, although many of the excised provisions came to pass regardless. Passage of the PSDA itself prompted several states to enact advance directive legislation. Many providers willingly document patients' treatment wishes. In addition, the education component was retained, although not as part of a specific obligation to establish an ethics committee.

As passed, the PSDA required the Secretary of Health and Human Services to "develop and implement a national campaign to inform the public of the option to execute advance directives and of a patient's right to participate and direct health care decisions," develop or approve nationwide informational materials, and assist state agencies in developing state-specific documents. To date, the federal government has provided little help to the states or health-care facilities in this regard. There has been no coordinated "national campaign," and the offer of the Health Care Financing Administration (HCFA) to give assistance to states was sent out four months after the 1991 PSDA effective date. HCFA issued final interim regulations regarding the PSDA in early March 1992.[10]

The case of Nancy Cruzan brought national attention to the need for widespread education about the use of advance directives. Nancy Cruzan, a 23-year-old Missouri woman, was left in a persistent vegetative state as a result of a single-car accident. After her parents accepted the fact that their daughter would never regain either consciousness or any level of meaningful existence, they petitioned a Missouri court for permission to have her removed from artificial nutrition and hydration. Nancy Cruzan had never completed an advance directive of any kind, had left no written evidence of her treatment preferences in case of future incapacity, nor had she legally appointed a surrogate decision maker for her health care. A local probate judge, accepting oral testimony from her parents and personal friends that Nancy would not have wanted her life to be sustained under such conditions, granted her parents permission to have her removed from life supports. The attorney general of Missouri appealed the matter to the supreme court of Missouri, and the case was eventually heard by the U.S. Supreme Court.

The only question put before the U.S. Supreme Court—the first time that court had considered the issue of the "right to die"—was: Can the state of Missouri require "clear and convincing evidence" of Nancy's own wishes in deciding whether to grant permission to Nancy's parents? "Clear and convincing" is one of the highest levels of evidentiary proof required by the law in order to prove as true a statement or event. In a criminal trial, for example, a person can be found guilty only if a judge or jury finds him or her culpable "beyond a reasonable doubt"—the highest standard required in a court of law. "Clear and convincing," a slightly lower standard, is often taken to mean written evidence, such as could be shown by an advance directive, letter, diary, or other document written by the person.[11] The Supreme Court ruled that although such a high level of proof is not required in such cases, states are indeed permitted to set the standard at that level.

The case was returned to the trial court, where additional witnesses testified that Nancy herself had told them that she would not want to live in the condition she now was in. Finding that this new evidence met the clear and convincing standard, the judge ruled in favor of Nancy Cruzan's parents on December 14, 1990. No further appeal was filed. Nancy Cruzan died several days after her healthcare providers agreed to withdraw artificially-supplied food and water.

In an important side note to the Cruzan case, Supreme Court Justice Sandra Day O'Connor wrote in her concurring opinion:

> Few individuals provide explicit oral or written instructions regarding their intent to refuse medical treatment should they become incompetent. States that decline to consider any evidence other than such instructions may frequently fail to honor a patient's intent. Such failures might be avoided if the State considered an equally probative source of evidence: the patient's appointment of a proxy to make health care decisions on her behalf. . . . These procedures for surrogate decision making, which appear to be rapidly gaining in acceptance, may be a valuable additional safeguard of the patient's interest in directing his medical care.[12]

STATEMENT OF STATE LAW

The PSDA requires that states develop written statements of local law concerning advance directives that would be distributed by covered providers or organizations to patients, residents, members, or clients. Efforts to meet this requirement have varied considerably. In a recent evaluation of each state's response, researchers sought to identify the process used to comply, the difficulties encountered, and the effects of the PSDA on the effort itself.[13]

Most states read the language of the statute narrowly: The drafting effort was led by a state agency in 33 states and by a hospital or legal association in another 12. Massachusetts Health Decisions, a nonprofit health education and public opinion organization, was the sole consumer group taking a lead role by convening a statewide task force of 16 professional, provider, and education associations and state agencies. Most states worked collaboratively with a variety of concerned groups and organizations. Typical representation came from professional associations (hospital, medicine, nursing, hospice, long-term care, social work, chaplaincy, and law), interested state agencies (health and human services, attorney general, elder affairs), and, to a lesser extent, consumer organizations (illness support, aging, health promotion). It is interesting to note that only one state had a minority group involved, though 19 states had plans to translate the state law description.

Although the statute requires only a description of advance directive law, most states included related information about informed consent, decision making in the absence of an advance directive, and competency (to complete a directive) and capacity (to make one's own healthcare decisions). Most also addressed the role of health providers in counseling patients' decisions to forgo or withdraw life-sustaining treatments and the kind of information generally needed to make healthcare decisions.

In the survey, 40 states reported problems or concerns with their own state law. These fell into five categories: (1) concerns about living will laws, (2) concerns about durable power of attorney legislation, (3) decision making absent advance directives, (4) nutrition and hydration, and (5) witnessing procedures. Ten states introduced new legislation to remedy the problems or clarify ambiguities. Fifteen simply noted the uncertainty in their public description of the law (e.g., "If you have no family, or if there is disagreement about what treatment you would want, a court may be asked to appoint a guardian to make those decisions for you"). Other states did nothing or sought clarification from their attorney general.

As all states now have a written statement, was the required process a total success? No, but all states have the opportunity to modify their statement and must inevitably do so as federal and state laws change. For instance, only ten states included information about updating the directive. Just over half of the states advised discussion with family or friends. Only six described the process for determining incapacity (in order to invoke the advance directive). Less than half addressed the issue of having the directive honored in other states.

From a layperson's point of view, these omissions might be critical. Many, if not most, people will first learn about advance directives on admission, just as envisioned by the PSDA. Easy access and quick comprehensibility might determine whether the concept is worth a second thought—then or at a later time. Because health facilities are not required to distribute advance directives, the statement of state law might be the only introduction to advance directives offered by a facility to new patients. It is important, then, that the document convey not only the letter of the law, but its spirit. The intent of the PSDA is to educate and foster communication. If the initial exposure to information does not promote those goals, then subsequent efforts might prove starkly ineffective.

Collaborative efforts to refine and improve the statement of state law might also point out inconsistencies and vague areas in the law. Rose Gasner, former legal director at Choice in Dying, points out that the law regarding treatment refusal has "developed very haphazardly in many states, as the legislatures and the courts have responded to the fast-paced development of the issue. . . . Coalition work can create opportunities for law reform and bring together those interested groups that need to be involved in the political process to ensure passage of amending or substitute legislation."[14]

"ON ADMISSION . . ."

Providers must give inpatients, on admission, written information about their healthcare decision-making rights, including the right to complete an advance directive. Presumably, this statement will be taken verbatim or adapted from the statement of state law, also required by the PSDA, and discussed previously.

Providers must also give to inpatients, on admission, written information about the provider's policies respecting the implementation of patients' healthcare decision-making rights. In most cases, this has not required a burst of administrative development by institutions. Facilities have routinely added policies concerning informed consent protocols, advance directives, and decision making in the absence of family or advance-planning documents. Where this has not yet been done at all, or has not been modified to reflect current law or practices, many professional associations and private organizations have excellent resources for developing such policies.[15]

It is essential that policies reflect both the reality of professional interaction in the facility and the moral philosophy guiding the provision of care (conscientious objection to advance directives is covered in a later section of this chapter). For example, most proxy laws require a determination of capacity to be made by an attending physician before the patient's named healthcare agent is legally authorized to act. If frequent or lengthy visits by an attending physician are not the general rule, as is often the case in long-term care facilities and hospice and home care, then policies should clearly indicate how the facility would honor advance directives completed by patients, residents, or clients.

Providers must document in the patient's medical record whether the patient has executed an advance directive. For most facilities, this also means filing a copy of the advance directive itself in the patient's medical record, according to state law. The PSDA is silent, as are most state laws, on the extent of the provider's responsibility to secure a copy of the directive once a patient says he or she has completed one. Providers should be encouraged to use reasonable efforts to emphasize the importance of having a copy of the directive in the medical record where the person is or is planning to be a patient or resident. Yet consumers have the final responsibility of making sure that their completed directive is filed and has been discussed with their provider, surrogate, and any other person who may have an interest in their health care.

For supporters and critics alike, these three required items are the "heart and soul" of the PSDA. Without them, the act is all gums and no teeth. But it has become abundantly clear that providers will comply with the law in a variety of ways, from the marginally legal and painfully superficial to the exemplary. Anecdotal evidence has some providers handing out photocopies of articles about advance directives from the popular press. And that's all. Other providers have given directives and decision-making rights top billing in comprehensive pre-admission packets, complete with state law, instructions, and blank forms plus a referral number for more information.

Facility staff should be encouraged to develop presentation skills that both meet the letter of the law and promote the kind of careful consideration needed to make advance directives work as intended. For example, nursing intake personnel at the University of Minnesota Hospital asked patients on admission the following questions:

1. Have you discussed your current medical condition with a family member or close friend?
2. Has a family member or close friend been told what medical treatment you want or do not want if you are unable to speak for yourself?

3. Have you told your doctor what medical treatment you want or do not want?

4. Have you written a living will? If yes, have you discussed it with your doctor?[16]

Who will present the required information is an important concern in many facilities and organizations. Typically, information is included in pre-admission packets for people voluntarily admitted into service. This is especially true of health maintenance organizations (HMOs), nursing homes, and hospice and home care agencies. It is important to note that every Medicare and Medicaid provider has the obligation to query patients and provide information, even though many patients will have been exposed to the information from a previous provider.

In large institutions, however, the task has proven more difficult. Admissions clerks often are the first employees to give out information, with information or counseling backup provided variously by social service staff, chaplains, patient care representatives, or nurses. Unless patients are already familiar with the facility and its staff, they may find it very difficult to make the necessary connection between printed information received as a small part of a typical admissions packet and an identified staff resource. Both printed information and initial information providers should point to further sources of information and conversation.

Whomever provides required information and asks patients if they have completed an advance directive should stress that completing an advance directive is a voluntary act. It is too easy for advance directives to be included in a stack of forms to sign, and most experts agree that admission is an inappropriate place to complete advance directives. Admission personnel must also be familiar with:

- The process for completing advance directives under state law.
- Institutional policy on having employees witness advance directives, as well as other legal documents.
- The general elements of a valid advance directive under state law.
- Institutional policy on honoring or dishonoring advance directives.
- Answers to the most commonly asked questions or the name and phone number of the person identified as a primary resource on advance directives (see also the section "Staff Education").

ENSURING COMPLIANCE

The PSDA requires that covered providers will ensure compliance with state laws on advance directives. Compliance will be a logical extension of efforts to educate the medical and professional staff involved with implementing advance directives in any facility. Rose Gasner believes that "this section of the PSDA may serve as a basis for a new federal legal argument placing responsibility on the facility for knowledge of the law, as well as holding facilities responsible for the actions of staff."[17] She cites the example of a physician who refuses to comply with the decision of an authorized agent. In this case, many state statutes require the physician to transfer the patient to another physician who is willing to honor the request. Gasner argues that the PSDA compliance section might put the burden on the facility, as well as the physician, to ensure the prompt transfer of the patient.

OBJECTION ON THE BASIS OF CONSCIENCE

The PSDA, as it was passed as part of OBRA 1990, does not "prohibit the application of a State law which allows for an objection on the basis of conscience for any health care provider . . . which, as a matter of conscience, cannot implement an advance directive." Most state directives do include provisions for conscientious objection on religious, moral, or professional ethical grounds.

The interim final regulation issued by HCFA in March 1992 tries to clarify the provider's obligation to alert patients on admission of any conscientious objection—as a matter of written policy—by the facility. It states that the provider must inform the person in writing of state laws regarding advance directives and of the policies of the provider regarding the implementation of advance directives, including a clear and precise explanation of the provider's conscientious objection to implementing an advance directive.

Charles Sabatino, assistant director of the American Bar Association's Commission on Legal Problems of the Elderly, pointed out that providers and consumer advocates have very different views of the "clear and precise" requirement. Providers contend that it is better to adopt general, flexible policies so that objections can be handled on a case-by-case basis and that the standard itself is unrealistic. A facility's policies rarely take into account the personal values of each member of the professional staff. Consumers, however, feel that the requirement does not go far enough: The too-general language could be used to thwart any treatment option raised by a patient or agent that the facility objects to—whether or not as a matter of conscience.

The Commission suggested that provider policies:

1. Clarify any differences between institution-wide conscientious objections and those that might be raised by individual physicians.
2. Explain the basis for any facility objection (e.g., religious, moral, professional).
3. Identify the state legal authority permitting the objection.
4. Describe the range of medical conditions or procedures affected by conscientious objections.
5. Describe what steps will be taken to transfer or otherwise accommodate people whose wishes are impeded by the institution's policy.[18]

NONDISCRIMINATION

Under the PSDA, providers may not condition care or otherwise discriminate against a person based on whether that person has completed an advance directive. Indeed, many state statutes and statements of state law have already made note of this requirement. The Massachusetts statement, for example, reads, "You are not required to complete a Health Care Proxy on admission or at any other time in order to receive medical care from any health care providers. You have the right to receive the same type and quality of health care whether or not you complete a Health Care Proxy."[19]

Providers are cautioned that this provision might inadvertently be violated if admissions staff gives the impression that an advance directive, included as just one of a number of required forms to be completed at or before admission, is part of the regular admissions routine. Staff must alert patients that advance directives are voluntary documents that require significant prior thought and conversation to be truly effective. In addition, some providers have the mistaken impression that the requirements of the PSDA apply only to Medicare or Medicaid patients rather than to all admitted inpatients in facilities that accept Medicare or Medicaid payments.

Some people will never sign an advance directive, and that right must be respected. Patients might have family constellations upon whom they depend utterly and might have confidence in the family's efforts to make appropriate decisions. Some might come from cultures where naming as an agent someone other than a family leader would be an unforgivable affront. Still others are resigned to live and die fatalistically, either unwilling or unable to choose a surrogate. These are strictly personal choices for the patient, however frustrating or burdensome they might be for ultimate decision makers. It is altogether appropriate, however, to let patients know that if they do not make choices about their future health care and healthcare decision makers, the choices may still have to be made. However, they may be made by total strangers.

EMERGENCY ADMISSIONS

Nonvoluntary admissions may require special consideration in the development of facility policy, professional practice, staff education, and statewide protocols. Emergency admissions are addressed in the HCFA final regulations, but only with regard to the timing of informing patients of decision-making rights:

> If a patient is incapacitated at the time of admission . . . , then the facility should give advance directive information to the patient's family or surrogate to the extent that it issues other materials about policies and procedures. . . . This does not, however, relieve the facility of its obligation to provide this information to the patient once he or she is no longer incapacitated or unable to receive such information.[20]

Anecdotal evidence indicates that institutional emergency departments will not honor an advance directive unless it is absolutely clear that the incapacitated patient's preference would have been to refuse emergency care. Some emergency departments have begun keeping card files or other records of advance directives, though this is practical only in smaller facilities. Most difficult are emergency admissions where an appointed healthcare agent has accompanied the now-incapacitated patient to the facility and demands that his authority be honored in directing treatment on behalf of the patient. Many emergency medical staff believes that the emergency room is not the time or place to make a critical judgment call. They feel that one should spend time making a written determination of patient incapacity, validate the integrity of the written advance directive, verify the identity of the authorized agent, and engage in the required informed consent procedures with the agent or treat the patient. Supporters of this view argue that they would opt to treat the patient under typical implied consent protocols, at least to the point of stabilization, and then follow advance directive procedures—even if that meant withdrawing life-sustaining treatment.

Some consumer groups, as well as providers, have already begun efforts to educate consumers about the appropriate use of emergency services. Most laypersons are unaware of the legal requirements to "activate" a healthcare agent's decision-making authority, assuming that simply being a holder of a validly signed document is sufficient to direct treatment decisions. In addition, most laypersons are unaware of state laws that require emergency medical service staff to provide life support at the scene. Hospice home care presents a typical situation. A person cares for a dying spouse at home, supported by hospice services. Though counseled about the actual events of dying and death, the caregiver and appointed healthcare agent (who is, however, not yet authorized by a physician's determination of incapacity) panics at the onset of a terminal seizure and calls emergency services. Emergency personnel arrive and begin treatment despite the caregiver's protests that the dying patient wanted no heroic measures.

In response to frequent episodes such as the one just described, several states have taken the lead in establishing pre-admission "do not resuscitate" (DNR) procedures, either through legislation, regulation, or statewide adoption of protocols.[21] Although the situations covered by DNR orders are far fewer than those usually addressed in advance directives, emergency service personnel nevertheless believe the new guidelines help to recognize patient autonomy in treatment preferences. Several states now employ a dated DNR bracelet as a way of notifying emergency service staff. It is hoped that these tentative steps will encourage wider observance of more comprehensive advance directives among emergency services and institutional emergency departments.

PSYCHIATRIC ADMISSIONS

At admission, some patients are not capable of receiving or comprehending information or of completing advance directives. Many, as described earlier, are emergency admissions and can receive the required information at a later time. Other people, however, are neither emergency admissions nor adjudicated legally incompetent. Such cases are common in long-term care facilities, where up to one-half of all admissions can be persons who are mentally and functionally incompetent, but who have not been declared so by a court and do not have a legal guardian. Because the law assumes that all persons are competent to conduct their own affairs until a court determines otherwise, and because many advance directive laws presume the validity of signed directives, facilities with significant admissions of "questionably competent" persons will need to get good counsel in developing effective but legally sound policies.

It is useful to remember that, as a general rule, competency is something determined by a judge in an impartial court hearing. The law presumes competence until proven otherwise. Capacity to make healthcare decisions is frequently determined (as allowed and required by law) by an attending physician in following an advance directive state statute. Indeed, the two concepts may be quite separate and distinct: A person involuntarily committed to a psychiatric facility might still be legally capable of making his or her own healthcare decisions—so long as the person can participate meaningfully in the traditional informed consent or refusal process.[22] To the extent that any person can engage in significant discussion about his or her own health care, treatment preferences, quality of life, or personal values, that person cannot only help shape future options, but also help providers become aware of his or her wishes.

Most proxy and durable power of attorney statutes do not specify a time period during which an attending physician must determine that a person has either lost or regained decision-making capacity. The danger exists that the act of determining capacity can be misused as a management tool. For example, if a physician is uncomfortable with treatment preferences being expressed by a still competent patient, or if dealing with the designated agent seems to be easier or more consistent with his or her own values, then the physician has the option (albeit unprofessional, illegal, and unethical) to determine the patient incapacitated for the purpose of seeking consents or refusals from the agent. Conversely, if the physician believes that the designated agent will make treatment choices inconsistent with either his or her professional values or the known wishes of the already incapacitated patient, the physician might postpone making a determination of incapacity and rely temporarily on other vehicles for securing treatment consents or refusals.

To be sure, these are gross abuses of professional authority and would open the physician to substantial liability. Yet in the often hazy area of capacity determination, where hesitation, caution, and prudence are more often the rule than the exception, the law provides little direction for physicians, who may be guided at a practical level by their good professional instincts and their desire to take "the long view." In becoming familiar with advance directives, many physicians are still uncomfortable dealing with designated agents, who often are strangers to them but who hold the authority of consent and refusal no less certainly than their competent patients. The obligation of a physician to get to know an agent should be shared by both the physician and the patient. The agent deserves to be brought into conversations between doctor and patient well before the agent may be required to consult with the doctor in making choices on behalf of the patient. Should misuses of capacity determination as a management tool become anything more than isolated incidents, legislatures might consider modifying statutes to require that patient assessments and reassessments be made within specified time periods.

STAFF EDUCATION

Throughout 1991 and early 1992, healthcare facilities, education and training organizations, lawyers, bioethicists, and others held thousands of seminars, conferences, video-linked teleconferences, and in-service sessions concentrated on advance directives and the PSDA. By late 1992, however, the bloom was clearly off the rose. Staff development personnel typically reported, "We did that last year. All our staff know about the living will; we had an in-service and put a sample will in everyone's mailbox."

Regular and periodic education should be provided to all healthcare staff with direct patient contact, including physicians, nurses, social service professionals, patient care representatives, chaplains, admissions clerks, and others who may be in a position to talk with inpatients about directives. Even if their obligation is only to refer the patient to a more knowledgeable resource, staff should be aware of the basics. Because of staff turnover, especially among physicians, nurses, and nursing aides, facilities should include information on advance directives and policy in the basic orientation process.

Passage of the PSDA has prompted a deluge of clinical articles and educational information on advance directives as well as on the law itself. Much of this material is generic and not specific to any one state's law. Healthcare professionals are obliged to have not just a general knowledge of advance directives, but a solid understanding of their own state's law and their facility's policies to implement it. Educational materials for staff and the public should contain information specific to the state and facility.

Many physicians have been reluctant to honor advance directives for fear of liability. Some simply ignore directives entirely.[23] Even the advantage of having an identified decision maker was not enough to persuade them to accept a surrogate, legally appointed or not. Because most education efforts have been aimed at consumers, not providers, some physicians are still unaware that state statutes offer full immunity from criminal or civil prosecution if the physician follows the wishes of a validly-appointed healthcare agent in good faith. Although this does not totally insulate providers, it does give some assurance that a physician's reasonable efforts to secure informed consent through conversations with an agent will not lead to the devastating consequences of a successful suit for malpractice, or worse, wrongful death.

Admissions and records staff should be aware of basic form requirements as specified or allowed by state law. Many providers believe that the only advance directives submitted to them will be the ones they themselves distribute to patients and the public. This certainly is not so and will become less true as time passes. People will be introduced to directives from a variety of sources: lawyers, doctors, financial planners, insurance agents, senior organizations, illness support groups, religious organizations, and libraries, to name a few. In states with a prescribed form, nonconforming documents might be less of a problem than in states with either no form or only suggested language. Gatekeepers of the medical record ought to be able to spot a faulty document before it is filed and flag it without referring the document to the legal department or administration.

Patients will naturally assume that if they complete a document in good faith and submit it to the facility for filing they can depend on the terms of the document being honored. Although the PSDA does not address the issue of filing the form itself, many state statutes do. I believe that facilities that do not object to honoring advance directives (by conscience and as an explicitly-stated policy) have a moral obligation to tell patients whether the form submitted will be honored in the event of future incapacity. There can be no guarantees, understandably. But of what use to a patient is a directive dismissed as nonconforming or defective when pulled from a medical record just at the time it might be of use—that is, after the patient has become incapacitated and is unable to redo the directive?

Should facility staff help patients complete advance directives? This might depend, in part, on whether the facility has formal policies that support conscientious objection to advance directives. In general, however, facilities should be encouraged to provide the means for a patient to complete an advance directive while in the facility. The facility should have an adequate supply, not only of the required materials to provide at admission, but also additional information to be considered at a later time, appropriate and state-specific forms, a personal resource person, and at least several people who can serve as witnesses to signing (if allowed by local law).

PUBLIC EDUCATION

Long-term health education campaigns, such as those on smoking cessation, substance abuse, human immunodeficiency virus (HIV) prevention, nutrition, and women's health, have taught us a valuable lesson. We know that education works, but it takes a long time. The legal requirements of the PSDA will certainly result in many people being given information on their rights to accept or refuse recommended treatment and on advance directives. But the real change occurs when completing a living will or healthcare proxy comes to be perceived, quite simply, as the right thing to do, like giving up smoking or cutting back on prime rib and pizza in favor of grilled chicken and pasta salad. Systemic changes cannot be forced. They can be facilitated by persuasion, perhaps eased by suggestion. But transformations happen when all participants in the system begin to operate as if the change had already taken place. In the case of PSDA, the 15 to 20 percent rate of completion of advance directives will jump to 50 or 60 percent when both providers and consumers of healthcare agree that having a directive makes life easier and more certain for everyone.

The PSDA requires healthcare facilities to provide information to patients, residents, clients, or members on admission. Real change will occur when physicians in private practice routinely ask their 18-year-old patients, "Say, now that you can vote and you have your own place, did you ever give any thought about who would make healthcare decisions for you if you got in a skiing accident and were unconscious for a few weeks?" Real change will occur when lawyers give out free copies of advance directives to clients, perhaps as part of an overall estate planning discussion. Real change will occur when colleges and universities include advance directives in admission packets sent to incoming freshmen that include language like the following:

> Dear Freshman Parent:
> We look forward to welcoming Carmen to our beautiful campus in early fall. During these summer months, we hope you and your daughter will give some thought to what it means for a young person to make the transition into adulthood. Moving away from home into a new environment is certainly part of that change. But making one's own choices, especially about matters as personal as health care, is also a matter for adults. We have enclosed a pamphlet on the Massachusetts Health Care Proxy . . .

Physicians can be the best primary source of information. Written materials for the professional office are now available in every state from a variety of sources. Virtually every professional healthcare association in the country has some kind of PSDA or advance directive publication for general use. Videos on advance directives are available; healthcare power of attorney forms are available in Braille, large type, and in dozens of non-English languages; and books are sold in shopping mall bookstores on all facets of healthcare decision making for the lay as well as professional reader.[24] Trained medical office staff can be good sources of information and responsive to patient questions. But nothing will substitute for the sincere suggestion from a trusted doctor to consider the issue. Physicians must reclaim their roles as teacher and counselor in this regard.

Any public education program must emphasize the importance of talking with one's chosen healthcare agent and family members. Most advance directive forms are easy to complete and take little time. The discussions needed to give substance to those forms are not. But there are good resources here as well. The values history—an in-depth assessment of personal values, activities, goals, and preferences—has become a useful teaching tool as well as personal supplement to any kind of advance directive.[25] Initiating a discussion with family members is perfect for role-play exercises and is especially useful in settings where family members are actually present. The American Hospital Association, American Medical Association, American Association of Retired Persons, and most of the community health decisions programs have suggested guidelines for holding conversations with one's family, chosen agent, or physician.[26]

Any print materials distributed by your facility should be in a language, format, and style appropriate to your community.[27] If you have the chance to develop your own materials, make sure the drafting committee represents a cross section of interested people. Members might include a physician, a nurse, a lawyer, an ethicist, a clergyperson, a records administrator, the lay community, and maybe even a visiting English or humanities professor. Before you go to press, test a draft with your own staff, patients, and community members.

Many providers have discovered that inviting the public into a healthcare facility to hear a talk about advance directives rarely attracts an overflow crowd. Following are suggestions for fulfilling the PSDA community education requirement:

1. If you invite the public, do whatever you need to ensure your facility is known to be the sponsor, but unless you have a well-established reputation for holding lively, community-based meetings and events at your facility, hold the event somewhere else.

2. Work with other healthcare or social service providers in your area to present programs. If you work for a long-term care facility, join with staff from other nursing homes, a local hospital and hospice, or the local town nurse. A shared program will attract more people, reduce the staff burden on each facility, and provide economies of scale for print materials. It also reassures laypeople that this is not a competition for new clients: If several institutions and agencies are working together, with common materials, it must be okay.

3. Develop a linguistic or cultural minority outreach program in collaboration with other neighborhood organizations.

4. Work with local secondary schools, junior and community colleges, and universities to present programs to the 18- to 24-year-old crowd. Remember, many of the major cases of healthcare decision making and incapacity have involved young people, not elders (Karen Ann Quinlan, Nancy Cruzan, Paul Brophy, and Elizabeth Bouvia). Teachers in civics, health, healthcare administration, social work, and even government would appreciate your willingness to help with an occasional class.

5. Offer your help to classes of entering students in local medical schools, nursing schools, and schools of the allied health professions.

6. Adopt the "train the trainers" model of education. Develop a program to train office staff of physicians in your area. And make sure the physicians are invited, too.

7. Develop a program to train local parish clergy on the use of advance directives.

8. Develop a program to train a group of your best facility volunteers—the people who make you feel guilty because you never seem to have enough challenging tasks for them. Many facilities are using their volunteers rather than paid staff to provide community education.

9. Offer an intergenerational program, or one for your patients and their families, or for family members only. Offer a program for patients and their chosen agents.

10. Offer a program for employee assistance professionals in your area. How about benefits managers or staff in human resources?

11. Develop a program that provides "brown bag" seminars for employees in local corporations. (California and Massachusetts Health Decisions both have active programs for corporate employees. Almost without exception, employees are grateful to have the opportunity to consider the topic when they are healthy and making other kinds of future plans.)

12. If your facility does not have its own video production studio, do a program for your local community access cable station. Six months later, you can sponsor a repeat showing.

13. Invite your board president, mayor, governor, or one of your legislators to sign an advance directive at a public event.

14. At every public event, make sure two items are given out without fail: free copies of an advance directive and a simple three- or four-question evaluation to be returned anonymously. If you do not know what went wrong, you will never get it just right.

The PSDA is one of those rare pieces of legislation that gives us a good sense of things, as we know they ought to be in the best of all worlds but few specifics on how to construct that world. No healthcare facility runs quite like another, and no two healthcare professionals share identical values. In a healthcare system strained by legislation and public opinion from all sides, the requirements of the PSDA remind us that the enduring value of good health care comes not from legislated procedures but from the quality of human relationships born and nurtured in the system. The PSDA encourages healthcare providers and consumers to talk candidly with each other about matters of consequence: Will I get well? How will you treat me? What do you do here? Who will speak for me? Can I trust you? In a perfect world, all such questions merit straight and honest answers. Let us hope that the PSDA succeeds in encouraging both providers and consumers to ask the right questions and answer honestly.

5-YEAR IMPLEMENTATION UPDATE

In 1998, more than five years had passed since the PSDA became effective in December 1991, and the healthcare industry had undergone extraordinary change. During this period, there was an unprecedented and largely unsuccessful effort to reform the very nature of the delivery system, attention was refocused on the issue of physician-assisted suicide and euthanasia at state and national levels, and there was a massive shift toward managed care in both the private and public sector. Many smaller community hospitals had to close their doors, unable or unwilling to form alliances with other organizations. Large national chains assimilated extended-care facilities. Home care agencies engaged in repeated mergers, often as part of multisetting provider networks. Healthcare professionals—once among the most independent of workers—either had their jobs "reengineered" into extinction or became employees of newly-formed corporations. In short, apparently more pressing issues quickly overshadowed the PSDA.

Has the PSDA fulfilled its promise? Is it working? It depends where you look and whom you ask. It is important, however, to ask even more basic questions, some generated by the federal law itself, others stemming from the administrative changes required by the regulation (and by associated state laws), and still others emerging from case law and health professional practice. Certainly not all of these will be dealt with in this update, but the following questions warrant significant empirical research in their own right:

- How effective were state agencies in circulating the statement of state law required by the PSDA? Did every facility receive a copy, along with information about its use? If there have been subsequent changes in the statutory or case law, have state agencies been successful in notifying all covered organizations of the change(s)?
- What percentage of organizations covered by the PSDA have fully institutionalized the requirements of the PSDA? That is, are facilities giving patients, residents, and clients copies of their healthcare decision-making rights, including the right to complete an advance directive? Have all facilities developed written policies? Are facilities training all staff with relevant patient contact, including physicians? Are facilities providing education to the wider community?
- Are advance directives being recognized and honored?
- Is there an effective evaluation program in place? If there are flaws in the advance directive administrative system, who would know? How effective is the ongoing process of remediation? How are organizational policies being enforced, and by whom?

In the absence of any large-scale studies, some assessment must be limited to anecdotal evidence, though that itself is considerable. In general, the basic legal mandates of the PSDA have become institutionalized in healthcare agencies and institutions nationwide. To a greater or lesser degree, people admitted to facilities are asked, "Do you have an advance directive?" And there is some effort to provide information about healthcare decision making to admitted patients, residents, clients, and members.

It is far less certain, however, that the other PSDA requirements are being satisfied by organizations in any care setting. In my experience, few facilities have developed protocols for patient education beyond handing out a sheet of state law decision-making rights, though systematic follow-up has become a requirement of the Joint Commission on Accreditation of Healthcare Organizations (JCAHO). This will be discussed later in this five-year update. Given the large rate of staff turnover in health care generally, it has been surprising that staff education—at least among patient care representatives, nurses, social workers, and clergy—appears to have been consistent. Professionals, physicians, however, seem to be the least knowledgeable about advance directives. This may be due to the "point of contact" established by the PSDA itself. According to the regulation, persons are to be informed and queried on admission, which most often puts the responsibility for program administration on admissions clerks or social workers. Unless a person becomes terminally ill or incapacitated, it is highly likely that a physician would not even be alerted to the existence of an advance directive, much less its instructions or appointed agent. The Robert Wood Johnson Foundation sponsored the Study to Understand Prognoses and Preferences for Outcomes and Risks of Treatment (SUPPORT) which was comprehensive study to determine preferences in seriously ill patients. One of the lessons learned from the SUPPORT project is that communication between physicians and other professional care providers, especially with regard to prognostic information and family interaction, needs substantial improvement.[28]

Other than anecdotes and observations, what has happened to the PSDA? This update will focus on three areas of movement: (1) the Interim Final Rule (1992) and the Final Rule (1995) of the PSDA itself as published by HCFA, (2) new standards regarding advance directives established by the Joint Commission for all care settings, and (3) known case law challenges involving advance directives.

PSDA Interim Final Rule (Effective April 1992)

In March 1992, HCFA issued the Interim Final Rule of the PSDA. It officially implemented sections 4206 and 4751 of OBRA 1990, also known as Public Law 101–508. It described in general terms the provisions of the PSDA that had already become effective on December 1, 1991—several months previously. It also announced a 60-day public comment period, the results of which formed the basis for the Final Rule issued in 1995. And finally, the Interim Final Rule gave brief suggestions on how providers might meet the requirements of the PSDA, offered sample text for a public information document on advance directives, listed print and video resources, and assured providers that HCFA would provide technical assistance for providers in the PSDA implementation process.

PSDA Final Rule (Effective July 1995)

The Final Rule restates the original OBRA regulation with several minor changes based on HCFA's review and consideration of 85 comments submitted during the 60-day public comment period. The Rule reports on a public-education campaign conducted by HCFA in 1992, primarily by means of print materials, public service announcements on television and radio, and a toll-free Medicare hotline. The Rule specifically notes that

> the Office of the Inspector General (OIG) conducted an early implementation study in December, 1992, to determine compliance with the advance directive provision and facility and patient responses (OEI-06-91-01130 and OEI-06-91-01131). This study found that at that time two-thirds of the patients in the facilities studied had some understanding of advance directives. We believe that this finding indicates that HCFA, in concert with other members of the healthcare industry, has made significant strides towards educating the public on advance directives.

The large majority of the Final Rule, however, consists of the comments submitted by citizens and HCFA's responses. Although these are too numerous and lengthy to summarize, it is instructive to read the document if only to appreciate the caution and concern clearly shown by all parties. Issues range from conscientious objection to patient or agent treatment requests, facility exemption from PSDA requirements, public education definitions, and the costs of program administration. In general, HCFA tactfully disagrees with most commenters—many of whom wrote to seek exemption, modification, or simplification of the general rule. To critics of the regulation, the PSDA was yet another administrative requirement loaded onto an overburdened and overregulated industry. To supporters, it was reassuring to see the government say, as it does in several places: "While we recognize that preparing this material may be a challenge, the law requires that it be done. . . ."

Following are synopses of key issues discussed in the Final Rule, often at length. Where the Final Rule either affirms or modifies the regulation as it was first circulated in 1991, I note it at the end of each synopsis.

Information to Be Provided to Patients

The PSDA requires providers to give each adult individual admitted information concerning his or her rights under state law to make decisions concerning medical care, including the right to accept or refuse medical or surgical treatment and the right to formulate, at the individual's option, advance directives.[29] By December 1991, the effective date of the PSDA, almost all states had developed and circulated to providers statewide the required "statement of state law" regarding healthcare decision-making rights. In most cases, this statement is a brief summary of statutory and case law specific to that state describing the elements of informed consent, advance directives, and perhaps involuntary treatment, emergency care, and protective services. Many facilities, however, seem to have neglected this statement and, instead, opted to inform patients that they have a simple, but unexplained, right to accept or refuse treatment and complete an advance directive. This is insufficient to meet the requirements of the PSDA, and providers should secure copies of the statement of state law for their state to incorporate or modify as appropriate.

In addition, many providers, especially those serving large populations of elders, seem to have confused the PSDA-required statement of state law with the statement of patient's rights required separately under Medicare provisions. The two are not the same, and both are required. (Affirm)

Informing on Admission

Each organization or facility bears responsibility for informing patients of their healthcare decision-making rights, including the right to complete an advance directive. If a patient is being transferred from one care setting to another, it is suggested that the transferring facility include copies of completed directives in order to ensure a smooth coordination of care. The receiving facility, however, still has the responsibility of informing the newly admitted patient or resident and asking whether a directive has been completed.[30] (Affirm)

In the case of hospitals, information must be given to patients on admission, unless they are incapacitated. Information is not required for patients in an outpatient setting, except for home health, hospice, and personal care services.[31] (Affirm) For these providers, it is permitted to give information at the time of the first home visit as long as the information is given before actual care is provided.[32] (Affirm)

Incapacitated Admissions

If a patient or resident is incapacitated at the time of admission, the facility should give information to the family or surrogate. However, the facility is still obliged to inform the patient once he or she regains capacity.[33] (Modify) Providers will need to develop appropriate follow-up procedures (see also Joint Commission update, below). There is no "good faith" exception for persons involuntarily admitted for psychiatric treatment. Such a determination must always be made on a case-by-case basis.[34] (Affirm)

Community Education

Providers must be able to document their community education efforts. This could be done by maintaining copies of any materials used as part of its community education programs.[35] (Modify) Educational materials used to inform the community about advance directives must be written and must include a description of a person's rights under state law to make healthcare decisions, including the rights to accept or refuse treatment and to complete an advance directive. The materials must also include the provider's or organization's implementation policies concerning an individual's advance directive.[36] (Affirm)

Providing written materials to individuals who come to a facility to investigate admission or to visit family members is not sufficient to meet the community education requirement.[37] (Affirm)

In response to one commenter who asserted that enforcement of the community education requirements would violate a provider's First Amendment rights to freedom of religion, and hence would warrant an exemption from the requirement, HCFA responded:

> We believe it would be appropriate for a provider to register that objection as it conducts its community education requirement. That is, the provider must meet its obligation to conduct community education on advance directives, but may inform the community that the State law offers a choice that, because of a conscientious objection, it would not honor. We believe that this information is valuable for community members to have since it may affect their choice of a provider.[38]

Facility or organization public relations offices might be used to inform the community about advance directives, and the associated costs generally would be related to patient care rather than to advertising to the general public. As such, the costs of advance directives activities could be considered an allowable cost related to patient care under existing Medicare policy. And to the extent that states make additional payments to providers for their costs of advance directives, federal financial participation is available at the federal Medicaid Assistance Percentage.[39] (Affirm)

What is "the community"? It relates to the catchment area of the individual providers, which means that an HMO and a hospital, for example, would likely have community areas very different in scope. For managed care plans, *community* is defined as the organization's service area.[40] (Affirm) For all other organizations—hospitals, home care agencies, extended care facilities, and personal service organizations—the definition of *community* is left to the discretion of the organization but generally is meant to be the catchment area and community-at-large. (Affirm)

Providers should distribute materials that are clear and understandable to each patient. If the patient's knowledge of English or the common language of the facility is inadequate for clear understanding, then a means to communicate the information concerning patient rights and providers' responsibility and practices must be available and implemented. For foreign languages commonly encountered, the provider should have written translations of its description of state law and its statement of protocols, and should, when necessary, make the services of an interpreter available.[41] (Affirm)

In the same vein, providers should be sensitive to cultural differences that might make a discussion of even the remote possibility of death awkward or difficult. The law does not make any exception, however, for these cases: Patients must still be offered information about their rights to enhance control over medical treatment decisions. (Affirm)

Conscientious Objection

When a provider, as a matter of conscience, cannot implement an advance directive, the provider must now provide in its written policies (and, hence, to patients) a "clear and precise statement of limitation." Regardless of any religious affiliation, that statement should (1) clarify any differences between institution-wide conscientious objections and those that might be raised by individual physicians, (2) identify the state's legal authority permitting such objection, and (3) describe the range of medical conditions or procedures affected by the conscientious objection.[42] (Modify)

It is important to note that many states adopted language found in the first statutory advance directive, the California Natural Death Act of 1976. This act said that if providers could not, as a matter of conscience, honor an advance directive, the physician bore responsibility for facilitating the patient's transfer—not just to another healthcare provider, but to one who would honor the request. Providers are encouraged to check state law before assuming either that the patient's desire for transfer is the patient's sole responsibility or that it is sufficient for the physician or facility to arrange transfer to any other willing provider.

Enforcement Procedures

Providers must now inform individuals that complaints concerning noncompliance with the advance directives requirements can be filed with the state survey and certification agency. To comply, providers could post a notice of an individual's rights and the name, address, and telephone number of the appropriate state survey and certification agency. This information must also be included in the written description of a resident's rights. The Medicare Hotline (1-800-638-6833) and the home health hotline can also be used to lodge complaints.[43] (Modify)

Joint Commission Standards

Effective June 10, 1996, the Joint Commission clarified the Advance Directive standard RI.1.2.4. Previous Joint Commission standards on advance directives—based on the PSDA and most state statutes—required facilities and agencies only to ask patients on admission or enrollment into service whether they had completed an advance directive. If so, and if presented, the facility was required to place a copy in the patient's medical record. The new standard applies when a patient reports not having an advance directive. The Joint Commission now gives facilities three options:

1. The facility can make arrangements to immediately obtain a copy of the existing—but not currently present or available—advance directive.
2. The facility can offer assistance to complete a new written advance directive.
3. A facility/agency designee can inform the patient that she or he may verbally specify treatment preferences, explaining the substance of any original advance directive, including preferred surrogate decision maker and specific wishes. If the patient chooses this option and verbalizes the information, the conversation must be documented in the patient's record, and the physician must be informed.

Facilities are strongly cautioned about the third option, because most state advance directive statutes require written documents with formal witnessing and possible notarization for either living will or proxy-type directives. But certainly the facility ought to be as proactive as possible in either seeking out an existing directive or offering to help complete (but not requiring) a new directive.

It is also clear that Joint Commission inspectors have been unusually forthright about encouraging facilities to develop follow-up strategies. Reasonable policies might describe ways: to remind or encourage patients to bring copies of directives for scheduled inpatient stays, record number and timing of follow-up phone calls to family members, and provide clear protocols for facilitating on-site completion, including providing persons who can serve as witnesses and, if required, a notary public. Many facilities, especially in extended care, have policies prohibiting any employee from serving as a witness to a resident's will or other legal matter. Advance directives ought to be given special consideration. It is to mutual benefit that a facility can provide the conditions under which a person can thoughtfully and calmly complete an advance directive.

Case Law Challenges to Advance Directives

In the more than 20 years since California enacted the first statutory advance directive, there have been very few cases involving advance directives in the courts. If a case made it to court at all, the matter was usually resolved through mediation or settlement before proceeding to trial. Trial court cases are rarely published except as reported in the popular press, because they do not set precedent: Cases that do not go on to appeal or to the state's highest court do not make law. Nor is it easy to go back and review the case.

Disputes frequently occur around a very narrow range of issues:

- Is the document valid and binding? Was the person who signed it mentally competent at the time of signing to do so? Was the signing forced in some way? Has the document been revoked, either through an automatic statutory revocation, such as divorce, or by some statement or action of the person?
- What does the document say? What is the appointed agent authorized to do, either by law or by the terms of the document? What treatment choices has the person made, as spelled out in the document or as told to the named surrogate?
- If legal and valid, is the document being honored? Has a facility or agency produced the document entrusted to it in the medical record? Is a healthcare provider abiding by the terms of the document or following the directions of the named agent? Is there a valid conscientious objection by a provider to follow the directions of the patient or surrogate? Is there any other reason for a provider to ignore the directions of the patient or surrogate?

Generally speaking, most of these questions are resolved in discussions between the patient and provider or between the surrogate and provider. An administrator or risk manager might become involved, perhaps even a lawyer for the agency or family. But cases specifically involving advance directives that proceed to open court usually follow one of very few courses:

1. The patient's request for treatment has been ignored or overridden, and as a result of a failure to treat, the patient is now dead.
2. The patient's request to forgo treatment has been ignored or overridden, and despite having requested the right to die the patient is still alive and charged for treatment given over his or her objection.
3. The patient's request to forgo treatment has been ignored or overridden, and as a result of unwanted treatment the patient is still alive but is either in a worse condition or simply doesn't want to be alive.

The first case, exemplified by Gilgunn v. Massachusetts General Hospital, indicates that medical professionals may refuse to provide requested care when that care is clearly not medically appropriate or is actually harmful to the patient.[44] Persons do not have a right to demand what a provider honestly believes will not be a benefit. But providers must be open and proactive in developing so-called futility policies so that honest respect for the limits of the medical profession is not construed as a shield of professional arrogance or economic advantage. In developing such policies, it may prove very useful to involve other organizational providers and residents of the community, as has been done in several metropolitan areas nationwide.[45] Among the three examples, this appears to be most easily resolved through traditional actions for professional malpractice, or through more recent discussions of "medically inappropriate care."

The second and third examples are more difficult, primarily because courts have traditionally ruled that being alive is always better than being dead, no matter how burdensome or unwanted the living. The trend may be changing, however.

In Elbaum v. Grace Plaza of Great Neck, Inc., the second example, a nursing home resident sued when the home billed the family for care provided after the patient specifically refused that treatment.[46] An early decision favoring the family was later reversed on appeal.

The third example comes from a distressing Michigan case reported on the front page of the New York Times in 1996.[47] In that case a young woman developed a seizure syndrome. Advised by her physician that the condition would only become progressively worse, she named her mother as her health-care surrogate in a valid Michigan Health Care Proxy. When she later became fully incapacitated from an unusually strong seizure, the mother instructed the attending physician and hospital to do what her daughter wished: forgo the extraordinary treatment, the ventilator, and allow her to die. The directive and mother were allegedly ignored, and the daughter remains profoundly disabled following a two-month coma during which time she was tube fed and on a ventilator. In a suit against the hospital and physician on behalf of the young woman, a jury awarded her $16.5 million.

A recent Ohio case, however, indicates that the consequences of failing to honor valid advance directives are far from settled and certainly not uniform across the country. In 1988, an 82-year-old man entered a hospital for treatment of a coronary problem. Despite a valid DNR order, the man was resuscitated when tachycardia caused him to stop breathing. He later suffered a stroke that left him partially paralyzed and in a nursing home. He sued for damages for his pain, suffering, emotional distress, and medical and other expenses of his "wrongful life." He died two years after entering the hospital.

The trial court initially held for the defendant hospital, stating that Ohio did not recognize a cause of action for wrongful life. After several appeals, the case was heard by the Ohio Supreme Court, which finally dismissed the action. It ruled that even though the hospital might be accused of committing a battery (legally defined as any unconsented touching, such as unrequested medical treatment), unless the plaintiff could show that the battery actually caused a further impairment such as the man's stroke and paralysis; there was no harm from treating a person against his wishes.[48]

Other cases are presently in the courts, and many have gone before, each seeking to confirm what many scholars and attorneys often take for granted: that competent persons have the constitutionally protected right to accept treatment or to refuse any unwanted treatment.[49] Causes of action (the legal basis on which a lawsuit can be brought to court) vary somewhat: battery, right of privacy, common law right to refuse treatment, negligence, wrongful death, wrongful life, as well as simple medical malpractice. However, the issues under consideration are even more complex: persons who are competent, incompetent but conscious, never competent, semicomatose, or permanently comatose; substituted judgment; and the clear and convincing standard for evidence brought before the court. Even with 97 advance directive laws—at least 1 in each of the 50 states—and the PSDA, it seems to remain questionable whether those rights can be exercised in advance of incapacity and with confidence.

If the intent of the PSDA was to introduce a concept to the general public by means of an education program having little oversight of content, delivery, evaluation, and enforcement, then the regulation is working. As the Inspector General found, many people have "some understanding" of advance directives. And healthcare professionals and organizations have largely institutionalized protocols designed to meet minimum thresholds set by the law. But if the intent of the law was to increase substantially the number of advance directives completed, discussed, submitted, and honored, then it can be described as a law that has had a good beginning, with the better part of the race yet to be run. Both empirical research and anecdotal evidence indicate that the percentage of persons with signed advance directives remains somewhat constant at 15 to 20 percent.[50]

As with preventive medicine, education leading to behavioral change is a long-term enterprise. Just ask the people in the smoking cessation movement who have worked and waited for almost 50 years for positive feedback from one of the longest education efforts in history. Not smoking is, at last, becoming the norm. Will it take 50 years for the PSDA to have more than a superficial effect on how healthcare providers and their patients relate to each other? One hopes not.

Further regulation and promotion of the education process, either by the Joint Commission or by changes in state law, will inevitably result in greater adherence to the prescribed PSDA regimen. So, too, might lawsuits like the ones described. But legal remedies for violations of distinctive state laws will have only a gradual effect on behavior in other jurisdictions. As far as we know, no suits have been filed alleging violations of the federal PSDA requirements—only violation of state advance directive laws or federal constitutional law regarding the right to refuse treatment are on record. With the PSDA modified by the Final Rule to require notification to patients of a state-based complaint process, it will be interesting to see whether this path to enforcement will be used by persons who believe their advance directive rights have been violated.

Will providers be the primary source of information about healthcare decision making and advance directive rights? They may be in a good position to do so, but many people argue that admission to a healthcare facility is a profoundly poor time to think carefully about one's treatment preferences, possible incapacity, and naming a surrogate decision maker—better to consider those weighty issues when healthy and curious. The more effective efforts will likely come through innovative education programs developed by professional associations, nonprofit organizations, and volunteer associations who want to promote wider use of advance directives and interact more frequently with healthy constituents.

Will the PSDA ever result in having all persons complete advance directives, just as we all apply for driver's licenses and credit cards? Doubtful. Many citizens find the concept of personal autonomy strange, even highly objectionable. Self-disclosure, one of the necessary components of completing any of the proxy documents, is not a valued skill to many people. And is it, in fact, desirable that as many people as possible exercise as much control as possible over their health care? What is there to lose? What is at risk if we do not? Skeptics will answer that we do not need to have control over treatment options that we might not be offered anyway. They argue that health care is so technologically advanced that the choice we are authorized to make is illusory: Our doctor cannot explain the choice in words we know, and we cannot comprehend the true range of options we really have. So why choose at all?

Choice is, after all, one of the enduring American values. Pity the grocer who stocks only one brand of anything. That grocer will soon be out of business. Put choice on the shelves, and the register will ring all day. And so it is with the PSDA. At the insistent request of the American public, the federal government has enacted legislation that urges, encourages, pushes, and nudges us to be choosy. Inspect, assess, evaluate, weigh, discuss, and deliberate—then choose. I will not settle for health care that someone else selects for me. I want to choose it myself, in my own time. It has to suit me. I will have that one, please.

15-YEAR IMPLEMENTATION UPDATE

After 15 years, the PSDA is working, though certainly not so vigorously or effectively as many advocates had hoped. The following provisions of the act are largely institutionalized in most healthcare organizations:

1. A process of providing written information about one's healthcare decision-making rights under state statutory and case law, including the right to complete an advance directive
2. A process of providing a copy of the organization's institutional policy regarding its observance of Number 1 above
3. Education of staff on advance directives
4. Education of members of the general public and documentation of those efforts

Has the PSDA fulfilled its goal of encouraging members of the healthcare-consuming public to complete advance directives in larger numbers? Generally speaking, no. It is estimated that 15 to 20 percent of the population has completed an advance directive, figures that have remained static for more than two decades. This is not a failure of the statute, however, but rather a measure of presumptions that simply have not materialized. Many people presumed that the PSDA would:

- Encourage more people to exercise a greater degree of self-determination with regard to their treatment options.
- Encourage physicians to talk with their patients about advance directives, not only in internal medicine or routine office encounters, but in any encounter where a physician has a large and regular exposure to competent patients.
- "Encourage" (because it was a stated requirement of the law) large-scale and regular public education.
- Encourage discussion between persons and their named proxy decision makers.

Related and Contentious Issues

If the many supporters of the PSDA presumed that some of the most difficult decisions in end-of-life care and care for people without decision-making
capacity would be resolved quickly, they were mistaken. Difficult ethical,
social, medical practice, and policy issues remain. Others are newly arisen. It
is unlikely that consensus will develop quickly, if ever, about these matters.
The active and ongoing debates they engender among members of the public
and healthcare professionals are healthy and robust. Among the more contentious are the following:

Physician-Assisted Suicide

May a competent, terminally ill person enlist the help of a willing physician
to secure drugs that would enable the person to end his or her life? In 1997,
Oregon became the first state in this country to allow physician-assisted suicide. Though challenged vigorously several times, the statute remains in
effect. Since its passage in 1997, approximately 240 terminally ill people have
used the law to end their lives as they wished—hardly the flood of suicides
feared by critics.[51]

Treatment Refusal by Surrogate

May the legally-authorized representative of a person refuse medical care
that is keeping the person alive? The affirmative answer to this question is
well settled as a matter of law. But this has not prevented lengthy and heated
confrontations, perhaps most notably in the Florida case of Terri Schiavo. In
1990, Ms. Schiavo suffered cardiac arrest, apparently caused by a potassium
imbalance, that led to irreversible brain damage due to lack of oxygen. She
spent the next 15 years in a persistent vegetative state. Ms. Schiavo had
never completed an advance directive, and her husband was appointed her
legal guardian by a Florida court. After several years of seeking further treatment for his wife, and several confirming assessments of her vegetative state,
Mr. Schiavo ultimately sought to have his wife's feeding tube removed. This
refusal of life-sustaining care would, he believed, give effect to his wife's own
wishes under the circumstances.

Ms. Schiavo's parents and a growing list of third parties, including religious
leaders; local, state, and federal legislators; representatives of the community
of physically disabled persons; and others, all sought to challenge not only the
decision made by Mr. Schiavo on behalf of his wife, but also his right to make
those decisions. The legal dispute over Ms. Schiavo's care, dying, eventual
death, and burial persisted for more than 12 years.[52]

Prospective signers of advance directives regularly ask: "If I sign this document, is it certain that I won't have to have a treatment I don't want, or get a
treatment I do?" It would simplify matters if the answer could be a simple yes
or no. But it is seldom a simple matter. Rather, it sometimes depends on the
treatment sought or forgone and the legal competence of the signer. The
signer's decision-making capacity at some future decision point also influences whether the treatment decision can be made at relative leisure and

deliberation or in an emergency and whether other persons believe or wish they had the authority to intervene.

Mr. Schiavo did not derive his decision-making authority on his wife's behalf through a healthcare proxy or healthcare power of attorney. As a court-appointed guardian, however, his legal responsibilities and obligations to act on his wife's wishes or in her best interests were virtually identical. The saga of the Schiavo family demonstrates the tremendous uncertainty of the deci-sion-making process, notwithstanding what many believed was a solid foun-dation for choosing and trying to give effect to a preferred outcome. Clinicians would be well advised to be cautious in guaranteeing outcomes envisioned by means of an advance directive.

Refusing Treatment Absent Terminal Illness

May people refuse unwanted medical care, even if they are not terminally ill and refusing care will result in their death? The affirmative answer to this question, too, is long settled in the law, and most recently affirmed by the United States Supreme Court in the Nancy Cruzan case.[53] In public percep-tion and clinical practice, however, many people view a total refusal of all care—especially in the absence of a terminal illness—as immoral or a form of suicide, or both. Although refusal of all care does not constitute suicide, in the legal sense some religions and moral systems condemn the practice or disal-low it. Clinicians, too, often are reluctant to honor total treatment refusals, either because they believe the person could benefit from additional treat-ment, or because they believe such a refusal could only be made irrationally by an incompetent or incapacitated person, or because their personal values are inconsistent with those of their patient or surrogate.

Issues Raised by Changes in State and Federal Law

The following are some of the issues raised by changes in state and federal law. Note that the PSDA itself has not been changed since its implementation date of December 1, 1991.

State Advance Directive Laws

What began more than 35 years ago as a novel proposal to allow citizens the opportunity to refuse unwanted care in the final days of life has evolved quickly given the sensitivity of the topic and the traditional pace of legislative activity. All states now have at least one form of advance directive, either a proxy designation or narrative living will, and some have both. The large majority of states have statutory forms, a frustrating turn of events for many lawyers who believed they could draft more effective documents. As might be expected, the individual state laws continue to differ significantly, even though a model Uniform Health-Care Decisions Act has been available for more than a decade.[54] A few states require notarization, though most do not. Some require "clear and convincing" evidence of a signer's intent to refuse artificial nutrition and hydration or to refuse other life-prolonging care. Oth-ers give agents full authority to make any and all healthcare decisions that the signer could, if able, including decisions about life-sustaining treatment.

Some recognize documents from another state, whereas others would enforce only those documents that do not violate their own requirements. In short, in the 30 years since California became the first state to legislate into law the original notion of a "Living Will," first suggested by Louis Kutner in 1969, we have yet to develop a nationally uniform way of recognizing personal choice in matters of health treatment.

Is a uniform, nationally recognized statute and accompanying form likely in the near future? No, in this writer's opinion. In many states, the legislative process of developing locally acceptable law involved serious, often bitter debate among advocates for the right to life, the right to die, various religious perspectives, the integrity of the medical and nursing professions, and the rights of people with disabilities, among others. As with most legislation, compromises were made. But the original polar positions and prices paid were not entirely forgotten. Any effort by one group to modify existing law may be met by former opponents equally eager to maintain the status quo or revive the original debate that once ended in a barely acceptable compromise.

But a uniform law, adopted by all states, would remove one significant barrier to wider use of advance directives: the current lack of portability for persons who move frequently, spend significant time in other states, reside in one state but receive regular health care in another, have no fixed residence, or who seek specialized care out of state.

Default Surrogate Consent Laws

As of 2006, 38 states have enacted laws that prescribe a list of persons from whom a clinician can seek informed and voluntary consents to or refusals of care when the patient has not completed an advance directive. Generally, the laws specify a range of possible surrogates, for example, a spouse, adult child, parent, sibling, nearest relative, or friend. They set a priority ranking of the potential surrogates and give detailed information on the kinds of decisions allowed, preconditions for their appointment, and solutions for conflict resolution.

Proponents of surrogate consent laws, mainly physicians and healthcare organizations, have welcomed laws that specify a legal decision maker and minimize or avoid time spent mediating family disputes or seeking court-ordered temporary guardianships. As clinical management tools, surrogate consent laws are useful.

As a mechanism of patient preference and civil rights, however, the value of surrogate consent laws is less clear. Surrogate consent, as a means to give voice to the values and preferences of a now incapacitated person, is useful only insofar as the surrogate has knowledge of those values and preferences. Without that knowledge, the surrogate is "flying blind." It makes no difference whether the surrogate is an agent acting by means of a validly completed healthcare proxy or simply the next available person appearing on a list of potential surrogates authorized by a well-meaning state statute. A useful surrogate is one who knows the patient's wishes or knows the patient well enough to decide—with some measure of confidence and assurance—in the patient's best interest.

One unanswered question of decision-making authority under both advance directive and surrogate consent laws concerns consent to research. Because many advance directive laws were enacted in "piggyback" fashion, with one state borrowing language from others, the authority to make "healthcare" decisions is almost universally defined as the right to make "decisions regarding the diagnosis, prognosis and treatment of a mental or physical illness." But does this mean that a chosen agent or statutorily selected surrogate could enroll the patient in a clinical trial or other form of research? If the clinician cannot provide clear and proven information about the likely benefits, burdens, and possible side effects of the proposed intervention, then the minimum provisions of legal informed consent cannot be satisfied. That is, what is being proposed is something *other than* treatment? Yet clinical trials might, in fact, be a route chosen by the presently incapacitated patient seeking aggressive if unproven care. Should not the patient's own selected decision maker be legally allowed to make the same choice?

This unresolved issue becomes more pressing as clinical trials of unproven therapies become more commonly applicable to persons in terminal or end-stage conditions. Healthy persons who would favor such aggressive, experimental, or unproven care and are presently either completing advance directives and/or engaging potential surrogate or family members in advance planning conversations might consider adding a provision that gives his or her agent specific authority to enroll the principal in clinical trials or other research if available and appropriate. Many people would seek to avoid such a scenario. Indeed, the fear of a long, lingering illness; physical or mental deterioration; loss of control; and burden on others all prompt many people to insist on "no heroic measures." For those few who want "everything possible," however, the chosen agent may need additional authorization to facilitate the preferred course of events.

HIPAA

The Health Insurance Portability and Accountability Act (HIPAA) of 1996 is a broad-spectrum federal law designed, in part, to safeguard the privacy of a person's health status and healthcare information. Implementation of the law has changed dramatically the level of communication among a person's clinicians, caregivers, family members, insurers, and other interested third parties. HIPAA does not affect state advance directive laws, however. A person's designated healthcare agent under a healthcare proxy or healthcare power of attorney continues to have full authority to secure access to any and all information about the principal. Indeed, in the legal sense, the appointed agent *is* the patient and is entitled to be given all information that the patient would receive, including confidential information. There simply is no provision in HIPAA that contradicts, supersedes, or overrides the 50 state laws governing the appointment of substitute decision makers by means of healthcare proxies, healthcare powers of attorney, or the equivalent.

In practice, however, some clinicians and organizations wrongly refuse information to legally-appointed surrogates. Instead, they first require the patient to sign a separate, and wholly unnecessary, "HIPAA Waiver." It is hoped that through JCAHO or internal policy reviews, or other periodic quality assurance mechanisms, such unnecessary barriers to a person's legally recognized advance planning will be modified to conform to federal law.

The privacy section of HIPAA became effective on April 14, 2003, following a lengthy public comment period during which the federal Department of Health and Human Services (DHHS) received more than 11,000 comments from healthcare professionals and organizational providers, insurers, and members of the public. So complex is the law, in both its privacy and security aspects, that a virtual industry evolved to help the healthcare field comply with its requirements. More than three years after implementation, the DHHS continues to maintain a comprehensive section of its Web site devoted to this important statute that affects virtually every aspect of the healthcare delivery system, as well as the persons served by it.

Remaining Barriers to Implementation

There continue to be significant barriers to more widespread use of advance directives in planning ahead for time of possibly incapacity or imminent death. Most concern professional medical practice patterns, institutional or organizational will, or personal values.

Physician Practice Patterns

As was pointed out earlier, physicians are best positioned to be effective promoters of advance directives. After all, they share in the benefits of successful completion by their patients. Having an identified surrogate can save considerable time in securing consents to or refusals of care. Knowing the patient's own preferences for care at the end of life allows both the physician and family to proceed with confidence and comfort, secure in the knowledge that both are carrying out the patient's wishes. Virtually all advance directive statutes insulate physicians from civil or criminal liability in following the patient's express wishes or the surrogate's decisions, so long as the physician acts in good faith. Such legal protection is generally not available to physicians whose actions are not governed by his patient's or legal surrogate's fully informed and voluntary consent. In those states without a surrogate consent law, turning to a spouse, family member, or friend for consent may be a time-honored tradition, but it does not fulfill the legal requirement that informed and voluntary consent can only be secured from someone with the legal authority to grant it.

Many physician advocates of advance directives also cite the personal and professional satisfaction that comes from enhancing their relationships with patients to a level of trust and confidence well beyond the "find it and fix it" mode of service. However, the PSDA obligation of patient education applies only to organizations and institutions, not individual physicians. Nor do most insurers reimburse for time spent providing education or eliciting personal preferences. Until conversations about advance care planning are accepted as a standard of care, with appropriate reimbursement, physicians will continue to be reluctant to be primary information providers.

Some physicians incorrectly believe that all advance directives concern only treatment choices for end-of-life care. They think it is inappropriate to raise the topic unless the patient is gravely or terminally ill, or very old. Although the PSDA requires regular staff education, anecdotal evidence suggests that

comprehensive education on advance directives is often limited to nonphysician staff: nursing, case management, admitting, chaplaincy, and patient
advocacy. It would be helpful if PSDA-covered institutions included all clinical
staff with patient contact, including both employee and community physicians, in their regular education programming.

Many physicians still fail to distinguish between decision-making capacity
and competency. Although the concepts are related, they are not synonymous.
Capacity is a clinical term, whereas *competency* is a legal term and can be
determined only by a judge in a court setting, albeit with information provided
by professionals familiar with a person's mental status and ability to conduct
his or her affairs with safety and independence. As a general rule of thumb,
persons are presumed to be competent to do any legal act—sign advance directives, make contracts, marry, vote, bring suit in court, retain and dismiss
health professionals—unless or until a judge determines otherwise. Decision-
making capacity, however, refers to a person's present ability to make healthcare treatment choices. In many states, it is the patient's attending physician
who is obligated to assess decision-making capacity as part of advance directive
law dealing with informed consent. Even a person who has been adjudicated
incompetent by a court may still have the capacity to make fully informed and
voluntary choices about proposed health care. It is crucial for physicians not to
confuse these concepts. Doing so may wrongly deny patients important civil liberties, including the right to complete and have honored a valid healthcare
proxy, as well as subject the physician and the physician's institution to liability. One of the better discussions of competency and capacity is found in a
report "Ten Myths about Decision-Making Capacity" issued by the National
Ethics Committee of the Veterans Health Administration in 2002.[55]

Organizational Will

Healthcare facilities, the target entities of all PSDA requirements, have
fallen short in two ways. First, the overwhelming majority have either failed
to develop a meaningful community education program or have let the program lapse. In the past 10 years, I have not seen one newspaper article or
news story on the topic; not one notice of an advance directive informational
program held at a local library, community hall, or senior center; not a single
promotional piece in my health plan newsletter. The PSDA requires public
education, as does JCAHO (see the section on "Public Education"). It is time
someone offered a prize for the most creative and effective program. With no
federal enforcement of the provision, it may be the last, best incentive.

However, before the towel is thrown in, it must be said that several programs have proven successful in reaching the public and increasing the skills
of clinicians. "Respecting Choices" is a thoughtfully designed and robust program of the Gunderson Lutheran Health System based in Wisconsin. Using a
train-the-trainer model, the advance directive promotion includes pre- and
postprogram evaluations; clinical staff, patient, and community education;
patient follow-up; and engaging task-oriented materials. Completion rates in
communities adopting the program have risen to 80 to 90 percent from the
standard 15 to 20 percent.[56]

EPEC, an acronym for Education in Palliative and End-of-Life Care (and formerly, Education of Physicians in End-of-Life Care), is a rigorous professional training program for physicians and other clinicians in all aspects of palliative and terminal care. The comprehensive program addresses disparate aspects of the field, including legal issues, pain management, communicating "bad news," futility and conflict resolution, depression, and other topics.[57]

The Institute for Healthcare Communication, based in New Haven, Connecticut, specializes in helping clinicians work more effectively with patients by enhancing their communication skills around many traditionally difficult issues. "Care, Not Cure" and "Conversations at the End of Life" are superb continuing medical education programs that can be presented by trained Institute faculty at any organization nationwide. Other programs help clinicians work with "difficult" patients, move creatively beyond the informed consent form to mutual decision making, work better with patients who must make behavior changes as part of a treatment regimen, and disclose unanticipated outcomes and medical errors. It is important to note that all programs of the Institute are intensive and interactive skill-building workshops, not lectures.[58]

Second, some organizations have taken the letter of the PSDA too literally. Where the PSDA calls for organizations to provide written information on advance directives and their state's healthcare decision-making rights, that might be the upper limit of materials provided. Many facilities confuse the Medicare Statement of Patient's Rights with the PSDA requirement of providing information about their individual state law (statutes and cases) regarding informed consent, advance directives, and related topics of decision making. In the initial rush to PSDA implementation, some institutions never received copies of the state-specific rights as required by the law. Or if they did, the content was reduced to statements so overly simplistic as to be unhelpful. For example, "You have the right to give your consent to treatment as allowed by law and to fill out an advance directive." No available forms. No trained staff with time available to give information to people with limited reading proficiency. No interpreters to speak with patients or their families in their own language. Hopefully, internal or external licensing or quality assurance mechanisms will ultimately raise the standards for these organizations.

The Public

It is the healthcare consuming public, however, that poses the greatest challenge to PSDA advocates and promoters. The U.S. healthcare system is based largely on autonomy—the capacity of people to be self-directed in life's goals and activities. Indeed, it is at the core of our notion of informed consent that underlies the entire advance directive movement. Autonomy, as a principle, is responsible for much of the conversation between doctors and patients. Choice and personal autonomy are so firmly rooted in our contemporary culture that it is difficult to imagine that many people just do not value them highly. In our hospitals and nursing homes, home care services and clinics, it is the individual who has the right—arguably, the obligation—to choose among options for a preferred treatment.

For many people, in many families and cultures, that is simply not how important decisions are made. People have differing ideas, such as:

"Grandfather will decide."

"Mother and father will choose for me."

"I couldn't make that choice—the decision's not mine to make."

"If I signed that myself, my family would disown me."

"How mean spirited can you be? If you tell our mother that she's dying, she'll lose hope. We'll take her out of this hospital and take her somewhere where the doctors respect us."

"What do you mean 'plan ahead for dying'? We don't talk about things like this in our family. If we talk about them, they will happen. Do you want someone in our family to die?"

With the U.S. immigrant population growing quickly, it is essential that clinicians develop effective "workaround" strategies so that the idiosyncrasies of the patient's culture and familial decision-making process are respected, while at the same time fulfilling the legal obligations of informed consent. Many good resources are available, both in hard copy and online, to help clinicians learn more about how people from many non-Western cultures generally view the clinician-patient relationship, the value of maintaining good health through prevention, and the sources of illness and wellness.[59] Many organizations have taken proactive steps to assure that trained medical interpreters are available for any clinical encounter. For smaller organizations, or in cases where small populations of non-English speakers make it unfeasible to have an interpreter for that language on staff, there are several commercial organizations that specialize in telephone-based language services.[60] Although some administrators might view providing interpreter services as an unnecessary luxury, it is, in fact, a necessary element of legal informed consent. Most state informed consent laws require physicians to provide patients or their surrogates information about recommended treatments *in language they can understand.* That does not mean simply explaining information to patients in nontechnical language, it also means providing it in their spoken language of comprehension. It is a significant breach of confidentiality, as well as practically ineffective, to have a patient's family member intercede as an interpreter.

The PSDA has been a significant milestone in the movement to safeguard patients' rights and to encourage more frequent conversations about one's preferences for health care in the event of future incapacity or terminal illness. At the outset, proponents knew that the PSDA's effect on the healthcare system would be limited because the identified targets of the act were limited: healthcare organizations and institutions that participated in Medicare and Medicaid. At a practical level, it would have been impossible to include mandates that applied to those healthcare institutions and professionals who are arguably much better positioned to be effective advocates of advance directives. A short list of people and organizations that could "get the word out" more effectively and efficiently would include internal and family medicine physicians in private and group practices, nurses, physician assistants and nurse practitioners, case managers, physical and occupational therapists, and the many thousands of outpatient and ambulatory care centers nationwide. And in fact, there seems to be steady progress in this direction. Although these organizations and people are not required under the PSDA to do anything, many are taking up the cause. Why? Because patients ask for information, and because many professionals find that a brief conversation about substitute decision making is a useful way to learn more about their patients and families and to engage with their patients with empathy and understanding. Comprehensive training programs continue to be developed and refined. Innovative community promotion programs and materials have appeared recently. Some organizations have been creatively reaching out to minority populations for whom the notions of advance directives, advance care planning, and personal choices are uncommon.

In these respects, the PSDA and its requirements have exceeded all expectations by becoming an informal standard of care—the "right thing to do" as the TV ad says. It is hoped that this trend toward universal acceptance and promotion, without legislative mandates or punitive enforcement, continues well into the future.

SUMMARY

This chapter provides a detailed overview of the reasons for the enactment of the PSDA and how it has been implemented in medical practice with varying degrees of success. It details key features of this important act including its implementation for emergency, psychiatric, and general hospital admissions. The JCAHO clarifications on advanced directives are also presented. Finally, the chapter makes the case that much more can be done to educate both healthcare professionals and the public about the choice to have advanced directives.

QUESTIONS FOR DISCUSSION

1. Why do only 15 to 20 percent of patients have advance directives?
2. What are healthcare organizations' ethical responsibilities with respect to the PSDA?
3. What is needed for healthcare professionals to be advocates of the PSDA?
4. How do you think the Schiavo case impacted surrogate consent laws and public attitude toward the PSDA?
5. Why would an ethics-based professional support the PSDA?

NOTES

1. L. Kutner, "Due Process of Euthanasia: The Living Will, A Proposal," *Indiana Law Journal* 44 (1969): 537-554; Omnibus Budget Reconciliation Act of 1990, Sections 4206 and 4751, Public Law 101-508, signed by President George H. W. Bush on November 5, 1990, and effective December 1, 1991.

2. However, as of June 1992, 30 states had passed "family consent" statutes that give a priority by which certain family members (e.g., one's spouse, adult children, etc.) are authorized to act for the incapacitated person. Only four states—Arizona, Florida, Illinois, and New York—include "close friend" in the list of permissible surrogates. Traditional guardianships and protective service proceedings are available, although courts are reluctant to become involved in large numbers of healthcare decisions. For a complete listing, see C. P. Sabatino, "Surrogate Decision Making in Health Care," in *Health Care Decision-Making in the 1990s: The Surrogate and Advance Directives at the Bedside* (Chicago: American Bar Association Section of Real Property, Probate and Trust Law, 1992). For full discussion of the issues, see New York State Task Force on Life and the Law, *When Others Must Choose: Deciding for Patients Without Capacity*, 1992: 304. Order from Health Education Services, PO Box 7126, Albany, NY 12224.

3. *Choice in Dying, Refusal of Treatment Legislation: A State by State Compilation of Enacted and Model Statutes* (New York: Choice in Dying, 1991; with annual updates).

4. See, for example, the draft "Health-Care Decisions Act" proposed by the National Conference of Commissioners on Uniform State Laws, 676 North St. Clair Street, Suite 1700, Chicago, IL 60611. See also T. A. Eaton and E. J. Larson, "Experimenting with the 'Right to Die' in the Laboratory of the States," *Georgia Law Review* 25 (1991): 1253–1326.

5. In "the battle of the forms," a number of articles have appeared in which authors not only urge the use of a particular kind of advance directive over another, but also question the effectiveness of the PSDA in achieving its goals by means of promoting advance directives. For a sampling, see G. J. Annas, "The Health Care Proxy and the Living Will," *New England Journal of Medicine* 324 (1991): 1210–1213; A. S. Brett, "Limitations of Listing Specific Medical Interventions in Advance Directives," *Journal of the American Medical Association* 226 (1991): 825-828; L. Emanuel and E. Emanuel, "The Medical Directive: A New Comprehensive Advance Care Document," *Journal of the American Medical Association* 261 (1989): 3288–3293; R. S. Olick, "Approximating Informed Consent and Fostering Communication," *Journal of Clinical Ethics* 2, no. 3 (1991): 181–195.

6. S. M. Wolf et al., "Sources of Concern about the Patient Self-Determination Act," *New England Journal of Medicine* 325 (1991): 1666–1671.

7. J. Lynn and J. Teno, "After the Patient Self-Determination Act: The Need for Empirical Research on Formal Advance Directives," *Hastings Center Report* 23, no. 1 (1991): 20–24.

8. M. M. Handelsman, "Federal Policy Regarding End of Life Decisions," in *Euthanasia: The Good of the Patient, the Good of Society*, R. Misbin, ed., (Frederick, MD: University Publishing Group, 1992).

9. Ibid.

10. Department of Health and Human Services, Health Care Financing Administration, Medicare and Medicaid Programs, Advance Directives, 42CFR Parts 417, 431, 434, 484, 489, 498.

11. The "clear and convincing" standard adopted by Missouri and New York has prompted concern that relatives or caregivers of persons in persistent vegetative states might never be able to have treatment withdrawn, no matter how futile the present or proposed treatment.

12. *Cruzan v. Director, Missouri Department of Health*, 110 S.Ct. 2841 (1990), concurring opinion.

13. J. M. Teno et al., (Center for Evaluative Clinical Science, Dartmouth Medical School; and American Bar Association, Commission on the Legal Problems of the Elderly), *Evaluation of the Impact of the Patient Self-Determination Act: State Response to Write Description of State Law*, presented at Choices and Conversations (National PSDA conference sponsored by the

Pacific Center for Health Policy and Ethics, University of Southern California Law Center, Pasadena, Calif., January 8–9, 1993).

14. M. R. Gasner, "The PSDA: A Next Logical Step," *Journal of Clinical Ethics* 2, no. 3 (1991): 173–177.

15. See, for example, *American Association of Homes for the Aging, Patient Self-Determination Act of 1990: Implementation Issues* (Washington, D.C.: American Association of Homes for the Aging, 1991); California Consortium on Patient Self-Determination, *The PSDA Handbook*, hospital edition (Los Angeles: Pacific Center for Health Policy and Ethics, University of Southern California Law Center, 1991); J. F. Monagle and D. C. Thomasma, *Medical Ethics: Policies, Protocols, Guidelines and Programs* (Gaithersburg, MD: Aspen Publishers, 1992).

16. R. Jackson and A. Carlos, "Getting Ready for the PSDA: What Are Hospitals and Nursing Homes Doing?" *Journal of Clinical Ethics* 2, no. 3 (1991): 177–181.

17. Gasner, op. cit.

18. C. P. Sabatino, "Surely the Wizard Will Help Us, Toto? Implementing the Patient Self-Determination Act," *Hastings Center Report* 23, no. 1 (1993): 12–16.

19. Massachusetts Health Care Proxy Task Force, Consensus Report (Sharon, MA: Massachusetts Health Decisions, 1992).

20. Department of Health and Human Services, Health Care Financing Administration, Medicare and Medicaid Programs, Advance Directives, 42CFR Parts 417, 431, 434, 484, 489, 498.

21. Examples of programs designed to recognize pre-admission DNR orders include Connecticut (Emergency Medical Services), Virginia (EMS-initiated legislation), North Carolina (county-by-county adoption of EMS guidelines), California (EMS; guidelines adopted county by county; legislation introduced), New York (State Department of Health; 1992 legislation), and Montana (legislation). Also, MedicAlert® (2323 Colorado Avenue, Turlock, CA 05380) has initiated a national pre-admission DNR project.

22. For a model policy for implementing living wills and medical durable powers of attorney for the Virginia Department of Mental Health, Mental Retardation and Substance Abuse Services, see K. H. Swisher, "Implementing the PSDA for Psychiatric Patients: A Commonsense Approach," *Journal of Clinical Ethics* 2, no. 3 (1991): 199-205. See also New York Task Force on Life and the Law, *When Others Must Choose: Deciding for Patients without Capacity* (New York: New York Task Force on Life and the Law, 1992; order from Health Education Services, P.O. Box 7126, Albany, NY 12224). On the nature of competency in general, see especially B. Chell, "Competency: What It Is, What It Isn't, and Why It Matters," in *Medical Ethics: A Guide for Health Professionals*, J. Monagle and D. Thomasma, eds. (Gaithersburg, MD: Aspen Publishers, 1988).

23. M. Z. Solomon et al., "Decisions Near the End of Life: Professional Views on Life-Sustaining Treatment," *American Journal of Public Health* 83, no. 1 (1993): 14–23.

24. In my experience, three of the best are G. J. Annas, *The Rights of Patients: The Basic ACLU Guide to Patient Rights*, 2d ed. (Carbondale, IL: Southern Illinois University Press, 1989); N. Dubler and D. Nimmons, *Ethics on Call* (New York: Harmony Books/Crown Publishers, 1992); and T. Scully and C. Scully, *Making Medical Decisions* (New York: Fireside Books/Simon & Schuster, 1989).

25. P. Lambert et al., "The Values History: An Innovation in Surrogate Medical Decision-Making," *Law, Medicine and Health Care* 18 (1990): 202–212. The values history is published without copyright and may be reproduced and adapted as necessary.

26. See, for example, B. Mishkin, *A Matter of Choice: Planning Ahead for Health Care Decisions* (Washington D.C.: American Association of Retired Persons, 1986); American Hospital Association, *Put It in Writing: A Guide to Promoting Advance Directives* (Chicago: American Hospital Association, 1991).

27. T. C. Davis et al., "The Gap between Patient Reading Comprehension and the Readability of Patient Education Materials," *Journal of Family Practice* 31 (1990): 533-538; J. Klessig, "The Effect of Values and Culture on Life-Support Decisions," *Western Journal of Medicine* 157 (1992): 316–322.

28. SUPPORT Principal Investigators. "A Controlled Trial to Improve Care for Seriously Ill Hospitalized Patients: The Study to Understand Prognoses and Preferences for Outcomes and Risks of Treatments (SUPPORT)." *JAMA* 274, no. 20 (Nov. 22/29, 1995): 1591–1598.

29. United States Department of Health and Human Services, Health Care Financing Administration, 42 CFR Parts 417, 430, 431, 434, 483, 484, 489. Medicare and Medicaid Programs—Advance Directives (Patient Self-Determination Act, Final Rule). Federal Register 60 (June 27, 1995): 33262–33292.

30. Ibid., 33265.

31. Ibid., 33277.

32. Ibid., 33278.

33. Ibid., 33265.

34. Ibid., 33279.

35. Ibid., 33274.

36. Ibid., 33266.

37. Ibid., 33274.

38. Ibid.

39. Ibid., 33275.

40. Ibid., 33290.

41. Ibid., 33277.

42. Ibid., 33280.

43. Ibid., 33285.

44. *Gilgunn v. Massachusetts General Hospital, et al.*, Suffolk (Mass.) Superior Court, 92–4820, April 1995.

45. See, for example, *ECHO (Extreme Care, Humane Options): Community Recommendations for Appropriate, Humane Medical Care for Dying or Irreversibly Ill Patients*, (Sacramento, CA: Sacramento Healthcare Decisions, 1997). Similar projects have been carried out in Denver and other urban areas.

46. *Elbaum v. Grace Plaza of Great Neck, Inc.*, 148 AD2nd 244, 544 NYS2nd 840 (2d Dept 1989).

47. "Ignoring 'Right to Die' Directives, Medical Community Is Being Sued," *New York Times*, June 2, 1996.

48. *Anderson v. St. Francis–St. George Hospital, Inc.*, No. 95–869 (Ohio, Oct. 10, 1996), as reported by Choice in Dying, New York.

49. *Cruzan v. Director, Missouri Department of Health*, 497 US 261 (1990).

50. E. J. Emanuel et al., "How Well is the Patient Self-Determination Act Working?: An Early Assessment," *American Journal of Medicine* 95, no. 6 (Dec. 1993): 619–628.

51. The State of Oregon maintains a section of its official Web site devoted to the Death with Dignity Act. The site includes the entire text of the law, a comprehensive section on frequently-asked questions, and complete copies of all Annual Reports to date. See: www.oregon .gov/DHS/ph/pas.

52. The Bioethics Programs at the University of Miami has maintained a timeline of the events in the life and case of Terri Schiavo. Visitors to the site can use hotlinks to view legal filings and rulings of the court, reports by various court-appointed guardians ad litem, and a copy of the autopsy report.

53. *Cruzan v. Director, Missouri Department of Health*, 110 S.Ct. 2841.

54. The National Conference of Commissioners on Uniform State Laws (NCCUSL) is a nonprofit organization that has for more than 100 years provided states with nonpartisan, well-conceived, and well-drafted legislation that brings clarity and stability to critical areas of the law. NCCUSL's work supports the federal system and facilitates the movement of individuals and the business of organizations with rules that are consistent from state to state. The Uniform Health-Care Decisions Act was proposed as a advance directive law that could be adopted by all states, thereby avoiding the significant differences that now exist among the

many state laws. The entire text of the law can be found on the NCCUSL site. See: www.nccusl.org. Click on "Final Acts & Legislation,," then choose "Health-Care Decisions Act" from the pull-down search menu.

55. See www.ethics.va.gov/ETHICS/docs/necrpts/NEC_Report_20020201_Ten_Myths_about_ DMC.pdf.

56. Gunderson Lutheran Health System, "Respecting Choices." See www.gundluth.org/web/ ptcare/eolprograms.nsf.

57. EPEC Project: Education in Palliative and End-of-Life Care (formerly Education of Physicians in End-of-Life Care). See www.epec.net/EPEC/webpages/index.cfm.

58. Institute for Healthcare Communication. "Care Not Cure: Dialogues at the Transition" and "Conversations at the End of Life." See www.healthcarecomm.org. Under "Courses," choose "Continuing Education Workshops."

59. "CultureMed: A resource center of print materials promoting culturally competent health care for refugees and immigrants." State University of New York, Institute of Technology, Utica, New York. See: http://culturedmed.sunyit.edu.

60. Certainly the oldest and most well-known of these is Language Line, originally a service of AT&T. Over-the-phone interpretation is available 24/7 in 170 languages and dialects. Translation services for written information is also available. See www.languageline.com.

ADDITIONAL RESOURCES

American Bar Association, Commission on Law and Aging. *Consumer's Tool Kit for Health Care Advance Planning*, 2nd ed., 2005. 26pp. See www.abanet.org/aging/publications/docs/consumer_ tool_kit_bk.pdf.

____. "Making Medical Decisions for Someone Else: A Maryland Handbook." 2006, 23pp. See www.abanet.org/aging/publications/docs/proxy_guide_long_final_2.pdf.

____. "Surrogate Consent in the Absence of an Advance Directive." (Chart of surrogate consent laws, by state, as of July 1, 2004, available as PDF or Microsoft Word document.) See www.abanet.org; in search box, enter "surrogate consent," with or without quotes.

American Bar Association, Commission on Law and Aging; American Psychological Association; National College of Probate Judges. "Judicial Determination of Capacity of Older Adults in Guardianship Proceedings." 2006, 93pp. See www.abanet.org/aging/docs/judges_book_ 5-24.pdf.

American Health Decisions. "The Quest to Die with Dignity: An Analysis of Americans' Values, Opinions and Attitudes Concerning End-of-Life Care." B. A. Tyler et al., research team. 1997. Contact: Beverly A. Tyler, Executive Director, Georgia Health Decisions, 14 Marietta Street, Ste 127, Atlanta, GA 30303.

P. S. Appelbaum, "Commentary: Psychiatric Advance Directives at a Crossroads—When Can PADs Be Overridden?" *Journal of the American Academy of Psychiatry and the Law*. 34, no.3 (2006): 395-397. See www.jaapl.org/cgi/reprint/34/3/395.

M. E. Baker, "Cultural Differences in the Use of Advance Directives: A Review of the Literature." *African American Research Perspectives* 6, no. 3 (Fall 2000): 35–40. See http://rcgd .isr.umich.edu/prba/perspectives/fall2000/mbaker.pdf

C. Barnette, "Advance Directives: Implementing a Program that Works." *Nursing Management* (October 1994): 58–56.

Bazelon Center for Mental Health Law. "Advance Psychiatric Directives." See www.bazelon.org/ issues/advancedirectives/index.htm.

J. T. Berger, "Patients' Interests in their Family Members' Well-Being: An Overlooked, Fundamental Consideration within Substituted Judgments." *Journal of Clinical Ethics* 16, no. 1 (Spring 2005): 3–10.

J. M. Breslin, "Autonomy and the Role of the Family in Making Decisions at the End of Life." *Journal of Clinical Ethics* 16, no.1 (Spring 2005): 11–19.

A. S. Brett, "Limitations of Listing Specific Medical Interventions in Advance Directives." *JAMA* 266 (1991): 825–828.

L. L. Brunetti, et al., "Physicians' Attitudes Toward Living Wills and Cardiopulmonary Resuscitation." *Journal of General Internal Medicine* 6 (1991): 323–329.

A. E. Buchanan and D. W. Brock, *Deciding for Others: The Ethics of Surrogate Decision-Making.* New York: Cambridge University Press, 1990.

L. L. Emanuel, et al., "Advance Care Planning as a Process: Structuring the Discussions in Practice." *Journal of the American Geriatrics Society* 43 (1995): 440–446.

____. "Advance Directives: Stability of Patients' Treatment Choices." *Archives of Internal Medicine* 154 (January 24, 1994): 209–217.

A. Fagerlin, and C. E. Schneider, "Enough: The Failure of the Living Will." *Hastings Center Report* 34, no. 2 (March-April 2004): 30–42.

"Five Wishes." See www.agingwithdignity.org/5wishes.html.

L. Ganzini and S. K. Dobscha, "Clarifying Distinctions between Contemplating and Completing Physician-Assisted Suicide." *Journal of Clinical Ethics* 115 no.2 (Summer 2004): 119–122.

Hastings Center, "Advance Care Planning: Priorities for Ethical and Empirical Research" (Special Supplement). *Hastings Center Report* (Nov.-Dec. 1994): 1–36.

____. "Dying Well in the Hospital: Lessons of SUPPORT (Special Supplement)." *Hastings Center Report* (Nov.–Dec. 1995): S1–S34.

D. Hoffmann, et al., "The Dangers of Directives or the False Security of Forms." *Journal of Law, Medicine & Ethics* 24, no. 1 (Spring 1996): 5–17.

E. G. Howe, "Patients May Benefit from Postponing Assessment of Mental Capacity." *Journal of Clinical Ethics* 17, no. 2 (Summer 2006): 99–109.

B. Jennings, et al. (Eds.), "Improving End of Life Care: Why Has It Been So Difficult?" *Hastings Center Report Special Report* 35, no. 6 (2005).

R. C. Kolarik, R. M. Arnold, et al., "Advance Care Planning: A Comparison of Values Statements and Treatment Preferences." *Journal of General Internal Medicine* 17, no. 8 (August 2002): 618–624. See www.pubmedcentral.nih.gov/articlerender.fcgi?artid=1495096.

E. J. Larson and T. A. Eaton, "The Limits of Advance Directives: A History and Assessment of the Patient Self-Determination Act." *Wake Forest Law Review* 32 (1997): 249–293.

E. Loewy and R. Carlson, "Talking, Advance Directives, and Medical Practice." *Archives of Internal Medicine* (Oct. 24, 1994): 2265–2267.

T. R. Malloy, et al., "The Influence of Treatment Descriptions on Advance Medical Directives." *Journal of the American Geriatrics Society* 40 (1992): 1255–1260.

L. Markson, et al., "Implementing Advance Directives in the Primary Care Setting." *Archives of Internal Medicine* (Oct. 24, 1994): 2321–2328.

S. V. McCrary, "Physicians' Legal Defensiveness in End-of-Life Treatment Decisions: Comparing Attitudes and Knowledge in States with Different Laws." *Journal of Clinical Ethics* 17, no. 1 (Spring 2006): 15–26.

K. M. McIntyre, "On Advancing Advance Directives: Why Should We Believe the Promise (Editorial)." *Archives of Internal Medicine* 155 (Nov. 27, 1995): 2271–2273.

A. Meisel, "Legal Myths about Terminating Life Support." *Archives of Internal Medicine* 151 (1991): 1497–1502.

J. A. Menikoff, et al., "Beyond Advance Directives: Health Care Surrogate Laws." *New England Journal of Medicine* 327 (1992): 1165–1169.

R. S. Morrison, et al., "The Inaccessibility of Advance Directives on Transfer from Ambulatory to Acute Care Settings." *Journal of the American Medical Association* 274, no. 6 (Aug. 9, 1995): 478–482.

____. "Physician Reluctance to Discuss Advance Directives: An Empiric Investigation of Potential Barriers." *Archives of Internal Medicine* (Oct. 24, 1994): 2311–2318.

E. H. Moskowitz and J. L. Nelson (eds.), "Dying Well in the Hospital: The Lessons of SUPPORT." *Special Supplement, Hastings Center Report* 25, no. 6 (1995).

National Reference Center for Bioethics Literature (at Georgetown University, Kennedy Center of Ethics). See www.georgetown.edu/research/nrcbl/nrc/index.htm.

National Resource Center on Psychiatric Advance Directives. See www.nrc-pad.org/index.php.

D. Neumark, "Providing Information about Advance Directives to Patients in Ambulatory Care and Their Families." *ONF* (April 1994): 771–775.

New York State Task Force on Life and the Law, *Life-Sustaining Treatment: Making Decisions and Appointing a Health Care Agent.* New York: New York State Task Force on Life and the Law, 1987.

____. *When Others Must Choose: Deciding for Patients Without Capacity.* New York: New York State Task Force on Life and the Law, 1992.

K. Oleson, et al., "A Quality Improvement Focus for Patient Rights: Advance Directives." *Journal of Nursing Care Quality* (April 1994): 52–67.

Oregon Department of Human Services, "Death with Dignity Act Annual Reports." Annual state reports on physician-assisted suicide law, 1999–2006. See http://egov.oregon.gov/DHS/ph/pas/ar-index.shtml.

D. Orentlicher, "The Illusion of Patient Choice in End-of-Life Decisions." *JAMA* 267 (1992): 2101–2104.

____. *Making Health Care Decisions: The Ethical and Legal Implications of Informed Consent in the Patient-Practitioner Relationship.* Washington, DC: U.S. Government Printing Office, 1982.

President's Commission for the Study of Ethical Problems in Medicine and Biomedical and Behavioral Research, *Deciding to Forgo Life-Sustaining Treatment: Ethical, Medical and Legal Issues in Treatment Decisions.* Washington, DC: U.S. Government Printing Office, 1983.

T. E. Quill, "Initiating End-of-Life Discussions with Seriously Ill Patients: Addressing the 'Elephant in the Room.'" *Journal of the American Medical Association* 284, no. 19 (2000): 2502–2507.

B. Reilly, et al., "Promoting Inpatient Directives about Life-Sustaining Treatments in a Community Hospital." *Archives of Internal Medicine* 155 (Nov. 27, 1995): 2317–2323.

B. Reilly, et al., "Can We Talk? Inpatient Discussions about Advance Directives in a Community Hospital: Attending Physicians' Attitudes, Their Inpatients' Wishes, and Reported Experience." *Archives of Internal Medicine* 154 (Oct. 24, 1994): 2299–2308.

S. W. Salmond and E. David, "Attitudes Toward Advance Directives and Advance Directive Completion Rates." *Orthopaedic Nursing* 24, no. 2 (March-April 2005): 117–127.

R. Schouten, "Commentary: Psychiatric Advance Directives as Tools for Enhancing Treatment of the Mentally Ill." *Journal of the American Academy of Psychiatry and the Law* 34, no. 1 (2006) 58-60. See www.jaapl.org/cgi/reprint/34/1/58.pdf.

A. B. Seckler, et al., "Substituted Judgment: How Accurate are Proxy Predictions?" *Annals of Internal Medicine* 115 (1991): 92–98.

M. J. Silveira, et al., "Deciding How to Decide: What Processes Do Patients Use When Making Medical Decisions?" *Journal of Clinical Ethics* 15, no. 4 (Fall 2004): 269–281.

W. Smucker, et al., "Elderly Outpatients Respond Favorably to a Physician-Initiated Advance Directive Discussion." *Journal of American Board of Family Practitioners* (Sept.–Oct. 1993): 473–482.

J. Sugarman, et al., "Catalysts for Conversations about Advance Directives: The Influence of Physician and Patient Characteristics." *The Journal of Law, Medicine, & Ethics* (Spring 1994): 29–35.

D. P. Sulmasy, et al., "More Talk, Less Paper: Predicting the Accuracy of Substituted Judgment." *American Journal of Medicine* 96 (1994): 432–438.

S. W. Tolle, et al., "Characteristics and Proportion of Dying Oregonians Who Personally Consider Physician-Assisted Suicide." *Journal of Clinical Ethics* 115, no. 2 (Summer 2004): 111–118.

R. F. Uhlmann, et al., "Physicians' and Spouses' Prediction of Elderly Patients' Resuscitation Preferences." *Journal of Gerontology* 43 (1988): M115–M121.

United States Department of Health and Human Services, *Omnibus Budget Reconciliation Act of 1990, Sections 4206 and 4751*, Public Law 101–508 (Patient Self-Determination Act).

____. Health Care Financing Administration, 42 CFR 417, 431, 434, 483, 484, 489, and 498, Medicare and Medicaid Programs—Advance Directives (Patient Self-Determination Act, Interim Final Rule). Federal Register 57 (March 6, 1992): 8194–204.

____. Health Care Financing Administration, 42 CFR Parts 417, 430, 431, 434, 483, 484, 489. Medicare and Medicaid Programs-Advance Directives (Patient Self-Determination Act, Final Rule). Federal Register 60 (June 27, 1995): 33262–92.

United States Department of Health and Human Services, Office of Civil Rights. "Does the HIPAA Privacy Rule Change How a Person Can Grant a Health Care Power of Attorney?" See http://hhs.gov/ocr/hipaa. Under "Educational Materials," click "Your frequently asked questions on privacy," then enter the search text term "health care power of attorney," with or without quotes.

University of Miami, Ethics Program, "Schiavo Case Resources: Selected Bibliography." See www6 .miami.edu/ethics2/schiavo/terri_schiavo_bibliography.html.

____. "Schiavo Case Resources: Key Events in the Case of Theresa Marie Schiavo." See www6 .miami.edu/ethics/schiavo/timeline.htm.

J. Virmani, "Relationship of Advance Directives to Physician-Patient Communication." *Archives of Internal Medicine* 154 (April 25, 1994): 909–913.

S. H. Wanzer, et al., "The Physician's Responsibility Toward Hopelessly Ill Patients." *New England Journal of Medicine* 310 (1984): 955–959.

____. "The Physician's Responsibility Toward Hopelessly Ill Patients: A Second Look." *New England Journal of Medicine* 320 (1989): 844–849.

N. R. Zweibel and C. K. Cassel, "Treatment Choices at the End of Life: A Comparison of Decisions by Older Patients and Their Physician-Selected Proxies." *Gerontologist* 29 (1989): 615–621.

CHAPTER 9

Older People and Long-Term Care: Issues of Access

*Jan Gardner-Ray**

OVERVIEW

This chapter presents a historical view of issues of access in long-term care; unfortunately, this situation has not improved. Gardner-Ray, an executive in the long-term care industry, reviewed Binstock's original article and supports his premises. The issue of access to long-term care promises to be even more critical given the imminent influx of the baby boomers and their potential need for elder care. The ethical issues posed by both Binstock and Gardner-Ray are certainly not limited to the past, but will challenge our thinking for years to come. In fact, the issue of access to long-term care will loom large in the twenty-first century. Therefore, it is important to understand the issue's history and potential and begin to address its ethics.

INTRODUCTION

During the last decades of the twentieth century, there was increasing evidence of the public's interest in improving access to humane and appropriate long-term care services in the United States. Opinion polls indicated that a substantial majority of Americans—in all adult age groups—feared the financial, familial, psychological, and social consequences of dependence on long-term care. Most Americans favored the general principle of expanding government financing for such care as the principal means of increasing access to it.[1] A number of bills to provide new programs of public funding for long-term care were introduced in Congress in the late 1980s and early 1990s, with estimated annual price tags ranging up to $60 billion in the first year.

Why did long-term care begin to emerge from the dominant shadows cast in the healthcare arena by the more dramatic treatments and cures offered by acute-care medicine? One major element is the enormous growth of our older population, those aged 65 and over, which doubled from 16 million in 1960 to 32 million in 1990. Persons in this age category are presently 12.5 percent of our population and are expected to constitute 20 percent in the year 2030.[2]

Another element has been the growing constituency of adult children of elderly patients who are perceiving the importance of long-term care services because of their direct contact with providing or arranging for the care of their aged parents. Over 13 million adults in the United States who have disabled elderly parents or spouses are potential providers of long-term care, financial assistance, and emotional support; 4.2 million of them provide direct care in

---

*Revised from R. H. Binstock, "Older People and Long-Term Care: Issues of Access," in *Health Care Ethics: Critical Issues for the 21st Century*, Original ed., 1998, edited by John. F. Monagle and David C. Thomasma. Sudbury, MA: Jones and Bartlett, 2005.

home settings.[3] Disabled children, younger disabled adults, and their families, respectively, are additional potential constituencies to the support of greater access to long-term care.

Despite the underlying needs and hopes of these constituencies, enactment of a government program to expand access to long-term care in the immediate future is problematic because of the substantial funds that would be required. Achieving a "balanced budget" is a rhetorical mainstay of contemporary national politics, and containing government expenditures on healthcare costs is one of the major means for balancing the federal and state budgets.

The challenges of ensuring adequate access to long-term care for all who need it are substantial. The number of Americans requiring some form of long-term care is already large and will grow significantly over the next few decades. Financing such care is already very difficult for individuals, their families, and governments. Yet, indications are that the prices for services and their aggregate national costs will continue to escalate, while the role of governments in paying for care of an expanded disabled population could be curtailed.

This chapter focuses on issues of access for older people, although it also considers the need for long-term care for younger disabled persons and the political role they might play in improving access for persons of all ages. First, an overview of the growing population that needs long-term care is provided. Second, issues of access to care are discussed. Third, the chapter briefly recounts how proposals to expand public funding for long-term care rose to the national policy agenda in the early 1990s and then abruptly fell from it. Finally, the chapter presents the political and moral prospects for improving access in the years ahead.

THE GROWING POPULATION NEEDING CARE

In 1994, the U.S. General Accounting Office reported that more than 12 million Americans required long-term care. *Long-term care need* is defined as people who are functionally dependent on a long-term basis due to physical and/or mental limitations. Two broad categories of functional limitations are widely used by clinicians to assess need for care. One category is dependence in basic *activities of daily living* (ADLs)—getting in and out of bed, toileting, bathing, dressing, and eating. (Persons who have cognitive impairment, who need cueing from someone else to be able to perform their own ADLs, are called *ADL dependent*.) The other category is limitations in *instrumental activities of daily living* (IADLs)—taking medications, preparing meals, managing finances, doing light housework and other chores, being able to get in and out of the home, using the telephone, and so on. (Professionals use other criteria to assess children and people with mental illness, such as the ability to attend school or problems in behavior.)

The range of services needed by those who have difficulties in carrying out their ADLs and IADLs, as well as those needed by their primary caregivers, is extensive. Table 9–1 presents a list of such services. Almost all of the services can be provided for individuals regardless of where they reside—at home, in a nursing home, or in residential settings, such as retirement communities, board-and-care facilities, adult-foster homes, assisted-living facilities, and various other forms of sheltered-housing arrangements.

Table 9–1 Services that May Be Needed for Disabled Individuals and Their Families

Acute medical care	Homemaker	Personal emergency
Adult day care	Hospice	response system
Audiology	Legal services	Physical therapy
Autopsy	Medication and elimination	Protective services
Chore services	of drugs that cause	Recreation/exercise
Dental care	excess disability	Respite care*
Diagnosis	Mental health services	Shopping
Escort service	Multidimensional	Skilled nursing
Family support groups	assessment	Special equipment (ramps,
Family/caregiver counseling	Nutritional counseling	hospital beds, etc.)
Family/caregiver education	Occupational therapy	Speech therapy
and training	Ongoing medical	Telephone reassurance
Financial/benefits	supervision	Transportation
counseling	Paid companion/sitter	Treatment of coexisting
Home health aide	Patient counseling	medical conditions
Home-delivered meals	Personal care	Vision care

*Respite care includes any service intended to provide temporary relief for the primary care giver. When used for that purpose, homemaker, paid companion/sitter, adult day care, temporary nursing home care, and other services included on this list constitute respite care.
Source: Adapted from Office of Technology Assessment. *Confused Minds, Burdened Families: Finding Help for People with Alzheimer's and Other Dementias* (Washington, DC: Office of Technology Assessment, 1990).

Popular perception is that most of the long-term care population is elderly and resides in nursing homes. However, this is not the case. In 1994, people aged 65 and older comprised but 55 percent of the long-term care population. Working-age adults accounted for 42 percent of the total, and children the remaining 3 percent. Moreover, only 22 percent of the elderly population needing long-term care, and 19 percent of the total disabled population, resided in nursing homes and other institutions. More recent data indicates that these percentages are changing partially due to the increase in alternatives in elder care.

Although it seems apparent that the number of people needing long-term care will grow substantially in the future, reasonably precise predictions regarding the size of that population and its composition are difficult to generate because of the many factors that are involved. New and improved medical treatments and technological developments could help to prevent, delay, and compensate for various types of functional difficulties. Moreover, health-related lifestyle changes and environmental protection measures could markedly reduce rates of disabling diseases and injuries. To the contrary, medical advances could increase the need for long-term care. Lower death rates from heart disease and stroke, for example, could mean that more people will live longer with disabling conditions and into the pathway of late-onset illnesses such as Alzheimer's disease. Similarly, improvements in dealing with the complications of acquired immune deficiency syndrome (AIDS) could engender longer periods of care for patients with this condition.

Demographic factors might also affect future needs for providing and financing long-term care at older ages. For instance, the cohorts reaching old age in the next several decades will be better educated than their predecessors. Higher levels of education are associated with lower levels of disability and need for care.[4] Yet, the ethnic composition of these same cohorts suggests that the need for care and governmental subsidies for financing it might be even greater in the future than it is today. From 1990 to 2050, the proportion of non-white Americans aged 65 and older will more than double from 9.8 percent to 21.3 percent. When they reach old age, these racial minorities might be highly dependent on public subsidies for their long-term care if present patterns of economic resource distribution among racial and ethnic groups persist throughout the first half of the twenty-first century. Among persons aged 65 and older who have the lowest household incomes, nearly 40 percent are racial minorities, and their aggregate net worth is less than one-third that of older white persons.[5]

Even though precise projections are difficult, it is clear that there will be enormous increases in the number of disabled older people in the twenty-first century. When much of the baby boom—a large cohort of 74 million Americans born between 1946 and 1964—reaches the ranks of old age in 2030, the absolute number of people aged 65 and older will have more than doubled from about 31 million in 1990 to about 65 million. Moreover, the numbers of persons in advanced old-age ranges will also more than double. Those aged 75 and older will grow from 13 million to 30 million between 1990 and 2030, and those aged 85 and older will increase from 3 million to 8 million.[6] Rates of disability increase markedly at these advanced ages. One reflection of this is in the present rates (1996) of nursing home use in different old-age categories. About 1 percent of Americans aged 65 to 74 years are in nursing homes; this compares with 6.1 percent of persons ages 75 to 84, and 24 percent of persons age 85 and older.[7] Similarly, disability rates increase in older old-age categories among persons who are not in nursing homes, from nearly 23 percent of those aged 65 to 74 who experience difficulty with ADLs to 45 percent of those aged 85 and older.[8]

The tremendous future growth expected in the older population suggests that there will be millions more disabled elderly people in the decades ahead. Whether rates of disability in old age will increase or decline in the future, however, is a matter on which experts disagree, depending on their assumptions and measures.[9] Assuming no changes in age-specific risks of disability, Cassel et al. [10] calculated a 31 percent increase between 1990 and 2010 in the number of persons aged 65 and older experiencing difficulty with ADLs. Using the same assumption, the Congressional Budget Office projected that the nursing home population will increase 50 percent between 1990 and 2010, double by 2030, and triple by 2050.[11] But even those researchers who report a decline in the prevalence of disability at older ages in recent years, emphasize that there will be large absolute increases in the number of older Americans needing long-term care in the decades ahead.[12]

Predicting whether long-term care needs among people under age 65 will increase or decline is more difficult. One of the principal reasons is that reliable databases for making projections are limited as compared with well-developed national and longitudinal sources available regarding the older population. Data collected on a state basis vary widely with respect to state rates for various types of disabilities.[13] Moreover, the numbers involved with respect to various disabling conditions—such as spinal cord injury, cerebral palsy, and mental retardation—are relatively small and much more suscepti-ble to changing conditions.

Yet, experts agree that the number of younger disabled persons has grown in recent years, and this trend might well persist.[14] New technologies and increased access to medical care continue to enable more people to survive injuries and other conditions that were heretofore fatal, and thereby live for many years with ADL limitations. For example, biomedical advances have enabled many more children with developmental disabilities, as well as low-birth-weight infants, to survive much longer than in the past and to extend the years in which they need long-term care.

ISSUES OF ACCESS

Whether a long-term care patient is in a nursing home, living at home, or in another type of residential setting, certain aspects of care are desired. An ideal system of services would be amply available, of high quality, provided by well-trained personnel, easily located and arranged, and readily accessible through private and/or public funding. The present system, however, is far from ideal.

The supply of services is insufficient; service providers lack education and training; and the quality of many services is poor.[15] Moreover, the system is so fragmented that even when high-quality services are sufficiently available, many patients and families do not know about them and require help in defin-ing their service needs and in arranging for them to be provided.[16]

Underlying each of these problems, in turn, is the issue of financing. As is the case with most aspects of the U.S. healthcare delivery system, the charac-teristics of long-term care services have been substantially shaped by the nature and extent of policies for funding it.

The Costs of Care

Aggregate expenditures for long-term care are sizable and very likely to increase in the decades immediately ahead. The total bill in 1995 was $106.5 billion; 73 percent was spent on nursing home care and 27 percent on home and community-based care.[17] Out-of-pocket payments by individuals and their families accounted for 32.5 percent of the total. Private insurance benefits pay for 5.5 percent. Other private funds account for 4.6 percent. Federal, state, and local governments financed the remaining 57.4 percent. Medicaid paid for 85 percent of nursing home care.

Paying the costs of long-term care out-of-pocket can be a catastrophic finan-cial experience for patients and their families. The annual cost of a year's care in a nursing home averages more than $46,000, but can cost well over $100,000.[18] Although the use of a limited number of services in a home or other community-based setting is less expensive, noninstitutional care for patients who would otherwise be appropriately placed in a nursing home is not cheaper.[19]

For a high percentage of older people, the prices of long-term care are simply unaffordable. Among persons aged 65 and older, 40 percent have a pretax income of less than 200 percent of the poverty threshold—under $14,618 for an individual and $18,440 for a married couple in which the man is aged 65 or older.[20]

The costs of care will undoubtedly grow in the future. Price increases in nursing home and home- and community-based care have consistently exceeded the general rate of inflation. Trends in long-term care labor and overhead costs indicate that this pattern will continue.

Dozens of governmental programs are sources of funding for long-term care services, including Medicaid, the Veterans' Administration, Social Security's Title XX for social services, and the Older Americans Act.[21] Yet, each source regulates the availability of funds with rules as to eligibility and breadth of service coverage and changes its rules frequently. Consequently, persons needing long-term care and their caregivers often find themselves ineligible for financial help from these programs and unable to pay out-of-pocket for needed services. In one study, about 75 percent of the informal, unpaid caregivers of dementia patients reported that the patients did not use formal, paid services because the patients were unable to pay for them.[22]

Recent data on Medicare and Medicaid spending affirms the trends mentioned here. In 2006, these programs cost over $3 billion per day to run. In light of the fact that the first of the baby boomers (77 million) become eligible for Medicaid in 2008, the cry for reform is becoming even louder. However, even the 2003 prescription-drug benefit has not slowed down the increase in costs. Challenges lay ahead.[23]

The Caregiving Role of Families

A number of research efforts have documented that about 80 percent of the long-term care provided to older persons outside of nursing homes is presently provided on an in-kind basis by family members—spouses, siblings, adult children, and broader kin networks. About 74 percent of dependent community-based older persons receive all their care from family members or other unpaid sources; about 21 percent receive both formal and informal services; and about 5 percent use just formal services.[24] The vast majority of family caregivers are women. [25] The family also plays an important role in obtaining and managing services from paid service providers.

The capacities and willingness of family members to care for disabled older persons may decline, however, because of a broad social trend. The family, as a fundamental unit of social organization, has been undergoing profound transformations that will become more fully manifest over the next few decades as baby boomers reach old age. The striking growth of single-parent households, the growing participation of women in the labor force, and the high incidence of divorce and remarriage (differentially higher for men) all entail complicated changes in the structure of household and kinship roles and relationships. There will be an increasing number of blended families, reflecting multiple lines of descent through multiple marriages and the birth of children outside of wedlock through other partners. This growth in the incidence of step- and half-relatives will make for a dramatic new turn in family structure in the coming decades. Already, such blended families constitute about half of all households with children.[26]

One possible implication of these changes is that kinship networks in the near future will become more complex, attenuated, and diffuse,[27] perhaps with a weakened sense of filial obligation. If changes in the intensity of kinship relations significantly erode the capacity and sense of obligation to care for older family members when the baby boom cohort is in the ranks of old age and disability, demands for governmental support to pay long-term care may increase accordingly.

The Role of Private Insurance

Private, long-term care insurance, a relatively new product, is very expensive for the majority of older persons, and its benefits are limited in scope and duration. The best-quality policies that provide substantial benefits over a reasonable period of time, charged premiums in 1991 that averaged $2,525 for persons aged 65 and $7,675 for those aged 79.[28] About four to five percent of older persons have any private long-term care insurance, and only about one percent of nursing home costs are paid by private insurance.[29] A number of analyses have suggested that even when the product becomes more refined, no more than 20 percent of older Americans will be able to afford private insurance.[30]

A variation on the private-insurance-policy approach to financing long-term care is continuing care retirement communities (CCRCs) that promise comprehensive healthcare services—including long-term care—to all members.[31] CCRC customers tend to be middle- and upper-income persons who are relatively healthy when they become residents and pay a substantial entrance charge and monthly fee in return for a promise of "care for life." It has been estimated that about 10 percent of older people could afford to join such communities.[32] Most of the 1,000 CCRCs in the United States, however, do not provide complete benefit coverage in their contracts, and those that do have faced financial difficulties.[33] Because most older people prefer to remain in their own homes rather than join age-segregated communities, an alternative product termed "life care at home" (LCAH) was developed in the late 1980s and marketed to middle-income customers with lower entry and monthly fees than those of CCRCs.[34] However, only about 500 LCAH policies are in effect.[35]

A relatively new approach for providing long-term care in residential settings is the assisted-living facility. It has been created for moderately disabled persons—including those with dementia—who are not ready for a nursing home and provides them with limited forms of personal care, supervision of medications and other daily routines, and congregate meal and housekeeping services.[36] Assisted living has yet to be tried with a private-insurance approach. The monthly rent in a first-class nonprofit facility averages about $2,400 or higher for a one-bedroom apartment; the rent is even higher in for-profit facilities.

The Role of Medicaid

For those who cannot pay for long-term care out of pocket or through various insurance arrangements, and are not eligible for care through programs of the Department of Veterans Affairs, the available sources of payment are Medicaid and other means-tested government programs funded by the Older Americans Act, Social Service Block Grants (Title XX of the Social Security Act), and state and local governments. The bulk of such financing is through Medicaid, the federal-state program for the poor, which finances the care—at least in part—of about three-fifths of nursing home patients[37] and 28 percent of home and community-based services.[38] The program does not pay for the full range of home-care services that are needed for most clients who are functionally dependent. Most state Medicaid programs provide reimbursement only for the most "medicalized" services that are necessary to maintain a long-term care patient in a home environment. Rarely reimbursed are essential supports such as chore services, assistance with food shopping and meal preparation, transportation, companionship, periodic monitoring, and respite programs for family and other unpaid caregivers.

Medicaid does include a special waiver program that allows states to offer a wider range of nonmedical home-care services, if limited to those patients whose services will be no more costly than Medicaid-financed nursing home care. However, the volume of services in these waiver programs—which in some states combine Medicaid with funds from the Older Americans Act, the Social Services Block Grant program, and other state and local government sources—is small in relation to the overall demand.[39]

Although many patients are poor enough to qualify for Medicaid when they enter a nursing home, a substantial number become poor after they are institutionalized.[40] Persons in this latter group deplete their assets in order to meet their bills and eventually "spend down" and become poor enough to qualify for Medicaid.

Still others become eligible for Medicaid by sheltering their assets—illegally or legally with the assistance of attorneys who specialize in so-called Medicaid estate planning. Because sheltered assets are not counted in Medicaid eligibility determinations, such persons are able to take advantage of a program for the poor, without being poor. Asset sheltering has become a source of considerable concern to the federal and state governments as Medicaid expenditures on nursing homes and home care have been increasing rapidly—nearly doubling from 1990 to 1995.[41]

An analysis in Virginia estimated that the aggregate of assets sheltered through the use of legal loopholes in 1991 was equal to more than 10 percent of what the state spent on nursing home care through Medicaid in that year.[42] A study drawing on interviews with state government staff for Medicaid eligibility determination in four states—California, Florida, Massachusetts, and New York—found a strong relationship between a high level of financial wealth in a geographic area and a high level of Medicaid estate-planning activity. Most of these workers estimated that the range of asset sheltering among single applicants for Medicaid was between 5 and 10 percent and for married applicants between 20 percent and 25 percent.[43] A law enacted in

1996 made it a federal crime to shelter assets in order to become eligible for Medicaid. However, the law is so vague that, practically speaking, it has been unenforceable.

FORCES FOR IMPROVING ACCESS

From the mid-1980s until the mid-1990s, a number of national policy makers were sympathetic to these various dilemmas—the inability of individuals and their families to pay for services, the limitations of private insurance, and the anxieties of spending down. Since then, however, the main concern in Washington, D.C., as well as in the states, has been to limit Medicaid expenditures. In this new context, the most likely prospect is that public resources for long-term care will be even less available in relation to the need than they have been to date.

Public recognition of a need to improve access to long-term care has been building over the past two decades. The major initial impetus for this increased awareness has been successful advocacy efforts on behalf of older people, particularly the efforts undertaken by a political coalition formed in the mid-1970s concerned about Alzheimer's disease (AD).[44] This coalition was successful in getting Congress to earmark appropriations for AD research at the National Institute on Aging in the 1980s, and the amount of these funds has been increasing ever since.[45]

Advocates for victims of AD formally coalesced in 1988 with the broader constituency concerned for chronically ill and disabled older persons. The Alzheimer's Association, the American Association for Retired Persons (AARP), and the Families U.S.A. Foundation (a small organization originally established to improve the plight of poor older people) allied during the presidential campaign to undertake a lobbying effort organized under the name Long-Term Care '88.[46] The next year an explicit link was forged between advocates for the disabled and the elderly when Congressman Claude Pepper introduced a bill to provide comprehensive long-term home care coverage for disabled persons of any age who are dependent in at least two ADLs.[47] Although this bill was not voted on by Congress, it was a milestone in that it was the first major legislative effort to programmatically combine the long-term care needs of younger disabled adults with those of elderly people.

Following the Pepper bill, several dozen long-term care bills were introduced in Congress. The lobbying efforts for long-term care that were launched during the 1988 presidential campaign have broadened to encompass the needs of younger disabled people and have been carried forward by a coalition named The Long-Term Care Campaign. This Washington-based interest group claims to represent nearly 140 national organizations (with more than 60 million members), including religious denominations, organized labor and business groups, nurses, veterans, youth and women's groups, consumer organizations, and racial and ethnic groups, as well as older and younger disabled persons.[48]

In the early 1990s, advocates for the elderly and younger disabled persons were optimistic that the federal government would establish a new program for funding long-term care that would not be means-tested, as is Medicaid. A number of bills introduced from 1989 to 1994 included some version of such a program, including President Clinton's failed proposal for healthcare reform.[49] None of these proposals became law. The major reason was that any substantial version of such a program would cost tens of billions of dollars each year just at the outset and far more as the baby boomers reach old age.

By the mid-1990s, optimism regarding expanded governmental funding for long-term care was quashed. A new Republican majority in the 104th Congress reversed the focus on long-term care from expansion to retraction. It proposed to limit federal spending on Medicaid. Advocates for long-term care programs switched from offense to defense.

By 1995, Medicaid's expenditures on long-term care had been growing at an annualized rate of 13.2 percent since 1989.[50] As part of its overall effort to achieve a balanced budget, Congress initially proposed in that year to cap the rate of growth in Medicaid expenditures in order to achieve savings of $182 billion by 2002, to eliminate federal requirements for determining individual eligibility for Medicaid (as an entitlement), and to turn over control of the program to state governments through capped block grants. Such changes were vetoed by President Clinton. They resurfaced in 1996 with proposed reductions totaling $72 billion, but no legislation was enacted that year.

This approach remains on the policy agenda, strongly supported by the National Governors Association. According to one analysis,[51] the 1995 congressional proposals for limiting Medicaid's growth would have trimmed long-term care funding by as much as 11.4 percent by the year 2000 and meant that 1.74 million Medicaid beneficiaries would have lost or been unable to secure coverage. In addition, this analysis assumed that states would make their initial reductions in home- and community-based care services (because nursing home residents have nowhere else to go), and concluded that such services would be substantially reduced from their current levels. Five states were projected to eliminate home- and community-based services by the end of the century and another 19 were to cut services by more than half. If provisions to cap and block grant Medicaid do become law, they will almost certainly engender conflict within states regarding the distribution of limited resources for the care of older and younger poor constituencies.

WHAT PROSPECTS FOR IMPROVED ACCESS?

At the turn of the century, prospects for older people having better access to long-term care seem dim. Out-of-pocket payments for care are becoming larger and increasingly unaffordable for many. Only a minority of older persons—now about 5 percent, and perhaps 20 percent in the decades ahead—might be able to afford premiums for private long-term care insurance. Broad societal trends suggest that informal, unpaid care by family members might become less feasible in the future than it is today. Moreover, the safety net that government programs provide by financing long-term care for the poor is seriously threatened by contemporary federal and state budgetary politics.

How might the outlook improve in the future? The most promising seeds for change lie in the enormous projected growth in the number of older persons needing long-term care, outlined at the outset of this chapter. Moreover, leaders of the American Coalition of Citizens with Disabilities, representing 8 million disabled persons, have expressed for some years the hope that they might form a powerful political alliance with organizations representing 32 million older people to pursue this issue of mutual concern.[52]

As the demand for long-term care increases, while the means for access remain limited or become more restricted, a widespread and deeply felt popular demand for expanded government funding of long-term care could well emerge. Even as organized advocates for long-term care access brought the issue to the public policy agenda in the late 1980s and early 1990s, the entrance of the baby boomers into the ranks of old age may precipitate a grassroots movement that will revitalize political awareness of the issue as a major problem in American society.

However, even if a grassroots movement is able to elevate the principle of expanded government funding for long-term care to the top of the agenda, that general principle masks some basic value questions that, so far, have just begun to surface in public discussion. Widespread debate on and resolution of these questions will be required for a substantial proportion of Americans to understand and support the implications of any law that is to be enacted. Even if enacted, such legislation could be quickly repealed, as was the poorly understood Medicare Catastrophic Coverage Act of 1988.[53] Yet depending on the identity of the primary constituency seeking support for long-term care (the aged, the disabled, or a broader coalition of the aged, the disabled, and perhaps others), the configurations and primacy of the values involved might be very different, and the likelihood of generating widespread support might vary substantially.

From the perspective of older persons, long-term care is viewed as a problem besetting elderly people, categorically. The predominant, though not exclusive, element of interest in additional public insurance is generated by an economic concern. That concern is the possibility of becoming poor through spending down, depleting one's assets to pay for long-term care and then becoming dependent on a welfare program, Medicaid, to pay nursing home bills. There is a distinct middle-class fear—both economic and psychological—of using savings and selling a home to finance one's own health care. This anxiety reflects a desire to protect estates, as well as the psychological intertwining of personal self-esteem with one's material worth and independence.

The political weight of this type of concern, however, is not substantial in today's climate of public-policy discourse. The late 1970s, the political era in which categorical old-age entitlement programs were created and sustained with relative ease, appears to be over. The aged have become a scapegoat for a variety of America's problems, and many domestic-policy concerns have been framed as issues of intergenerational equity.[54]

If expanded public long-term care insurance is to be enacted as an old-age entitlement to serve older persons as a buffer against spending down, the American public will need to confront and resolve some fundamental moral and political issues, including the following: Assuming that we can improve laws for protecting spouses of long-term care patients from impoverishment, why shouldn't older people spend their assets and income on their health care? Why should government foot the bill? Why should it be government's responsibility to preserve estates for inheritance? In addition, should government take a more active role than at present in preserving economic-status inequalities from generation to generation? On what basis should some persons be taxed to preserve the inheritances of others? Should the taxing power of government be used to preserve the psychological sense of self-esteem that for so many persons is bound up in their lifetime accumulation of assets—their material worth? Widespread public debate on such issues might very well fail to resolve them in a fashion that supports a major initiative in long-term care to protect older persons from paying for their care.

Even if such questions were satisfactorily resolved, the challenge of bringing together the different perspectives of the elderly and the younger disabled population would remain. In contrast to older persons, younger disabled persons do not perceive long-term care funding as mostly an issue of whether the government or the individual patient and/or family pays for the care. Their main concern is the issue of whether such funding covers basic access to services, technologies, and environments that will make it feasible to carry forward an active life. They argue that they should have assistance to do much of what they would be able to do if they were not disabled.

The Americans with Disabilities Act of 1990, achieved through vigorous advocacy efforts, has helped to eliminate discriminatory as well as physical barriers to the participation of people with disabilities in employment, public services, public accommodations, transportation, and telecommunications. However, it will not provide the elements of long-term care desired by disabled younger adults, such as paid assistance in the home and for getting in and out of the home, peer counseling, semi-independent modes of transportation, and client control or management of services.

Although the disabled have advocated for long-term care services, they have rejected a "medical model" that emphasizes long-term care as an essential component of health services. This is understandable, given their strong desires for autonomy, independence, and as much "normalization" of daily life as possible. Similarly, disabled people have traditionally eschewed symbolic and political identification with elderly people, because of traditional stereotypes of older people as frail, chronically ill, declining, and "marginal" to society.

The efforts of disabled people to advocate on their terms for governmental long-term care initiatives, however, have made little progress. Rather, previous success in getting expanded public funding for long-term care on the national policy agenda—for persons of all ages—was due largely to advocates for the elderly and to broader concerns about the projected healthcare needs generated by an increasingly larger and, on average, older population of elderly people.

In any grassroots efforts to elevate long-term care funding to the top of the national policy agenda, advocates for the younger disabled would probably be well advised to suppress their objections to the healthcare model of long-term care. The challenge of gaining widespread popular support for long-term care funding is to overcome a long-standing cultural perception that long-term care is separate and detached from the arena of health care.

For most of this century, long-term care has been a comparatively neglected backwater in the overall American healthcare scene. Except for occasional nursing home scandals and fires—and subsequent ad hoc activities in response to these events—long-term care has received very little attention from the medical profession and society at large. It has been eclipsed by the glamour and prestige of hospital-based medical care that is inherently dramatic because it deals with acute episodes of illnesses and trauma, and their relatively high-tech and quick fix dimensions of diagnosis and intervention.

In effect, long-term care has not been perceived as part of health care. Long-term care has not even been covered through traditional health insurance mechanisms, such as employee benefit plans. When concerns are expressed about the fact that 40 million Americans are not covered by health insurance, coverage for long-term care is not part of the discussion.

Yet, there are good reasons to believe that long-term care will come to be perceived more widely as part of the continuum of health care that is needed by all of us.[55] As the baby boom cohort begins to approach the ranks of old age, the importance of long-term care, the formidable volume of need for it, the difficulties of financing it, and the challenges of delivering it effectively are likely to become increasingly accepted throughout American society. Such acceptance could bring with it a widespread understanding that long-term care is health care by another name. This perception may enfold long-term care into the shared understanding of justice in health care that dictates that access to long-term care is as much of a fundamental right as is access to other kinds of health care.

UPDATE FROM A PRACTITIONER'S VIEW

In reviewing Binstock's comments from my view, as an executive in a long-term care facility, I (Gardner-Ray) know that although the numbers and percentages may have changed, the trends and issues have not. Long-term care for the elderly and disabled continues to be problematic and the outlook for the future is bleak. Barriers to adequate long-term care, including cultural, social, and economic issues, are driven by the political climate that controls funding to specific minority groups.

More specifically, because the elderly and disabled have higher than normal healthcare needs, questionable healthcare status, and anticipated need for increasing services, funding is either capped or so costly that they cannot afford the insurance to cover services. Demand for long-term care will undoubtedly increase as the baby boomers age, but it is questionable whether the relationship between cost and accessibility will maintain the status quo as the budgets for Medicare and Medicaid programs are cut.

Although much was done to stall the cuts in Medicare and Medicaid in the 1990s, a rebirth in cost-cutting measures has proliferated since 1998 as responsibility for cost containment has been shifted from the federal government to the states. The effects of this shift create a push for alternative delivery methods in elder and disability care. Yet, alternative methods of care are generally not government funded.

If history judges a culture by how it treats its elderly and disabled, then what legacy do we wish to leave behind? Can we afford to be viewed as a society that values any human life more than another? If so, where do we draw the line; do we stop at 75 or 80 or what number? Is this determination made by level and degree of infirmity? Who will make the determination and what will their criteria be? Ultimately, is limiting and/or denying access equivalent to selective genocide? The implications are many, and the debate continues. What will public policy dictate and what will society tolerate? These are just a few of the ethical challenges in dealing with the issue of older people and long-term care.

SUMMARY

With the aging of the baby boomers and the increasing shortage of health-care professionals, access to long-term care promises to be a significant issue for the twenty-first century. This chapter identifies the population needing care and the type of services that will be needed in the future. It presents the issues surrounding access including cost, the role of insurance, the role of the family, and methods for improving access. Finally, the practitioner's view is expressed including challenges that must be met to address the ethics issues concerning access to long-term care.

QUESTIONS FOR DISCUSSION

1. Access to long-term care seems to be a problem for the elderly in general. However, it is even more difficult for those who represent minorities. Why do you think this is true?

2. Why do you think that long-term care insurance lacks popularity among older Americans?

3. How do you think the baby boomer generation will change access and delivery of long-term care services?

4. What ethical arguments can you make to answer the challenges posed by Gardner-Ray in the last paragraph of this article?

NOTES

1. S. McConnell, "Who Cares about Long-Term Care?" *Generations* 14, no. 2 (1990): 15–18.

2. F. B. Hobbs, *Sixty-Five Plus in the United States: U.S. Bureau of the Census, Current Populations Reports, Special Studies* (Washington, DC: U.S. Government Printing Office, 1996), 23–190.

3. R. Stone and P. Kemper, "Spouses and Children of Disabled Elders: How Large a Constituency for Long-Term Care Reform?" *The Milbank Quarterly* 67 (1989): 485–506.

4. U.S. Bureau of the Census, *Sixty-Five Plus in America: Current Populations Reports, Special Studies* (Washington, DC: U.S. Government Printing Office, 1992), 23–178.

5. S. Crystal, "Economic Status of the Elderly," in *Handbook of Aging and the Social Sciences*, 4th ed., R. H. Binstock and L. K. George, eds. (San Diego, CA: Academic Press, 1996), 388–409.

6. U.S. Bureau of the Census, *Sixty-Five Plus in America: Current Populations Reports, Special Studies*.

7. Ibid.

8. C. K. Cassel, M. A. Rudberg, and S. J. Olshansky, "The Price of Success: Health Care in an Aging Society," *Health Affairs* 11, no. 2 (1992): 87–99.

9. J. F. Fries, "The Compression of Morbidity: Near or Far?" *The Milbank Quarterly* 67 (1989): 208–232; K. G. Manton, L. S. Corder, and E. Stallard, "Estimates of Change in Chronic Disability and Institutional Incidence and Prevalence Rates in the U.S. Elderly Population from the 1982, 1984, and 1989 National Long Term Care Survey," *Journal of Gerontology: Social Sciences* 48 (1993): S153–S166; E. L. Schneider and J. M. Guralnik, "The Aging of America: Impact on Health Care Costs," *Journal of the American Medical Association* 263 (1991): 2335–2340; L. M. Verbrugge, "Recent, Present, and Future Health of American Adults," in *Annual Review of Public Health*, 10, L. Breslow, J. E. Fielding, and L. B. Lave, eds. (Palo Alto, CA: Annual Reviews, Inc., 1989): 333–361.

10. Cassel et al., op. cit.

11. U.S. Bureau of the Census, *Sixty-Five Plus in America: Current Populations Reports, Special Studies*.

12. Manton et al., op. cit.

13. M. P. LaPlante, *Disability Statistics Report: State Estimates of Disability in America* (Washington, DC: National Institute on Disability and Rehabilitation Research, U.S. Department of Education, Office of Special Education and Rehabilitative Services, 1993).

14. J. L. Ross, *Long-Term Care: Demography, Dollars, and Dissatisfaction Drive Reform. Testimony before the Special Committee on Aging*, U.S. Senate. U.S. GAO/T-HEHS 94-140 (April 12, 1994).

15. U.S. Congress, Office of Technology Assessment, *Losing a Million Minds: Confronting the Tragedy of Alzheimer's Disease and Other Dementias* (Washington, DC: U.S. Government Printing Office, 1987).

16. U.S. Congress, Office of Technology Assessment, *Confused Minds, Burdened Families: Finding Help for People with Alzheimer's and Other Dementias* (Washington, DC: U.S. Government Printing Office, 1990).

17. K. R. Levit, H. C. Lazenby, B. R. Braden, et al., "National Health Expenditures," *Health Care Financing Review* 7, no. 2 (1996): 175–214.

18. Ibid.

19. W. G. Weissert, "Strategies for Reducing Home Care Expenditures," *Generations* 14, no. 2 (1990): 42–44.

20. U.S. Bureau of the Census, *Poverty in the United States: 1995, Current Population Reports, Consumer Income* (Washington, DC: U.S. Government Printing Office, 1996), 60–194.

21. U.S. General Accounting Office, *Long-Term Care: Current Issues and Future Directions* (Washington, DC: U.S. Government Printing Office, 1995).

22. S. K. Eckert and K. Smyth, *A Case Study of Methods of Locating and Arranging Health and Long-Term Care for Persons with Dementia* (Washington, DC: Office of Technology Assessment, Congress of the United States, 1988).

23. J. Calmes, "Elephant in the Room: Budget Wish List Come and Go, but 'Entitlements' Outweigh All," *The Wall Street Journal* (February 3, 2006): A-1.

24. K. Liu, K. M. Manton, and B. M. Liu, "Home Care Expenses for the Disabled Elderly," *Health Care Financing Review* 7, no. 2 (1985): 51–58.

25. E. M. Brody, *Women in the Middle: Their Parent-Care Years* (New York: Springer Publishing, 1990); R. Stone, G. L. Cafferta, and J. Sangl, "Caregivers of the Frail Elderly: A National Profile," *Gerontologist* 27 (1989): 616–626.

26. National Academy on Aging, *Old Age in the Twenty-first Century* (Washington, DC: Syracuse University, 1994).

27. V. L. Bengston, C. Rosenthal, and L. Burton, "Families and Aging: Diversity and Heterogeneity," in *Handbook of Aging and the Social Sciences*, 3d ed., R. H. Binstock and L. K. George, eds. (San Diego, CA: Academic Press, 1990), 263–287.

28. J. M. Wiener and L. H. Illston, "Health Care Financing and Organization for the Elderly," in *Handbook of Aging and the Social Sciences*, 4th ed., R. H. Binstock and L. K. George, eds. (San Diego, CA: Academic Press, 1996).

29. J. M. Wiener, L. H. Illston, and R. J. Hanley, *Sharing the Burden: Strategies for Public and Private Long-Term Care Insurance* (Washington, DC: The Brookings Institution, 1994).

30. W. H. Crown, J. Capitman, and W. N. Leutz, "Economic Rationality, the Affordability of Private Long-Term Care Insurance, and the Role for Public Policy," *Gerontologist* 32 (1992): 478-485; R. Friedland, *Facing the Costs of Long-Term Care: An EBRI-ERF Policy Study* (Washington, DC: Employee Benefits Research Institute, 1990); A. M. Rivlin and J. M. Wiener, *Caring for the Elderly: Who Will Pay?* (Washington, DC: The Brookings Institution, 1988); Wiener et al. *Sharing the Burden*.

31. R. D. Chellis and P. J. Grayson, *Life Care: A Long-Term Solution?* (Lexington, MA: Lexington Books, 1990).

32. M. A. Cohen, "Life Care: New Options for Financing and Delivering Long-Term Care," in *Health Care Financing Review*, Annual Supplement (Thousand Oaks, CA: Sage Publications, 1988), 139–143.

33. T. F. Williams and H. Temkin-Greener, "Older People, Dependency, and Trends in Supportive Care," in *The Future of Long-Term Care: Social and Policy Issues*, R. H. Binstock, L. E. Cluff, and O. von Mering, eds. (Baltimore: Johns Hopkins University Press, 1996), 51–74.

34. E. J. Tell, M. A. Cohen, and S. S. Wallack, "New Directions in Life Care: Industry in Transit," *The Milbank Quarterly* 65 (1987): 551–574.

35. Williams and Temkin-Greener, op. cit.

36. R. A. Kane and K. B. Wilson, *Assisted Living in the United States: A New Paradigm for Residential Care for Older People?* (Washington, DC: American Association for Retired Persons, 1993); V. Regnier, J. Hamilton, and S. Yatabe, *Assisted Living for the Aged and Frail: Innovations in Design, Management, and Financing* (New York: Columbia University Press, 1995).

37. Wiener and Illston, op. cit.

38. American Association of Retired Persons, Public Policy Institute, *The Costs of Long-Term Care* (Washington, DC: American Association of Retired Persons, 1994).

39. R. B. Hudson, "Social Protection and Services," in *Handbook of Aging and the Social Sciences*, 4th ed., R. H. Binstock and L. K. George, eds. (San Diego, CA: Academic Press, 1996), 446–466.

40. E. K. Adams, M. R. Meiners, and B. O. Burwell, "Asset Spend-Down in Nursing Homes: Methods and Insights," *Medical Care* 31 (1993): 1–23.

41. Levit, Lazenby, Braden, et al., op. cit.

42. B. Burwell, *State Responses to Medicaid Estate Planning* (Cambridge, MA: SysteMetrics, 1993).

43. B. Burwell and W. H. Crown, *Medicaid Estate Planning in the Aftermath of OBRA '93* (Cambridge, MA: The MEDSTAT Group, 1995).

44. P. Fox, "From Senility to Alzheimer's Disease: The Rise of the Alzheimer's Disease Movement," *The Milbank Quarterly* 67 (1989): 58–102.

45. G. D. Cohen, "Alzheimer's Disease: Current Policy Initiatives," in *Dementia and Aging: Ethics, Values, and Policy Choices*, R. H. Binstock, S. G. Post, and P. J. Whitehouse, eds. (Baltimore: Johns Hopkins University Press, 1992).

46. McConnell, op. cit.

47. U.S. House of Representatives, *Long-Term Care Act of 1989, H.R. 2263*, 101st Congress (1989).

48. Long-Term Care Campaign, *Pepper Commission Recommendations*, released March 2, *Insiders Update* (Jan.–Feb. 1990): 1.

49. R. H. Binstock, "Older Americans and Health Care Reform in the 1990s," in *Health Care Reform in the Nineties*, P. V. Rosenau, ed. (Thousand Oaks, CA: Sage Publications, 1994), 213–235.

50. U.S. General Accounting Office, op. cit.

51. E. Kassner, *Long-Term Care: Measuring the Impact of a Medicaid Cap* (Washington, DC: Public Policy Institute, American Association of Retired Persons, 1995).

52. P. Rubenfeld, "Ageism and Disabilityism: Double Jeopardy," in *Aging and Rehabilitation: Advances in the State of the Art*, S. J. Brody and G. E. Ruff, eds. (New York: Springer Publishing, 1986), 323–328.

53. R. Himelfarb, *Catastrophic Politics: The Rise and Fall of the Medicare Catastrophic Coverage Act of 1988* (University Park, PA: Pennsylvania State University Press, 1995).

54. R. H. Binstock, "Policies on Aging in the Post-Cold War Era," in *Post-Cold War Policy: The Social and Domestic Context*, W. Crotty, ed. (Chicago: Nelson Hall, 1995), 55–90.

55. R. H. Binstock, L. E. Cluff, and O. von Mering, eds. *The Future of Long-Term Care: Social and Policy Issues* (Baltimore: Johns Hopkins University Press, 1996).

ADDITIONAL RESOURCES

AARP. (2006) *Policy and Research*. Available at www.aarp.org/research.

Alliance for Aging Research. (2006). *Ageism: How Healthcare Fails the Elderly*. Available at www.agingresearch.org/brochures/ageism/Index.cfm.

Consumers for Affordable Healthcare. (2006). Available at www.mainecahc.org/healthcare/healthcare forelderly.htm.

National Long-Term Care Ombudsman Resource Center. (2001). Available at www.ltcombuds man.org.

Medicare Budget Information. Available at www.cms.hhs.gov/CFOReport/Downloads/2006_CMS_ Financial_Report.pdf.

CHAPTER 10

Respecting the Autonomy of Old People Living in Nursing Homes

George J. Agich

OVERVIEW

This chapter examines an issue that will certainly become one of increasing importance in the twenty-first century as the population percentage of elderly increases. In his presentation, Agich reminds us that the definition of autonomy as just self-determination is too narrow when considering the frail elderly. It involves the consideration of the total person and the ability to choose and to be responsible for one's choices. He examines life in a nursing home from the resident's viewpoint instead of the caregiver's or administrator's and offers concrete suggestions for increasing respect for autonomy in actual practice.

INTRODUCTION

To respect autonomy is to treat someone as an adult, to expect him or her to act responsibly, and to acknowledge and support his or her capacity for self-determination. Old people who reside in nursing homes often exhibit incapacities that make these usual attributions of autonomy difficult. In this chapter, I explore why respecting the autonomy of old people living in nursing homes is so difficult and why a reconceptualization of autonomy is so critical to enhancing their dignity and quality of life. I first discuss the way that autonomy misleads us about which characteristics of nursing home residents require protection. I then discuss the way actual autonomy is founded on who the individual is and why identity precedes autonomy. I also discuss the institutional character of nursing homes and consider the conflict between the nursing home as a protective environment and a place to express autonomy.

In the context of this discussion, I consider the implications of identity for establishing a sense of home for people living in nursing homes. I conclude by arguing that the assumption that an old person lacks autonomy simply because the person lives in a nursing home is not supported by the reality that everyday autonomy is compatible with considerable degrees and kinds of dependence and incapacity. Hence, respecting the autonomy of people living in nursing homes requires that we allow ourselves to view them as individuals first. The features of autonomy that are most important line up on the side of dignity and self-expression rather than self-determination and independence.

INDEPENDENCE, RIGHTS, AND THE PARADOX
OF AUTONOMOUS LIFE IN A NURSING HOME

"Respecting autonomy" often is glossed over in terms of respect for individual self-determination or decision making. Respecting people's individuality or self-determination assumes that one allows people to exercise choices about how to live their lives. This often amounts to nothing more than noninterference or forbearance; it is what political theorists term *negative freedom*.[1] Furthermore, policies designed to protect autonomy in this sense are structured to afford individuals independence, relevant information, and the freedom to make choices. Such policies address autonomy abstractly in the way they approach individuality; it is primarily in abstraction from the concrete identity of the individual. Clearly, some individuals who live in nursing homes have chosen to do so and retain the capacity for choice.

Other individuals, however, live in nursing homes not by choice, but by circumstance. They feel they have no acceptable alternatives or the choice of institutionalized is thrust upon them by family members or health professions, because they are too impaired to make decisions rationally or to resist. They come to see themselves as having no other choice. This does not mean that there are no alternatives, but simply that the decision to live in a nursing home was influenced by economic, medical, and social circumstances that make the "decision" more a matter of acceptance or acquiescence than free choice. Indeed, in the face of pressure from physicians and family members, they might experience the decision to enter a nursing home as coerced.

In this light, a large body of literature characterizes the nursing home experience as a situation in which loss of personal freedom is prominent.[2] This loss begins with the decision to enter the nursing home. Remedial recommendations to deal with these circumstances include protecting patient rights through legal and policy mechanisms. Collectively, these approaches are designed to restore self-determination to dependent old people by correcting various autonomy-subverting features of nursing homes. These approaches, however, do not seem to recognize the complexity of the decision making surrounding institutionalization or the complexity of the situations that compromise the cognitive, communicative, physical, or emotional capacities of the majority of old people.

By not incorporating the concrete economic, medical, psychological, or social circumstances of old people who cannot care for themselves, such approaches oversimplify the ethical terrain where the decision making occurs. By minimizing the fact that incapacitated old people who are dependent on others actually lack the basic features of autonomy, namely, independence and self-reliance, critics assume that the solution is to correct or reform the situation by placing procedural remedies in place, such as extensive pre-admission agreements. Such remedies, however, presume a standard of autonomy that exceeds the capacity of most compromised old people needing nursing home care. These remedies are not only phenomenologically inept, but also ethically problematic. They divert attention from the difficult task of identifying the myriad practical and concrete ways that autonomy can be protected or enhanced in people who are frail, and channel it instead into the pursuit of the impossible ideal of full self-reliance and independence. Sorely needed is an approach that can accommodate the complex reality of the frail old person to correct these oversimplifications.

Although many people living in nursing homes are dependent, they are not completely dependent. Like competence, dependence is situated and instrumental. One is dependent for some particular need, dependent on a particular person, or dependent under particular circumstances. Generalizing from dependence in one area of life to other areas can lead to serious erosion of autonomy. Individuals who cannot ambulate might nonetheless be fully capable of deciding where and when they go, what they want to do, and with whom they want to spend time. Even people who are cognitively impaired can and do function on their own in many ways. Old people who wander might appear to do so aimlessly, but they are still doing so on their own. That means that many individuals retain some capacity for self-initiated action, and it is a mistake to think that they lack autonomy. Viewing the dependence of old people as situational therefore requires caregivers to rethink their approaches to patients and to reevaluate the ways that these approaches promote abstract considerations instead of encouraging a sustained analysis of the complex concrete circumstances of old people, whose need for care might not fully erase their autonomy.

Although there is a wide variation in the meanings and uses of the term *autonomy* in both public discourse and philosophical discussion, the core meaning of autonomy is usually understood to be related to the literal meaning of "self-rule."[3] To be autonomous means to be capable of self-determination and decision making. Furthermore, an autonomous person is characterized by the attributes of independence, self-reliance, absence of restraint on choice and action, and his or her own ability to reflect on preferences or desires, as well as to act in accord with them. These features collectively define autonomy as it is understood in the Western, liberal tradition.[4] In this tradition, autonomy points to an individual whose identity is constituted primarily by individual action, belief, and choice. Such an individual is typically regarded in isolation from others.

Influenced by the liberal vision of autonomy, it is natural to believe that the situation of nursing home residents is a problem that can be remedied by a strict observance of autonomy bolstered by insistence on the rights of nursing home residents. The motivation for such insistence is, of course, understandable. A long line of criticism of nursing homes views them as what Goffman called "total institutions," namely, institutions that comprehensively control the daily lives of "inmates."[5] As such, nursing homes are regarded as oppressive settings in which residents can be protected only if rights are affirmed.

There is good reason, however, to believe that simply insisting that rights be respected only deals with a set of concerns that are superficial from the standpoint of nursing home residents. These concerns include rights to full information, representation by surrogates or ombudsmen, security of personal property within the nursing home, privacy, and confidentiality.[6] These rights undeniably structure important ways that autonomy can be respected and provide a strong reminder to caregivers that old people deserve respect and deference despite their dependencies. Such insistence, of course, is defensible whenever the nursing home resident actually possesses the capacity to exercise the rights in question. However, the language of rights can befuddle the consideration of the everyday ethics of nursing home care, but limit attention to abstract rights.

Not all rights imputed to old people living in nursing homes can actually be exercised by them or, more importantly, are central to their day-to-day life. Some rights are simply too peripheral or require interests that nursing home residents seldom possess. For example, a right to full disclosure of nursing home policies, procedures, and rules is relevant only if the old person is able to understand the information and is able to use it in weighing the advantages and disadvantages of one nursing home over another. It adds little in situations where the person lacks the ability to understand or make choices or in situations where there are no realistic nursing home alternatives.

Taken to an extreme, the insistence on rights leads one to claim that people living in nursing homes have a right to be free of the shackles of the institution and to be free to live without supervision or professional health care. Such extreme insistence on liberating nursing home residents would seem to commit some of the follies that have occurred in the liberation of the mentally ill from institutions. As one commentator put it, the mentally ill were given, in effect, a right to rot, that should be respected with no further moral claim on our conscience.[7] A frail old person's right to deteriorate further is very much like the putative right to rot of the seriously mentally ill. No caring thinker would seriously defend such a "right," yet it seems to accompany the uncritical acceptance of a rights-focused approach. Such an approach should be defended only if we were prepared to accept with equanimity its effects on the quality of life of old people. Hopefully, we are not prepared to do so.

Making liberty rights the focus of our effort to respect dependent or incapacitated individuals is thus as problematic for frail people living in nursing homes as for seriously ill patients in psychiatric institutions. Many of these persons lack basic capacities to ambulate, to direct themselves according to a plan of action, or to meet their own daily care needs. Unlike a psychotic individual, who might seem able to act even if he or she does so on the basis of irrational or delusional schemes and plans, people with cognitive or memory impairments often cannot form or maintain a concept of a plan even if able to bodily enact it. Others are simply too frail to execute an action or plan. Although there is no denying that respecting the rights of old people is a common approach to the issue of respecting their autonomy, restricting our attention to a set of abstract rights tends to obscure the everyday struggles that many people in nursing homes have to undergo. The language of ideal autonomy and rights tends to encourage an oversimplified vision of the ethical problems associated with respecting autonomy on the ground. In doing so, it overlooks the everyday occasions in which autonomy might be advanced, enhanced, or thwarted as people receive daily care. Thus, a rights-dominated account of autonomy is not so much wrong as it is too blunt a tool to deal with the subtle concrete complexities associated with the practical caring of people in nursing homes. If autonomy is to be a guide to these everyday practical concerns, it will have to be understood in a fashion that is less familiar than the language of patient rights. It will have to connect with the day-to-day experience of nursing home residents.

ACTUAL AUTONOMY AND IDENTITY

Viewed in everyday terms, autonomy has to be compatible with dependence of varying sorts and with some kinds and degrees of external influence.[8] The concept of actual dimension of autonomy is contrasted with autonomy in the liberal sense, which, as mentioned earlier, is cast in terms of self-determination and self-reliance, and which raises the bar of autonomy to its ideal aspect. The demands of ideal autonomy are so rigorous that few human agents—and not simply frail old persons—would be autonomous for the simple reason that human agents often lack sufficient knowledge and experience to act without reasonable reliance on others. Whenever autonomous individuals rely on the advice of others or defer to experts or authorities (both ordinary practices, to say the least), they reveal their own lack of independence, and thus their own interdependence. In addition, no persons' possible capacities are such that they are fully intact across the wide range of human capacities, which means that all of us are in some senses and at some times dependent in various ways. This commonplace occurrence is, however, a problem only for those who insist that autonomy must be understood in terms of independent, rational decision making by individuals isolated from others.

Conceptions of autonomy that take seriously how autonomy is concretely enacted in everyday life will have no such difficulties. Such understandings of actual autonomy will see autonomy as compatible not only with reliance on others for advice, but also for actions and services that the individual is not able to accomplish alone. Indeed, to be actually autonomous is to behave in ways that essentially interacts with others.[9]

A concept of actual autonomy must recognize that individuals are not created as adults capable of rational decision making based on their own pre-given beliefs and values, but as entities who achieve autonomy in the course of their personal development in living with others. Autonomous persons are not fully formed in the world. They develop their distinct personalities and capacities through relationships with parents, family members, and others in important social settings, such as school or work. Autonomy as a personal capacity thus emerges and develops throughout one's life and is shaped in the course of lived interactions with others. As a result, autonomous persons acquire values and beliefs that connect with their life experiences. Some of those beliefs are background beliefs and values, with the help of which individuals exercise deliberation and rational choice. No rational deliberation about choices can occur without a taken-for-granted frame of reference. Such a reference points to the conditions that existentially define who the autonomous persons are and delineates the range of beliefs within which these persons realize themselves.

Self-realization is one of the most pedestrian forms of autonomy. It should not be confused with the attainment of ideals associated with psychological notions of self-actualization, but simply point to the processes through which a person's sense of self actually emerges in the course of a life. Such actualization occurs through myriad everyday actions and experiences. Such a self might embody widely-shared cultural, psychological, and/or ethical ideals. It might also deviate from these ordinarily-accepted values and beliefs. One's autonomous self is thus to be understood as an ongoing psychological process, far from being accomplished at some point once and for all, but being constantly shaped in the course of an individual's life. This means that respecting actual autonomy must involve recognizing and dealing with individuality as it engages with and experiences the world.

Individuality is consistent with constraints and responsibilities that arise, because our individual selves emerge as we interact with others in ordinary everyday life and in the communal setting of nursing home life. Autonomous individuals not only make themselves, but also discover and reveal themselves through their interactions with others. An autonomous person is thus fully autonomous only in terms of having an identity formed through these interactions. Another way of making this point is to say that an individual is not autonomous unless he or she is a person. Here, the concept of *person* is used not as a metaphysical category. It is used as a socio-psychological construct that provides a conceptual framework, or scaffolding, in terms of which the actions, choices, and experiences that we usually regard as autonomous are conducted.[10]

A person's identity is formed in interaction with others. One's identity always involves degrees of dependence on others—for example, parents, other authority figures, and contemporaries. In various ways, we learn to trust these individuals and to rely on them. From a certain point of view, trust implies that one must yield some degree of liberty to others, but it does not always follow that this surrender diminishes autonomy. Sometimes this yielding to others enhances our autonomy by linking our individuality with others, in sharing projects and experiences, and by allowing us to adapt or cope with anxiety. Respecting actual autonomy thus requires that we respect who the individual is, not simply the individual's abstract or concrete choices.

In everyday life, individuals can and do make choices that are unacceptable and indefensible. We accommodate action and choices that we do not accept by regarding individuals as responsible for their choices and actions. Awareness of responsibility introduces an entirely new sphere of ethical analysis that is often overlooked in standard discussions of the rights of old people.[11] In the context of a nursing home, where individuals live communally, and where they suffer from conditions marked by cognitive and other degenerations, awareness of responsibility defines a useful vantage from which to respect their actual autonomy.

Responsibility, after all, is linguistically dependent on the notion of *response*. All autonomous individuals are responsive, and responsivity is a basic feature for recognizing the capacity for responsibility. Seeing an individual as responsible to some degree is to accept that individual as a person, as a member of a moral community. Unfortunately, many dependent old people residing in nursing homes seem to be treated less as moral agents than as recipients of "bed and body" work by caregivers, who see their work more as tasks to be accomplished than care to be given.[12] Because these old people might not be responsive to language or oral statements of rules, there is a tendency to ignore their subjectivity even though they often are able to respond to perceptual and other cues in the environment. Caregivers might not appreciate that their behaviors are responsive, judging them to be meaningless or simply a risk to their safety. Yet, their capacity to interact with the environment, even when it involves wandering and incurs the risk of injury from falls, can provide a foundation for constructing strategies to protect their safety without thwarting the vestiges of their autonomous responsivity.

Locking doors and using restraints or other devices to limit movement can compromise basic expressions of autonomy by thwarting the person's urge to move. However, an environment structured to provide confused old persons with visual cues such as Velcro strips across prohibited doorways or the use of color instead of alarms or locks can help such persons negotiate the difference between permitted or prohibited spaces while minimizing the risk of injury.[13] These approaches recognize the capacity of wandering patients to be responsive to the environment. Because autonomy is essentially relational, treating persons as having the capacity to respond means that they receive respectful treatment consistent with their impaired capacities and not simply that they are expected to follow rigid rules or suffer punitive consequences. Rigidly-enforced rules can be counterproductive not only because the cognitive capacities of the old might be impaired enough to limit comprehension, but also because the situations and individual capacities of impaired old people are unique and dynamic.

To respect the autonomy of old persons who are significantly impaired first means that their residual capacities should be acknowledged by providing them with environments suitable to their incapacities. They should also be assisted to learn to adapt rather than imposing institutional rules they are simply expected to follow. Caregivers need to guard against the tendency to overlook the evidence of actual autonomous action. Whenever a gap between the lived experience of nursing home residents and that of daily caregivers is allowed to persist, rules proliferate, and respect for the fragile and fleeting moments of autonomy of compromised old people are sacrificed. This means that administrators and family who might not interact daily with individual patients should strive to be more in tune with the everyday activities of old persons in the nursing home.

If identity precedes autonomy, then the things and interests that are important for the old person should be respected. Some nursing home residents are subjected to myriad diagnostic or therapeutic interventions designed to enhance their well-being without seriously considering the effect on their compromised capacities for autonomy. Medical ethics permits surrogate decisions for people who are not able to make decisions for themselves.[14] This practice is defensible not only when decisions are made on the basis of an understanding of the person's past preferences and values, but also when the decisions reflect who the person actually is in their current situation. Because many of us do not have clear preferences or specific values about particular medical treatments, surrogates are not able to make decisions that reflect what we would truly decide. Instead, surrogate decision makers often are forced to rely on "best interests" judgments that tend to protect our physical well-being. Physical well-being, however, can be burdensome if it is bought at the price of thwarting the patient's own identity. Here, daily caregivers who are discerning might be more useful in forming a decision than family surrogates. Their distance from the daily actions of the patients can prevent them from seeing that a compromised individual can exhibit desires and preferences in their day-to-day activities. If autonomy is to be relevant at all, then paying attention to the current identity and quality of experience of the old person is essential. The sad reality is that only approximate understandings of such experiences, especially when old persons are not very communicative or are confused, might be the best that we can do.

NURSING HOMES

Respecting the autonomy of nursing home residents requires that we consider the institutional nature of the nursing home. Some nursing homes exclusively provide skilled care for the most physically-dependent individuals who are incapable of performing daily self-care activities or whose medical condition requires specialized services. Other nursing homes, however, provide minimal care for individuals who need a sheltered environment including basic services such as laundry, hygiene, food, and some custodial care. Still other institutions provide a mixture. Thus, the notion of a nursing home is a broad one. For present purposes, I limit discussion to nursing homes that provide skilled levels of care. Even with this limitation, these institutions are not uniform. Complicating matters further is the fact that there is wide variation in the capacities of the individuals living in nursing homes. This variability, more than any other feature, must be kept in mind, because respecting the autonomy of people in nursing homes is first and foremost a matter of acknowledging and respecting their individuality.

Although many residents of nursing homes require highly skilled care, the vast majority of people in nursing homes are there mainly because they lack family caregivers. Some lack financial resources to extend their living independently. Some are admitted from a hospital after an acute illness for skilled rehabilitative care. Some frail individuals are admitted for a wide but variable range of incapacities. Although many of these people have medical problems, their frailty is multidimensional and usually precludes their own self-care. For many, the nursing home is the last stage before death, and some even regard the nursing home as a fate worse than death. Like other total institutions, the nursing home is sometimes regarded as oppressive, but oppression here is as much determined by the frailty of the people who reside there. It does not take much to direct or influence an individual who is fundamentally incapable of daily self-care. Advocating the rights of nursing home residents, however, frequently overlooks the strikingly dependent and fragile nature of many of these people. Thus, respect for the autonomy of the old should be based on more commonplace and accessible features of autonomy than rights and must be focused on the everyday features of the nursing home environment that thwart or support autonomy. For present purposes, I focus on two aspects of the nursing home as the environment within which people live: first, as a place of safety and protection, and second, as a place that belongs to them as their "home."

Safety Versus Autonomy

Many nursing homes take an overprotective attitude toward residents. For example, believing that injuries from falls are preventable, staff restrain or confine frail old people who have any potential for falling.[15] Some suggest that this tendency is motivated by the nursing home's desire to avoid litigation, even though there is no good evidence to support this worry. Moreover, insisting on a frail old person's right to freedom of movement is far too abstract a response to the practice of restraining, because the problem of falls and related problems, such as wandering, are clinically too complex to be so conveniently resolved. Appealing to rights does not help much, because it raises the wrong kinds of questions.

Although old people certainly have rights, rights do not provide much guidance for caregivers, especially when old people cannot exercise them. The standard approach of turning to surrogates to make decisions for an old person instead of paying closer attention to the actual interests of the old person only respects autonomy as an abstract principle. Such an approach fails to respect the actual autonomy that the old person concretely possesses. A surrogate cannot exercise a person's right to freedom of movement, which may be of central importance fulfilling a vital need for a confused old person. Often, the surrogate is asked to consent to the imposition of constraints, which are couched in the person's interests as assuring their safety.

Safety is juxtaposed with the right to movement, which is itself abstracted from its vital relationship to the old people's own actual interests or autonomy. It is no wonder then that surrogates accept restraints when the risk of harm is stressed. The surrogate avoids the risks of injury due to falls as an expression of care for the person. In this situation, appealing to the right to movement is simply too abstract to outweigh the palpable need for safety. If the right to freedom of movement is not a sufficient ground, how can actual autonomy help us to address the problems associated with falls and wandering?

Actual autonomy focuses on how individuals experience and interact with the world. As such, autonomy is manifested in the spontaneous interaction with the world, because autonomous individuals create their world as they make their way in it. Making one's way in the world involves a wide range of activities in which individuals give meaning to their experience. As embodied beings, autonomous persons physically make their way in the world; they shape and reshape its meaning through their actions. This means that bodily movement is an important way by which people enact their autonomy. Restricting movement in order to protect old people, however, has two significant consequences. First, persons who are restrained are paradoxically prone to greater injury, and studies have shown that they require greater degrees of attention and care as a result.[16] Second, restraints not only limit movement, but also the chance to explore the world and to encounter opportunities to make sense of experiences. To appreciate this point, we must consider experience from the point of view of the wandering old person.

Assume that the old person is confused. The person does not know what she wants. She simply experiences a sense of things amiss or out of order. She longs for something, something that is missing in her life. As a result, the patient experiences anxiety and concern that naturally manifests itself in motor activity. She sets out to find what is missing. She acts not based on rational thought or deliberation, but simply out of a basic need. Her agitation moves her to action. Her action brings her into a wider range of experience outside of her room. Close observation of the movement of confused old people indicates that it is incorrectly described as purposeless. Although we do not explicitly know its intention or purpose for the old person, it does exhibit rational patterns.

Observational studies of institutionalized old people report that even seriously compromised and cognitively impaired old people actively work to fill up their time.[17] Indeed, the movement and activities of wandering old people change and are divided up, much like the institutional day, into three parts punctuated by meals.[18] One of the effects of movement is to keep the person attuned to the world and to others. Although cognitive and perceptual abilities may progressively deteriorate, the old person is actively engaged in the world around. Seeing the old person's everyday activities as attempts to make sense of one's experience, rather than as problems to be controlled or managed, is fundamental to respecting the actual autonomy of these people. Such a change of perspective involves much more than idealistically denying that cognitively impaired individuals are at risk for falling. Rather it recasts the problems of management in a new and, hopefully, more malleable form.

Uriel Cohen and Gerald D. Weisman argued that interest in the therapeutic potential of the physical environment has grown to the point that it is now possible to place the concept of autonomy in its proper environmental context.[19] They identified three environmental aspects of autonomy—mobility and independence, control and freedom of choice, and identity and continuity—that support a set of two dozen principles for the design of environments for people with dementia.[20] It has also been reported that the use of color-coordinated doorways or hallways and the use of color-coordinated barriers, including Velcro strips across doorways, can allow wandering individuals freedom of movement within the institution. It directs their movement to areas that are both supervised and safe. Restraints, however, stop movement, or limit it severely, because the movement itself is the problem.

Viewed from the perspective of actual autonomy, movement is not the problem but is an expression of the finite and fragile nature of actual autonomy. Humans are not normally stationary beings. They need opportunities for interacting with the environment around them. Artificially restricting the horizon of perception, by significantly limiting movement, increases agitation. Whenever the range of experiences is restricted, the opportunities for the old person to impart meaning to experiences are limited. Considering actual autonomy thus suggests new ways to understand movement. Movement can be viewed positively while, at the same time, recognizing that enhancing autonomy through movement is compatible with safety if the environment is structured in ways that prevent or limit the possibility of injury.

The world is a dangerous place, and it is impossible to rule out all risks. Parents cannot do so for their children, and children cannot do so for their aged parents. Placement in a nursing home, however, gives many family members the sense that the person is now fully protected. There is round-the-clock supervision, medical and personal care is provided, and so there should be no accidents. However, if autonomy is to be taken seriously, some kinds of risks need to be accepted.[21] Protection that insulates the individual from other persons, that keeps the old person from "dangerous" activities, such as walking, or that prevents visiting a library or church outside the safety of the nursing home needs to be reexamined. Overprotection can thwart autonomy by nipping it at its most basic level, namely in the everyday ways that people act in the world of the nursing home.

Identity and the Sense of Home

Being oneself is autonomous in terms of the particular values and beliefs that define who one is. However, the beliefs and values that are central to people's autonomy are not necessarily those that they articulate, but rather those that they live or enact in the everyday world. We identify with many things, and our orientation in the world is structured from a primordial identification with our own bodies. As people age, their bodies become resistant to them. In advanced old age, frailty can set in. Frail individuals require nursing home care mainly because of their own inabilities to care for themselves and because there are no resources for in-home care. They can no longer dress themselves, prepare food, or perform bodily cleaning and use the toilet. As a result, autonomy itself is threatened for these people. It would be absurd to think that according these people, substantial rights would make a meaningful difference to their everyday existence. Instead, we need to think about the important role that identification plays in assisting these people to maintain their sense of self. The most basic values that define the identity of a person are not abstract propositions or rights. Rather, basic values exist in a more concrete way—in everyday experiences and memories that define the personality. We develop our personalities in large part through our daily life in the world.

Through action in the world, personal values are expressed and discovered as components of who we are. In other words, one does not intellectually decide that one loves one's child based on a rational calculation or argument based on parental responsibilities, but one responds affectively to the child. Through myriad everyday interactions involving concern and caring, the child is valued and given a place within the identity of the parent. To speak here of free choice, especially where free choice is understood as a process of rational calculation, is to vastly oversimplify the complex, concrete reality of parental regard for children. Parental regard for children is a useful paradigm for understanding how it is that a person experiences and develops values integral to a sense of self, namely through basic body awareness, emotional interaction, and caring.[22]

Another component of identification involves not only the individual's body or bodily experience, but also the space immediately surrounding the body. That space, namely "the familiar," is a mobile environment in which we are "at home." "Home" not only has historical and social meaning for individuals, but it also has an evolving personal meaning throughout one's life in virtue of the space in which one lives. Insofar as people are able to define their space, they make it their own. For space to belong to someone does not imply a right of ownership, but rather a sense of self-definition. Thus, allowing nursing home residents and, indeed, encouraging them and their families to bring various personal items into the nursing home, to decorate the room, and to use their own clothes are important ways that they can be assisted in maintaining continuity with their identity. Maintaining a continuous sense of self is especially important for old people, because their frailty and incapacities already represent a significant loss not simply of capacity, but of who they are. In other words, we need to understand that the incapacities that bring people into nursing homes are not just physical, cognitive, or communicative inabilities, but also alterations in one's fundamental sense of self. As a result, nursing homes should provide an environment that encourages and permits a rebuilding of the compromised sense of self by allowing "space" for new identities to develop.

The identity of nursing home residents is not constituted simply by allowing them to have some "private" space, but in terms of the public ways that they are allowed and encouraged to comport themselves. Old people, despite their frailties, need to be accorded considerable latitude in defining relations with others in the nursing home. Too often, families try to secure private space for their loved one to ensure that there is no intrusion of others. If a nursing home is to be anything comparable to a home, it will develop only if a dynamically defined sense of "yours" and "mine" is allowed to occur. No matter what the motivation, be it concern for safety or protection of personal property, family members or administrators who insist on defining territory essentially violate a fundamental feature of actual autonomy. It is autonomy's prerogative to impart meaning to the world. Old people themselves should be allowed to define the limits and meaning of their world. Therefore, caretakers should attune themselves to the old persons' own definition and understanding of the environment. After all, the nursing home is the person's home. The caregivers are only working there, whereas the old person lives there.

Along with an identified space, nursing home residents should be permitted to reach out and to have visitors within their space. Both allowing and assisting them to entertain in their own personal space, for example, by providing and maintaining the ability to serve drinks and food, old people can maintain links with their past lives and preserve habitual or traditional acts of hospitality. All too often, however, nursing home administrators are motivated by concern to routinize and institutionalize life. As a result, a whole range of spontaneous interactions among (and between) old people, caregiving staff, and family or other visitors becomes strained. Ways need to be found to augment the old person's autonomous use of space if the nursing home is to be more a home than an institution. Unfortunately, space is often treated as fungible. A nursing home resident is admitted to the hospital for an acute illness and returns only to find herself placed in another room, with another roommate, with a different view out the window. Prohibiting such transfers can, of course, be secured by insisting on the person's rights, but rights alone will not help nursing home administrators to understand how important space is for respecting autonomy.

Communal spaces are not always shared equally. Some individuals congregate and form groups that exclude others. Care must be taken, of course, to prevent these natural groups from infringing on the rights of others. However, nursing home administrators should not forget the important role that communal or public space plays in our everyday lives. It is a space in which we feel capable of being ourselves with others. Sharing is an important human experience, but what constitutes good sharing cannot be decided abstractly. In nursing homes, a good deal of sharing occurs surrounding a television or before a window with a view. Clearly, not all residents in a nursing home will feel comfortable or even be welcomed into this space. Rather than insisting on equal access, multiple spaces amenable to different and creative uses should be provided. Wherever such options are not available, administrators must be careful not to arbitrarily define space by creating rules to regulate its use. Such rules can then promote labeling of those residents who cannot comply with the rules as "problems." A better approach would involve trying to foster creative and individual accommodation. Overregimentation of life within a nursing home curtails communal action, just as inflexible urban planning curtails rather than promotes creative use of space in cities. Rigid rules for particular spaces can thwart other spontaneous uses. If the actual autonomy matters, then spontaneous definition of space should be cultivated rather than controlled.

If autonomy is to be actually respected for residents of nursing homes, greater attention needs to be paid to the way that people have access to the private and communal spaces within the facility. One major problem with nursing homes in the United States is their tendency to be isolated from the surrounding community. Because administrators are concerned to prevent wandering and to "protect" confused old people, they tend to keep them indoors in confined spaces. With the perception of confinement, however, comes agitation and anxiety.[23] However, enclosed gardens or courtyards and public space with a variety of rooms can control movement, yet also afford experiential variety so important to many confused individuals.

CONCLUSION

Our tacit assumptions about autonomy lead to a number of misconceptions about old people in nursing homes. Because an old person is living in a nursing home, even a nursing home delivering skilled care, it does not follow that the individual is unable to make decisions. Some old people maintain high degrees of decisional capacity even though their medical conditions can limit their ability to execute or to act on their choices. For example, patients who are bedridden but otherwise cognitively intact can make decisions about not only their own medical care, but also about other important life matters. Nonetheless, these people might require assistance in carrying out their decisions. It is also important to note that decisional incapacity is seldom global. Decisional capacity is both an instrumental and local concept. It is good to remember that the kinds of inabilities in ordinary life that do not count against one's being regarded as autonomous should not count against a person just because the person is old and frail.

Decisional incapacity that is based on lack of information does not mean that patients cannot decide, but only that expert advice or information is needed. In similar fashion, a person might want to install a satellite television receiver, but not know how to do so. I am not normally regarded as decisionally incapacitated if I rely on a professional installer. In fact, for a whole range of services, it seems prudent that people do rely on specialists, because they can usually deliver a quality service or product better than an individual can provide for themselves.

People in nursing homes should not be regarded as nonautonomous simply because their decisional capacity is exercised under conditions of dependence. We are all dependent in a wide variety of ways. Thus, it may be too much to ask of a compromised or frail old person to articulate reasons reflective of deeply held beliefs or values, much less to defend these beliefs or convictions, because articulating reasons might be too stringent a demand. Ordinarily, we do not impose rigorous decisional standards on everyday decision making. Similarly, it has been argued that informed consent standards vary depending on the medical circumstances, the nature of the medical intervention, and the degree of risk and benefit.[24] Thus, how decisions are made, what impedes or thwarts self-expression and decision making, and what conditions are in place to augment or enhance it are themselves critically important points for respecting the autonomy of old people in nursing homes. The dependence of the old should not be contrasted with the independence of the young living outside nursing homes as if the simple need for nursing care defines a different class of individual, namely one who is not autonomous.

Consider adults living outside of nursing homes. Although we consider them independent, most well-functioning adults exist in highly dependent and interdependent relationships. They have spouses, children, parents, families, friends, coworkers, service providers, and others with whom they interact in everyday life and on whom they depend. Commuters rely on transit drivers and others to take them to work. Shoppers rely on supermarket managers, clerks, and others to replenish shelves and to assist them, for example, in taking groceries to the car. The need for help is hardly inconsistent with autonomy. Some kinds of help do conflict with some kinds of independence, but autonomy is compatible with the need for help. Similarly, dependence is compatible with autonomy. We need to reject the view that autonomy means independence, and that dependence is something to be avoided, because such a view obscures the concrete reality of everyday autonomy.

Consider the high level of autonomy that even frail individuals might exhibit. They might be able to engage in various kinds of activities, including maintaining social contacts with family or friends by telephone or having visitors. They might enjoy and participate in games or hobbies. Even individuals who seem to wander aimlessly do so in a way that attempts to define a space and to make a world for themselves. Such efforts are not dependent on others, although they require the cooperation of others. Such cooperation is not different in kind from that needed by most adults living outside of nursing homes.

In addition, nursing home residents are not necessarily dependent perceptually or communicatively. We think that people living in nursing homes exhibit deficient perceptual or communicative capacities only because of our reluctance to spend time in their world. Because individuals or groups exhibit different ways of seeing and experiencing the world, we cannot conclude that they lack perceptual or communicative capacity.[25] We simply should not forget the degree to which our own experience is culturally and socially determined. From the inside, our experiences are always full of meaning, but viewed from the outside they might appear to be senseless.

In ordinary and everyday experience, the actions and experiences of others are taken for granted as meaningful, because we see their actions as typical of those performed by other adults in situations that are similar or analogous to our own. We fail to do so in the case of old people living in nursing homes only because our society has tended to segregate dependent and frail old persons from our common experience. In part, this isolation is promoted by the abstract concept of autonomy that dominates American social and political discourse. If one is not robustly independent, then one must be dependent and not autonomous. The advantages afforded by the concept of actual autonomy in thinking about the ethics of nursing home residents are due largely to directing our attention away from the ideals of autonomy, and back to the everyday reality of autonomy. This everyday reality of autonomy in nursing homes is far more continuous with everyday autonomy outside these settings. Attention to actual autonomy importantly turns us away from the abstract language of ethics and redirects us to the concrete lives of the old people themselves.

SUMMARY

This chapter discusses why the preservation of autonomy for those living long-term care facilities is often difficult. Given the mission of nursing homes, a conflict can exist between protection of the resident and his or her autonomy. Therefore, in these situations, autonomy must be based on the identity of the elder. Agich points out that elders can have autonomy in nursing homes if we consider them as individuals. We must also provide them with the most important aspects of autonomy: dignity and self-expression.

QUESTIONS FOR DISCUSSION

1. Why do you think that it is important to use a broader definition of autonomy when dealing with nursing home residents?
2. What is the connection between autonomy and choice?
3. Why are the issues of safety and home-like environment so important for the ability to exercise autonomy as a nursing home resident?
4. Does dependence mean that you cannot have autonomy?
5. After reading this chapter, what advice would you give to a family member who needs to decide about institutional care for a loved one?

NOTES

1. I. Berlin, *Four Essays on Liberty* (Oxford, England: Oxford University Press, 1969), 118–172.

2. J. F. Gubrium, *Living and Dying at Murray Manor* (New York: St. Martin's Press, 1975); C. Laird, *Limbo: A Memoir of Life in a Nursing Home by a Survivor* (Novato, CA: Chandler and Sharp, 1979); C. W. Lidz, L. Fischer, and R. M. Arnold, *The Erosion of Autonomy in Long-Term Care* (New York and Oxford, England: Oxford University Press, 1992); M. O'Brien, *Anatomy of a Nursing Home: A New View of Residential Life* (Owings Mills, MD: National Health Publishing, 1989); J. S. Savishinsky, *The Ends of Time: Life and Work in a Nursing Home* (New York: Bergen & Garvey, 1991); R. R. Shield, *Uneasy Endings: Daily Life in an American Nursing Home* (Ithaca, NY, and London: Cornell University Press, 1988); M. Vesperi, "The Reluctant Consumer: Nursing Home Residents in the Post-Bergman Era," in *Growing Old in Different Societies: Cross-Cultural Perspectives*, J. Sokolovsky, ed. (Belmont, CA: Wadsworth, 1983), 225–237; and W. Watson and R. Maxwell, *Human Aging and Dying: A Study in Sociocultural Gerontology* (New York: St. Martin's Press, 1977).

3. J. Christman, "Constructing the Inner Citadel: Recent Work on the Concept of Autonomy," *Ethics* 99 (October 1988): 109–124.

4. G. J. Agich, *Dependence and Autonomy in Old Age: An Ethical Framework for Long-Term Care* (Cambridge: Cambridge University Press, 2003), 13–50.

5. E. Goffman, "Characteristics of Total Institutions," in *Identity and Anxiety: Survival of the Person in Mass Society*, M. R. Stein, A. J. Vidich, and D. M. White, eds. (Glencoe, IL: Free Press, 1960), 449–479; E Goffman, *Asylums: Essays on the Social Situation of Mental Patients and Other Inmates* (Chicago: Aldine Publishing Co., 1962).

6. B. F. Hofland, "Introduction," *Generations* 14 (Supplement, 1990): 5–8.

7. P. S. Appelbaum and T. G. Gutheil, "Rotting with Their Rights On: Constitutional Theory and Reality in Drug Refusal by Psychiatric Patients," *Bulletin of the American Journal of Psychiatry in the Law* 7 (1979): 308–317; T. G. Gutheil and P. S. Appelbaum, "The Patient Always Pays: Reflections on the Boston State Case and the Right to Rot," *Man and Medicine* 5 (1980): 3–11.

8. Agich, op. cit., 83–124.

9. G. J. Agich, "Reassessing Autonomy in Long-Term Care," *Hastings Center Report* 20, no. 6 (1990): 12–17.

10. F. Bergmann stresses that identity precedes autonomy in his book, *On Being Free* (Notre Dame, IN: University of Notre Dame Press, 1977).

11. A. Jameton, "In the Border Lands of Autonomy: Responsibility in Long-Term Care Facilities," *Gerontologist* 28 (Supplement, June 1988): 18–23.

12. Gubrium, op. cit., 123–157

13. Some research suggests that the physical activity is correlated with better quality of life in older adults. H. Elderly, et al., "A Randomized Trial Comparing Aerobic Exercise and Resistant Exercise with a Health Education Program in Older Adults with Osteoarthritis: The Fitness Arthritis and Seniors Trial (VAST)," *JAMA* 277, no. 1 (January 1977): 25–31; A. C. King, et al., "Moderate-Intensity Exercise and Self-Rated Quality of Sleep in Older Adults: A Randomized Control Trial," *JAMA* 277, no. 1 (January 1977): 32–37; D. M. Buchner, "Physical Activity and Quality of Life in Older Adults," *JAMA* 277, no. 1 (January 1977): 64–66.

14. A. E. Buchanan and D. W. Brock, *Deciding for Others: The Ethics of Surrogate Decision Making* (Cambridge, England: Cambridge University Press, 1989).

15. A. Jameton, "Let My Persons Go! Restraints of the Trade: Case Commentary," in *Everyday Ethics: Resolving Dilemmas in a Nursing Home Life*, R. A. Kane and A. L. Caplan, eds. (New York: Springer, 1990), 166-177; B. J. Collopy, "Safety and Independence: Rethinking Some Basic Concepts in Long-Term Care," in *Long-Term Care Decisions: Ethical and Conceptual Dimensions*, L. B. McCullough and N. L. Wilson, eds. (Baltimore: Johns Hopkins University Press, 1995), 137–152.

16. E. Capezuti, N. E. Strumpf, L. K. Evans, J. A. Grisso, and G. Maislin, "The Relationship between Physical Restraint Removal and Falls and Injuries among Nursing Home Residents," *Journals of Gerontology Series A: Biological Sciences and Medical Sciences* 53, no. 1 (1998): M47–M52; L. K. Evans, N.E. Strumpf, S. L. Len-Taylor, E. Capezuti, G. Maislin, and B. Jacobsen, "A Clinical Trial to Reduce Restraints in Nursing Homes," *Journal of the American Geriatrics Society* 45, no. 6 (1997): 675–681; R. R. Neufeld, L. S. Libow, W. J. Foley, J. M. Dunbar, C. Cohen, and B. Breuer, "Restraint Reduction Reduces Serious Injuries Among Nursing Home Residents," *Journal of the American Geriatrics Society* 47, no. 10 (1999): 1202–1207.

17. T. Diamond, "Social Policy and Everyday Life in Nursing Homes: A Critical Ethnography," *Social Science and Medicine* 23 (1986): 1287–1295; Gubrium, op. cit.

18. Gubrium, op. cit., 161–168.

19. U. Cohen and G. D. Weisman, "Environmental Design to Maximize Autonomy for Older Adults with Cognitive Impairments," *Generations* 14 (Supplement 1990): 75–78.

20. U. Cohen and G. D. Weisman, *Holding onto Home: Designing Environments for People with Dementia* (Baltimore: Johns Hopkins University Press, 1991).

21. Collopy, op. cit.

22. These points are central in recent feminist or care ethics. See, for example, E. Bushnell, Dana (ed.), *Nagging Questions: Feminist Ethics in Everyday Life* (Lanham, MA: Rowman & Littlefield Publishers Inc, 1995); M. A. Fineman, *The Autonomy Myth: A Theory of Dependency* (New York and London: The New Press, 2004); E. F. Kittay and E. K. Feder, *The Subject of Care: Feminist Perspectives on Dependency* (Lanham, MA: Rowman and Littlefield Publishers, Inc, 2002); C. Mackenzie and N. Stoljar, *Relational Autonomy: Feminist Perspectives on Autonomy, Agency, and the Social Self* (New York and Oxford: Oxford University Press, 2002); N. Noddings, *Caring: A Feminine Approach to Ethics and Moral Education* (Berkeley: University of California Press, 2005).

23. J. Cohen-Mansfield and N. Billig, "Agitated Behaviors in the Elderly I: A Conceptual Review," *Journal of the American Geriatric Society* 34 (1986): 711–721; "Agitated Behaviors in the Elderly II: Preliminary Results in the Cognitively Deteriorated," *Journal of the American Geriatric Society* 34 (1986): 722–727.

24. J. Drane, "Competency to Give an Informed Consent," *Journal of the American Medical Association* 282 (1984): 925–927.

25. Diamond, op. cit., 1289–1290.

CHAPTER 11

Death, Medicine, and the Moral Significance of Family Decision Making*

James Lindemann Nelson

OVERVIEW

In this chapter, Nelson examines some of the fallacies and facts about dying. He makes a case against the assumptions surrounding the romantic view of death, including that all patients experience transformation and have the need to be protected from the evils of family decisions. His chapter reinforces that the events in the well-publicized Terri Schiavo case are the exception, not the rule, in end-of-life events. Pay attention to his explanations for why advance directives are not well utilized and what alternatives might need to be considered. Consider the differing views of dying held by the individual, the family, and the hospital.

INTRODUCTION

The Death of Ivan Ilych is one of the best-known pieces in literature, a staple of undergraduate curricula.[1] Having access to the title, readers know what's going to happen right from the start: As though to eliminate any possible doubt, we watch the unfolding of Ivan's life, character, and relationships in flashback from his obsequies. Ivan himself, of course, is not so advantageously positioned. A good part of the story's drama consists precisely of his coming to understand that his illness is fatal. This task turns out to be complex and difficult, marked by ambivalence, insight, and denial.

Ivan's story offers us a powerful and particular image of what is involved in coming to grips with dying. It stresses the importance of the jobs we have to do as our lives come to a close and the value of the insights we can then gain. It also offers an equally forceful and vivid image of the place of the family at the end of life, one that highlights the falsity that permeates relationships and the unreliability of those who are closest to us.

Tolstoy wrote Ivan Ilych in 1886. We die differently now, many of us in hospitals, many in the aftermath of some deliberation and choice about using, withholding, or withdrawing therapies. Should a very-low-birth-weight, brain-damaged baby be removed from her ventilator, a step that will end her suffering, but also any chance she has at life? Should an elderly man with "multiple-organ failure" undergo the violence of cardiopulmonary resuscitation if his heart stops, trading a peaceful death for a tiny chance at staying

*Reprinted with permission from J. L. Nelson, "Death, Medicine, and the Moral Significance of Family Decision Making" *Michigan Family Review* 1, © (1995).

alive long enough to leave the hospital? Contemporary medicine has introduced new complexities into dying, complexities that often force patients and their families into making choices of a sort Ivan did not face. Yet current clinical practice and legal and ethical policy concerning those decisions reflect a very Tolstoyan construction of what is at stake and what is in danger.

The response of Ivan's family to his dying was not notable for its moral insight. This fact is most marked by the translucent curtain of deceit with which his family veils Ivan's descent to death. Ivan is dying, but his dying is a forbidden subject; Ivan in particular must not acknowledge or even allude to it. The terrible consequence is that he must suffer his dying without familial recognition:

> What tormented Ivan Ilych most was the deception, the lie, which for some reason they all accepted, that he was not dying but was simply ill, and that he only need keep quiet and undergo a treatment and then something very good would result . . . this deception tortured him—their not wishing to admit what they all knew and what he knew, but wanting to lie to him concerning his terrible condition and wishing and forcing him to participate in that lie.[2]

In this chapter, I pose a counter image to Tolstoy, in two parts. My leading idea will be that our most intimate connections—which is what I will take "family" to mean here—will often have very important constructive roles to play in the tasks we face as our lives come to a close. But I will also underscore the fact that families are often deeply involved in those tasks and significantly affected by how they are discharged. Accordingly, I will argue that families ought to have some say in how pertinent choices are made. Both these considerations should enrich and help direct our policy concerning end-of-life decision making.

THE STANDARD APPROACH: ROMANTICIZING DEATH, DEMONIZING FAMILIES

We enjoy a considerable measure of social consensus that treatment too burdensome for the benefits it promises may be withheld or withdrawn—even if rejection of treatment is tantamount to acceptance of death. This consensus was perhaps most clearly flagged by the Supreme Court's decision in *Cruzan vs. Missouri Department of Health*,[3] which upheld a patient's right to decide against life-sustaining therapy. There has also been wide agreement that such decisions are solely authorized by the principle of patient autonomy; that is, the moral claim that people enjoy a certain kind of sovereignty over what interventions in their bodies are consistent with their values, and which are not.[4]

This consensus has a certain instability packed in it. Economic pressures and a reassertion of the autonomy of healthcare professionals have led some to think that life-prolonging health care can in principle be withheld despite patient/family desires, if it is expensive enough,[5] or withdrawn over patient/family objection, or if the odds of it working are low enough.[6] But the major practical problem with the patient sovereignty view has been that when people are sick enough to require decision making of this kind, they are often too sick to make any decisions at all. For the past few decades, states have been experimenting with different means of extending a person's decision-making authority regarding health care, a movement culminating in the federal Patient Self-Determination Act of 1990, which mandates that all patients be informed of the procedures approved by their state for directing their health care even if they should become incapacitated.

Practically speaking, what this boils down to is allowing other people to convey a patient's treatment preferences if the patient cannot exercise this authority in his or her own voice at the time a decision is required. Others might assist in the interpretation of "living wills," or, more generally, written treatment directives, which are often both vague and ambiguous. They may simply make a decision as the patient's proxy, trying to judge as the patient would have judged. But in either case, the interpreter or proxy decision maker enjoys the position by virtue of relationship to the will of the patient: either because the proxy had been explicitly delegated to fill these roles, or in the absence of an explicit declaration made by the patient, because he or she is assumed to be able to transmit or reproduce the patient's preferences better than anyone else.

The natural assumption is that close relatives will typically be in the best position to decide. But there is an equally natural objection: Family members hardly count as disinterested parties. Because of their very closeness, relatives often have a sizable stake in how treatment decisions go, and if their interests influence the decision making, the orthodoxy regards the process as morally contaminated.

This "standard approach" to end-of-life decision making shares the suspicion about intimates found in Tolstoy's depiction of Ivan's decidedly nasty family, in which those who have some kind of relationship to the dying man—his wife and adult daughter—don't love him, and those who do—which is to say, his young son—seem to be permitted no relationship to him. Our thinking about end-of-life decision making, particularly concerning patients who cannot make decisions on their own behalf, seems to be haunted by specters closely resembling Ivan's wife and daughter, who saw him largely as a means to fulfilling their own desires. Therefore, judgments about starting or stopping life-sustaining therapy are carefully guarded to prevent such manipulation of vulnerable people.

Family members, then, have no standing simply as family members, but only as conduits to the preferences that the patient actually had, or would have had. If their interests influence whether medical treatment of various kinds continues or not, then the patient is at great risk of abuse: either suffering the continual burdens of invasive care for an inadequate goal, or forgoing desired care and with it the chance to extend life.

In fact, the picture for families is even darker. Not only are their motives suspect; it turns out that even their readings of the patient's desires are questionable. Recent studies of proxy decision making have indicated that families are, as it turns out, not very good at guessing the preferences of their relatives when it comes to the end of life.[7] In the standard view, then, their main claim to decision-making authority is undermined, while the main caution against them seems as strong as ever.

The picture for incompetent patients also appears grimmer than has yet been suggested. What they have at stake is not simply the possibility of undergoing extended discomfort or premature death because their families are either mistaken about their preferences or malignantly indifferent to them. Equally significant is the loss of the ability to invest their deaths with the kind of meaning that best comports with their sense of their life overall. Ivan Ilych provides us with a hint of this theme. Recall his painful examination of his life, his insight into how misdirected and trivial he had allowed his life to become, and how his final task is to accept himself, and his suffering, and hence to achieve salvation.

The idea that there is often a "terminal perspective" on life, from which we can get an especially accurate view of our lives, and the idea that how we end our lives, is crucial to the success or failure of those lives overall, strike me as at least loosely linked. Together they make up what might be called a romantic view of death, clearly present in Tolstoy, and not at all foreign to contemporary sensibilities. Consider this passage from *Life's Dominion*, by the influential philosopher and legal scholar, Ronald Dworkin:

> There is no doubt that most people treat the manner of their deaths as of special, symbolic importance: they want their deaths, if possible, to express and in that way vividly to confirm the values they believe most important to their lives.[8]

Whether or not Dworkin is right about "most people" on this point, he is, I think, surely right about what most ethical and legal theorists think when they take up the issue of how choices should be made at the end of life. We find here another significant reason why our evolving policy on this matter has, since the 1970s, been directed toward empowering patients. It isn't simply to defend them from assaults on what Dworkin would call their "experiential"[9] interests, or how things feel to them: It is also to protect their ability to live and die in accordance with their "critical" interests; that is, with their reflective sense of what is truly significant and characteristic about their lives. How we die is of particular significance to whether or not our critical interest in having lived a good life is achieved, and it is crucial to our achieving such a life that our deaths be as much as possible orchestrated according to our own ideas.

A REVISED ACCOUNT: DYING IN INTIMACY

The contemporary context of decision making in the face of death, then, is in very important respects much the same as it was in the late nineteenth century. We are cynical about families, romantic about death. What's wrong with this standard "Tolstoyan" concept of the significance of death and the suspicious character of families? In my view, pretty much everything.

This is not to say that there are no abusive and otherwise untrustworthy families out there. Nor is it to deny that for some people the process of dying is transformative, offering new and deep insights. Finally, I am not implacably hostile to the idea that the way we die can be crucial to the success or otherwise of our lives overall. Rather, my attitude toward these claims is that they are all overstated; they ought not to be taken as the predominating feature of either families or death. Many have families who are not decidedly nasty; many die without gaining deep insights into the nature of things. In addition, many can have bad deaths who had quite acceptable lives overall. Many have good deaths that are not good because they, personally or through carefully directed proxies, have orchestrated every step. The worst of the overstatement is what might be regarded as its cumulative implication: We face death alone most often as "vulnerable adults" whose chief need is protection from rapacious relatives.

General practice, as opposed to policy and theory, indicates that my misgivings about this tableau are not idiosyncratic. Relatively few people avail themselves of formal advance directives, despite the publicity given to the importance of advance healthcare planning; the few who do draw up such directives tend to be disproportionately white, well-off, and well-educated. While there are many possible explanations here, one plausible suggestion is that different subcultures within our nation have different views about how important it is to take a direct hand in end-of-life decision making.

Part of the problem may be that medical practice and legal policy regarding death correctly assume that most people want to die well, but that both practice and policy are confused about what dying well means to many of us. Doing something "well" does not necessarily mean doing it according to our own self-regarding desires; it may mean acting in accord with what strikes us as right, seemly, meet—where these notions guide us in ways that we believe to be good in themselves, and not simply because we happen to accept them. More particularly, many of us may believe that our deaths should cohere with a life lived in important connection with other people. The course of our dying should express concern about their burdens, not because doing so is the crucial task of our lives, nor because death has vouchsafed to us some special moral insight at the end, but because such concern is consistent with long-held views about how to live well, views that need not be abandoned when the job at hand is how to die well.

Not simply speculation, but data drawn largely from the work of High,[10] show that many people feel no need to file a formal document because they think of their families as their advance directives. The Harvard-based medical ethicists Linda and Ezekiel Emanuel[11] have wondered whether High's results do not simply reflect most people's uncritical acceptance of the view that families know best what we ourselves would want, and that this enthusiasm for relatives would not survive the growing evidence to the contrary. But their critique makes two crucial assumptions. First, it assumes that the kind of medical choices that are open to us as we die are typically such that we have considered preferences about them, preferences expressing something that matters to us deeply. It also assumes, perhaps even more significantly, that our choices rule the day, however they might affect the interests of those with whom we have been intimate.

But both these assumptions seem unwarranted. The legal theorist Patricia White, drawing on her experience in the presumably less emotionally charged area of estate planning, has pointed out that "people find it difficult to predict accurately how they would react to some hypothetical future crisis."[12] The idea, then, that the job of a proxy decision maker is to somehow elicit just what the patient would have wanted if the patient could speak in the present situation assumes that there is some one thing he or she would have wanted, and this assumption may well be false.

One of course could simply make determinations about one's future care, rather than predictions. That is, the decision maker would be exerting her autonomy now, reflecting her current preferences, rather than making a guess about what she would want in a future in which she is incapacitated, if, contrary to fact, she could make a considered decision at that time. But if we are to understand advance decision making as a determination rather than as a prediction, then it isn't clear that decision making at the end of life retains the kind of special moral significance the romantic perspective gave it. Dying "romantically"—i.e., in a way that reflects something crucially important about your life—might well require, not a blunt determination now of how a future event should be handled, but fine-grained sensitivity to the details of that future time. How much pain or discomfort is at issue? What are the chances that a medical intervention will achieve its end, and at what cost to the patient or to others the patient cares about? It is not implausible that making decisions of this kind could, in principle, allow the decision maker an opportunity to express and even develop her moral character. But, if so, what would allow her this opportunity is the ability to fit her decision precisely to the circumstances.

The result is that it is far from clear that all, or even many, of the preferences healthy self-aware people have about hypothetical future crises really count as considered or authoritative in any event. And we have yet to consider the point that, even if we assume incompetent patients typically have well-considered and well-ordered preferences that others might put into practice, the interests of their families remain morally relevant to decision making even if those interests run counter to patient preferences.

As John Hardwig[13] has powerfully argued, there is no good reason to think that the ill are totally excused from their moral obligations to their intimates simply because of their illness. Nor is it appropriate to think that family members are required to bear any imaginable burden to further any interest of a relative if that interest happens to be medical. Not a plea to endorse selfishness, the standard approach to decision making at the end of life proceeds as though selfishness were the appropriate standard. The patient's needs must be served, and the only way to assure they are met is to forbid family members to think of anything other than what the patient would.

However, families quite often have a different way of organizing the distribution of caring work that goes on within them. Sometimes that organization may be open to moral criticism—as when women are assigned an unequal share of caring labor simply because they are women—but the very fact that they distribute the family's resources in a way that is sensitive to many needs ought not to be regarded as beyond the moral pale simply on its face. Maintaining that proxy decision making by family members is to be censured is particularly ironic in the present context of healthcare delivery, in which the medical interests of patients are sometimes subordinated to the needs of the health maintenance organization in which they are enrolled, or the resources their state is willing to make available for Medicaid.

It is on the basis of considerations of this sort that I think that Ivan Ilych's sort of death ought to be seen as unusual—fit to be the subject of an immortal short story—rather than as a good guide to what challenges and choices people will regularly face as they die. We need not construct a policy that assumes families are to be carefully controlled, suspected of guilt until proven innocent. We need not think that putting our own stamp on the precise character of our death is a crucial determinant of the quality of our lives. Therefore, we need not be so enamored of systems that rely primarily on explicit advance directives, seeing their authority as stemming solely from the patient and, in effect, disadvantaging the many patients and families without advance directives to whom death will come. It seems to me both more realistic, as well as quite defensible morally, to reverse the burden of proof here. We ought to recognize that families have a certain kind of moral authority to serve as proxies, unless perhaps the patient has made an explicit declaration to the contrary, or unless that authority is misused to a point that constitutes abuse.

But this strategy is only part of what should be an overall rethinking of the contexts in which we die, and the assumptions that are prevalent in those contexts—assumptions that tend to undermine the kind of closeness that very ill patients can have with their families. Healthcare institutions should be set up to be as transparent as possible to these connections, which is not now the case. Hospitals, for example, remain places in which certain value commitments are evident and powerful. They are hierarchical, unfamiliar places that separate you from daily routines and common sources of identity affirmation, running all the way from your own clothes to your most intimate connections. Hospitals have their own clear agenda to which patients are strongly invited to subscribe. The notion that patients need to be empowered in such settings is exactly right; the mistake is in thinking this is likely to happen if patients are allowed to be alienated from their own sources of personal affirmation and authority in the name of giving such authority formal protection.

CONCLUSION

It might be alleged that, the institutional structure of healthcare systems apart, the decision-making system currently in place for incapacitated people is actually very well suited to accommodate just the values sketched out here. Many people have families in which there are people whom they trust. Many people do not think it essential that their death reflect precisely what their own decisions would have been, had they been able to make them directly. Such people can easily execute advance directives that say, in effect, "My spouse gets to decide any feature of my medical care, if I am not able to do so." For those people who either do not trust their families, or do not wish to burden them with the task of making end-of-life decisions, appointing non-family proxies will be possible. For people who think that it is crucial that the circumstances of their deaths fit as closely as possible some overriding concept of the integrity of their lives, more specific treatment directives are possible.

What really gets left out of the standard view? This very reasonable question has a pragmatic answer, to which I have already alluded, and a rather deeper answer. The pragmatic response is simply that the majority of people will, for the foreseeable future, die without a formal advance directive. At the very least, this fact suggests that we pay more attention to how to make health-care decisions for this group of people. The most reasonable response would seem to be a system of proxies arranged in descending order of priority: spouse, adult children, parents, siblings, and so on. This system would certainly not be without problems—for instance, understanding what "spouse" means in a society where people often live together without formal marriage—but it would at least have the right scope and the right slant. Individuals who felt uncomfortable with the ordering or wanted to leave specific instructions to their proxies would be within their rights to execute specific directives to change it.

The deeper reason is that the standard approach is not neutral among different views of what a person owes to his or her family, or more broadly, of the nature of intimate connections. It contains a certain expressive force suggesting that our intimate ties are insignificant unless formalized by an explicit exercise of our own sovereign authority. This view is neither self-evidently true, nor altogether innocuous with regard to its impact on how we think about family ties generally in this society. Rereading Ivan Ilych reminds us that skepticism about the family is not a new phenomenon, but should not distract us from the distinct possibility that new forms of defensiveness about intimate connections can make things worse, as well as better.

SUMMARY

In this chapter, Nelson first introduces the romantic view of death which tends to present families in a negative way. He then takes the position that this view is overstated and does not present the reality the dying process. Instead, he discusses the dying process as one which includes the family. He also suggests that the ill may even have a moral obligation toward them. Finally, he suggests that the healthcare system should rethink how it provides for people who are dying and honor role of the family in this process.

QUESTIONS FOR DISCUSSION

1. Consider the issue of autonomy as it applies to end-of-life decisions. Nelson says that selfishness is not the standard for autonomy at the exclusion of the family. What do you think autonomy means at the end of life?

2. If Nelson continues to be correct about advance directives, how should an organization handle end-of-life decisions when patients cannot articulate their wishes?

3. Do you agree with Hardwig that the ill have moral obligations to their family members? If so, what obligations do they have?

4. Some have said that we make policy based on the actions of a minority rather than for the majority. Given Nelson's argument, do you think advance directives as a policy are too limited?

5. What is your ethical obligation as a healthcare professional toward those who are at the end of their lives?

NOTES

1. L. Tolstoy, *The Death of Ivan Ilych and Other Stories*, trans. Alymer Maude (1866; reprint, New York: New American Library, 1960).

2. Ibid., 137.

3. *Cruzan v. Director, Missouri Department of Health* (1990) 110 Ct. 2841.

4. R. Faden and T. Beauchamp, *A History and Theory of Informed Consent* (New York: Oxford University Press, 1986); A. Buchanan and D. Brock, *Deciding for Others* (Cambridge: Cambridge University Press, 1989).

5. L. Fleck, "Just Health Care Rationing: A Democratic Decision Making Approach," *University of Pennsylvania Law Review* 140 (1992): 1597–1636.

6. T. Tomlinson and H. Brody, "Futility and the Ethics of Resuscitation," *Journal of the American Medical Association* 264 (1990): 849–860.

7. A. Seckler, et al., "Substituted Judgment: How Accurate Are Proxy Predictions?" *Annals of Internal Medicine* 151 (1991): 1276–1280; E. Emanuel and L. Emanuel, "Proxy Decision Making: An Ethical and Empirical Analysis," *JAMA* 267 (1992): 2067–2071; D. Shalowitz, E. Garret-Mayer, and D. Wendler, "The Accuracy of Surrogate Decision Makers: A Systematic Review," *Archives of Internal Medicine* 166 (2006): 493–497.

8. R. Dworkin, *Life's Dominion* (New York: Knopf, 1993), 211.

9. Ibid.

10. D. High, "All in the Family: Extended Autonomy and Expectations in Surrogate Health Care Decision Making," *Gerontologist* 28 (1988): 46–51; id., "Why Are Elderly People Not Using Advance Directives?" *Journal of Aging and Health* 5 (1993): 497–515; id., "Families' Roles in Advance Directives," *Hastings Center Report* 24 (Special suppl. 1994): 516–518.

11. Emanuel and Emanuel, op. cit.

12. P. White, "Appointing a Proxy under the Best of Circumstances," *Utah Law Review* (1992): 849–860.

13. J. Hardwig, "What about the Family?" *Hastings Center Report* 20 (1990): 5–10.

CHAPTER 12

Ethical Issues in the Use of Fluids and Nutrition: When Can They Be Withdrawn?

T. Patrick Hill

OVERVIEW

In his thoughtful chapter, Hill tackles the difficult question of when it is ethically sound to withhold or withdraw artificial nutrition and hydration. With the aging of America in the twenty-first century, this issue will certainly be one that will challenge us emotionally and ethically. Hill discusses the conflict between the right of the patient to control his or her dying process and society's right to preserve life. He also examines how the patient's rights can conflict with the medical staff's need for integrity. Using a discussion of balancing benefits and burdens, he demonstrates that providing these supportive actions, though viewed as merciful, may actually cause the patient harm.

INTRODUCTION

It has been some time since the landmark decisions regarding Karen Ann Quinlan[1] and Nancy Beth Cruzan[2] were handed down. Since then, it has been reasonable to think that the ethical issues central to these cases and others like them have been resolved and were settled matters. Conceptually that may be the case, but as the recent case of Terri Schiavo demonstrated, that is not true emotionally. There it seemed as though we were confronting the issues for the very first time without any precedent to guide us. And when dealing with a case that had finally exhausted our medically capacity to remedy, some tried literally to will a remedy out of conviction, regardless of credible clinical evidence to the contrary.

Conceivably, for this reason the issue of withholding and withdrawing artificial nutrition and hydration from dying and permanently unconscious patients remains contentious, deserving of renewed ethical consideration. It helps to measure the gravity of the problem when we remember that between 10,000 and 60,000 dying or permanently unconscious patients are actually maintained on sustenance supplied artificially by tubes.

In the case of one million recovering patients who annually receive artificial nutrition and hydration, no one doubts that artificial sustenance is a boon. But for those patients who, with or without artificially provided sustenance, have no hope of recovering from their illness, supplying nutrition and hydration might be as inappropriate as maintaining a brain-dead body on a ventilator. "Yet, perhaps because of the uniquely symbolic significance of nourishment in the minds of many, artificial feeding appears to be more difficult to discontinue than any other treatment. And this applies both to patients who are expected to die in a relatively short time, and to permanently uncon-scious and other patients whose death may not occur for months or years unless sustenance by tube is stopped."[3]

Is there something intuitively sound about this symbolism? If so, does it jus-tify the difficulty we feel when we consider discontinuing artificial feeding? Or is it possible on the basis of rational analysis to come to the conclusion that there are indeed sound ethical reasons why we should withhold or withdraw artificial nutrition and hydration? This chapter will attempt to show that in the case of dying and permanently unconscious patients, our intuitive sensi-tivity to the symbolism of nourishment notwithstanding, there are solid ethi-cal grounds for discontinuing artificial sustenance and permitting death from natural causes to occur.

The ethical questions surrounding the withdrawal of fluids and nutrition from a dying patient are more complicated in one significant respect than the withdrawal of any other life-sustaining treatment, such as antibiotics or car-diopulmonary resuscitation. The basic medical justification for the with-drawal of antibiotics, for example, is that under a particular set of clinical circumstances, they can no longer achieve their clinical purpose. When that happens, the fundamental ethical justification for withdrawal would come from the absence of any inherent value, again under these particular circum-stances, in continuing to provide antibiotics. The ensuing death of the patient is medically acceptable on the grounds that it results from an underlying pathology now no longer considered treatable. The death is ethically accept-able as something that has happened in the natural course of events, in this case, the inevitable progress of a fatal illness over which there is now no human control and for which there is no human responsibility. It is regret-table, but regrettable as a nonmoral harm.

Fluids and nutrition used in the care of a dying patient do not fit quite as readily into this line of medical and ethical reasoning because they are not therapeutic, in the strict sense of that term. But if not therapeutic, how are they to be understood? The question is basic and suggests two possible responses. The first, coming from the general perspective of the healthcare provider, is that fluids and nutrition function as a clinical scaffold to provide underlying support to a patient who cannot provide it from his or her own diminished resources. The second, coming from the perspective of family members and friends, is that fluids and nutrition serve as expressions of their instinct to be concerned and to care when hope for loved ones is exhausted. Neither medicine for the nurse and physician, nor food and water for the lay person, fluids and nutrition seem to confound us all and leave, as Quinlan, Cruzan, and Schiavo illustrate, their recipients at the mercy of an unavoidable ambiguity. Although public opinion polls suggest that the aver-age person is critical of the continued use of fluids and nutrition in medically hopeless circumstances,[4] that can change when it becomes a personal deci-sion to withhold or withdraw from a particular individual. Then the inherent ambiguity of fluids and nutrition can assert itself forcefully and painfully. When it does we have been inclined to respond first by saying that fluids and nutrition embody the natural instinct to care for the most vulnerable, the dying, when all hope of cure is gone. We can then go on to assert that they can serve to draw the distinction between cure and care in the medical setting. That is, a point might occur in the course of illness beyond which therapeutic treatment is useless and can, as a result, be stopped or withheld; it appears counterintuitive to say the same of care.

There is no medical justification for ceasing to provide care to a dying patient, and because there is always inherent value in providing care, there is no ethical justification for withholding it either. According to this line of reasoning, as long as fluids and nutrition are seen only as being a means of caring for, not curing, a dying patient, there would be no medical or ethical justification for withholding them in some form or another or in some degree or another. However, this line of thinking only confuses matters, because fluids and nutrition can hardly be thought of as therapy, except as a way to correct chemical imbalances in the body due to malnutrition and dehydration. As far as providing care goes, fluids and nutrition are not by definition care in themselves, but something we choose as an expression of our instinct to provide care. Ample evidence suggests, for example, in the coroner's report on Terri Schiavo that the continued provision of fluids and nutrition were more harmful to her than not.[5]

Consequently, it is of paramount importance to determine what fluids and nutrition are and when they can be regarded as having a medical purpose of maintenance in addition to that of providing human care. Beyond that, it is important to determine if and when the provision of fluids and nutrition to a dying patient serves no medical purpose and does not objectively constitute the provision of human care to that patient no matter how much we might subjectively like to think that it does.

To do this, it is necessary to acknowledge the difference between food and drink, on the one hand, and artificial nutrition and hydration, on the other. According to Devine,

> The common forms of eating and drinking are not at issue; this is not a matter of denying a person a lunch. At issue here is a range of medical technologies that vary in complexity, sophistication and, at times, danger. Total parental feeding is a world apart from dining on fried chicken, and the difference between them is obvious.[6]

There is a universal need for food and drink to sustain life. There is no such need for artificial nutrition and hydration to sustain life. As a universal need, food and drink might best be seen as a means of human care. Artificial nutrition and hydration, however, because they are designed to address a medical condition, such as a temporary or permanent inability to swallow, are better seen as a form of medical maintenance. Consequently, their use and purposes will be determined by the patient's diagnosis and prognosis.

Understood this way, according to Devine, artificial nutrition and hydration are an integral part of a larger medical effort to restore someone to health or maintain that person at a certain level of human functioning. But when that effort ceases overall to have a medical purpose, nutrition and hydration, as a constitutive part of the effort, also cease to have any purpose.[7] In other words, just as the purposes of the medical treatment plan for the patient justify the decision to provide nutrition and hydration, so, too, any eventual purposelessness of the same medical treatment plan can justify the cessation of treatment, including nutrition and hydration.

The difference between food and water and nutrition and hydration is then an important consideration when making an ethical decision to withhold the latter. So also is the difference between hunger and thirst and malnutrition and dehydration. A 1987 report by the Hastings Center draws the distinction by describing hunger and thirst as a need felt by the patient and defining malnutrition and dehydration as a chemical condition of the patient's body:

> Medical procedures for supplying nutrition and hydration treat malnutrition and dehydration; they may or may not relieve hunger and thirst. Conversely, hunger and thirst can be treated without necessarily using medical nutrition and hydration techniques, and without necessarily correcting dehydration or malnourishment.[8]

To support the validity of this distinction, the report observes that dehydrated patients, for example, can find relief from thirst by having their lips and mouths moistened with ice chips or a lubricant.[9] This observation gives additional weight to the argument that hunger and thirst are more appropriately the object of interventions to provide care, whereas malnutrition and dehydration are more appropriately the object of interventions to achieve a larger therapeutic goal in which nutrition and hydration play a supportive role. Once the case has been made for nutrition and hydration as a supportive element within a medical intervention, one can assume that the ethical criteria used in deciding to withdraw other medical life-sustaining treatments are applicable in deciding when to withdraw nutrition and hydration.

The core criterion around which all the others will congregate is the integrity of the patient as a person. Modern medicine operates by isolating symptoms and treating them accordingly. Although this discriminating methodology, which undeniably reflects the sophistication of contemporary medical practice, is highly effective, it runs the serious risk of atomizing the patient, organ by organ, system by system, particularly as a terminal illness runs its course and the body decompensates as a result. Under these circumstances, it is all too easy to lose sight of the person who is the patient and discount the personal control over treatment decisions without which it will be impossible for these decisions to be ethical.

This entails, on the part of those providing medical treatment, the utmost respect for the physical integrity of the body on which the patient has a fundamental claim. Central to any recognition of the physical integrity of the body as a necessary condition for ethical medical interventions is the patient's informed consent. Hence the need for the patient to consent to be treated and the need to respect the patient's refusal to begin or continue treatment. In other words, it must be a basic working assumption on the part of those responsible for treatment, in this case nutrition and hydration, that they may not withdraw them without the patient's consent.

Even more importantly, healthcare providers must recognize that the final authority in the patient-physician relationship is the patient. According to

J. E. Ruark, et al., "[a]lthough physicians must often be authoritative about the options available to patients, all involved must recognize that the actual authority over the patient never resides with the physician. Patients alone, or their legal surrogates, have the right to control what happens to them."[10]

All the requirements for an ethically satisfactory decision to withdraw or withhold nutrition and hydration will not be found in the patient's subjective preferences alone, significant as they are. Without direct reference to the clinical context, namely, the actual medical condition of the patient and its projected course, it would be ethically unacceptable to withhold life-sustaining treatment such as nutrition and hydration. Although it is true that ethical decisions are guided by principles, they are also rooted in the actual circumstances that suggest those particular principles and provide the justification for their use in a given case.

This observation is important because it illustrates an essential feature of ethical analysis, which, according to one ethicist, "is an exchange between the moral meaning found in the empirical context and the moral meaning found in the several principles contending for application in this concrete case."[11] The moral meaning of the empirical context will be measured in terms of bodily integrity and the extent to which withholding life-sustaining treatment will enhance or diminish that integrity. As we have already seen, bodily integrity is something to which the patient has a claim and something that the physician must respect.

The next question then is what is the strength of this claim? How forcefully can the claim to bodily integrity and its corollary, informed consent, be made to justify the decision to withhold or withdraw nutrition and hydration? In responding to this question, ethicists have resorted to the language of rights, saying that bodily integrity is so central to the patient that it can be claimed as a right.

Rights, according to philosophers such as Richard Wasserstrom, are "moral commodities" that automatically create obligations and duties.[12] Similarly, according to Hill, "[i]n other words, a right is a claim, the force of which derives, not from the physical strength or socioeconomic standing of the right holder but the inherent reasonableness of the right being claimed relative to the circumstances under which it is being claimed."[13] Relative to bodily integrity, this implies a patient's claim to discretion over his or her body.

In the context of deciding to withhold or withdraw nutrition and hydration, the implications of such a claim are troublesome, because they create obligations and duties for treatment providers. That could and does result in an adversarial situation as the patient or the physician seeks to control the outcome. In turn, this threatens the moral relationship between the patient and the physician presupposed by the patient's claim and the corresponding responsibilities of the physician. However, this problem has less to do with the concept of rights than it has to do with how we understand their function. Understood as a prerogative of the patient alone to be exercised against the physician, the right to bodily integrity can make it very difficult to achieve "the kind of joint decision-making of all the concerned parties that is required by a full theory of moral responsibility."[14] For this reason, philosophers such as John Ladd prefer to understand rights as claims to something rather than claims against somebody. A distinct advantage of this interpretation is that it presupposes cooperation rather than competition. Another is that rather than requiring particular obligations of particular individuals, rights entail collective responsibilities on the part of society at large. Ladd, therefore, refers to rights as ideal and argues that they "relate to things that a society ought to provide for its members so that they will be able to live a good life, that is, a moral life constituted by moral relationships of responsibility and caring."[15]

If we understand the right to bodily integrity as an ideal right on which the decision to withhold nutrition and hydration can be based, thereby permitting the patient to control the circumstances of his or her death, then the manner of the patient's dying becomes a moral enterprise in the same way that the manner of the patient's life has been a moral enterprise. Therefore, the decision to withhold or withdraw life-sustaining treatment, such as nutrition and hydration, might constitute the patient's most profound moral need at that stage in life. As expressed by Hill, "[a]s such it will be a necessary means to pursue whatever moral goals have been directing his life up to this point and should now be directing the circumstances and time of his death, if the two are to be consonant."[16]

However, rights have a habit of conflicting with other rights, and it is particularly important to understand what this might mean in the present context. The patient's claim to bodily integrity and its corollary, informed consent, in relation to the withdrawal of nutrition and hydration can and does, for example, conflict with society's right to preserve life as an interest central to the integrity of society itself. This conflict lies in one form or another at the heart of the decision to withdraw nutrition and hydration from the patient. As a decision taken in the interests of bodily integrity and informed consent on the part of one individual that leads inevitably to death, it is, potentially at least, a threat to the communal interests society has in the preservation of life in general.

At the same time, both claims can be justified. As a result, neither claim presumably is absolute. It follows then that one or the other claim can only be made legitimately when in doing so the individual does not essentially compromise society and society does not essentially violate the individual. Therefore, any patient decision to withdraw nutrition and hydration, if it is to be ethically acceptable, must not constitute a threat to society's legitimate interests in the preservation of life. The task then becomes one of establishing a working tension between the two claims so that when they do indeed conflict, there is a way to avoid paralysis and achieve a mutually acceptable way of determining which claim, the individual's or society's, should prevail in a given set of circumstances.

In its seminal decision in the case of Karen Ann Quinlan, the New Jersey Supreme Court was acutely conscious of the conflicting claims and of the need to provide a formula by which to resolve the conflict in a way that does justice to both individual and society at the same time: "We think that the State's interests [in the preservation of life] weakens and the individual's right to privacy grows as the degree of bodily invasion increases and the prognosis dims.

Ultimately, there comes a point at which the individual's rights overcome the State interest."[17]

In discussing the ethical criteria to be used in withholding nutrition and hydration, this statement is significant in the way it advances self-determination (or "privacy," as the court called it) by protecting the bodily integrity from futile medical treatment in the face of an increasingly dim prognosis. Where there is less and less hope that medical interventions will do anything for the well-being of the patient, there is a greater justification, should the patient wish it, to withhold life-sustaining treatment such as nutrition and hydration.

So far, this discussion has attempted to lay the ethical foundation for decisions to withhold or withdraw nutrition and hydration from a patient. When either decision is made, the patient will die eventually, raising the question whether such an outcome is, on the face of it, ethically acceptable. The assumption is that it is not. Thus, if death has occurred as a result of the decision to withhold or withdraw nutrition and hydration, it becomes necessary to show that someone has the right to make that decision. If someone does make that decision, what is the basis of that right? Assuming there is some basis for such a right, what circumstances and outcomes would justify its exercise?

The discussion, up to this point, has attempted to show that the individual with the rights to bodily integrity and self-determination would logically be able to exercise those rights by making decisions, for example, to withhold or withdraw medical treatment in general and nutrition and hydration in particular. In drawing the distinction between *care* and *cure* in order to show that nutrition and hydration have more to do with the latter, it becomes possible to see that under appropriate circumstances nutrition and hydration, like any other medical treatment, could be the object of such a decision. The individual is vested with moral authority to make decisions of this kind, and nutrition and hydration fall within the legitimate range of this authority. And even though this moral authority or right is not absolute, conflicting with a state interest in the preservation of life, in some circumstances the individual right to self-determination can take precedence over the state's interest.

It remains now to look at those circumstances as they appear in the clinical setting. Because nutrition and hydration are considered as a supportive element of a larger medical treatment, the decision to withdraw or withhold them will depend in some measure on whether, given the patient's condition, they can provide sufficient benefit without imposing a burden disproportionate to that benefit. Too frequently in this context the discussion of benefits and burdens is conducted in relation to clinical outcomes. Accordingly, the argument goes, when benefits to the patient's well-being are less than the burdens suffered to obtain those benefits, decisions to forgo such treatment are ethically acceptable, even when they hasten death as a result. This is a cogent argument as presented in terms of outcomes. However, the real strength of the argument is derived from the individual's right to bodily integrity and self-determination. Otherwise, what would ethically justify the opposite decision—to start or continue treatment even though its burdens outweigh the benefits?

This is a critical point, because on it rests the principle of self-determination and the correct relationship between the patient and the physician and the responsibility of the physician to provide for informed consent or refusal on the part of the patient. Independently of the patient, the physician can determine that, given the patient's diagnosis and prognosis, all treatment options entail greater burden than benefit. On the face of it then, withholding or withdrawing treatment can medically be the right thing to do. However, this would not be the ethically acceptable thing, at least minus any consideration given to the principle of patient bodily integrity and the principle of self-determination. Neither of these principles can be secure in the absence of consent or refusal from the patient, who realistically can only provide one or the other on the basis of an awareness of the treatment options and a clear grasp of their respective benefits and harms. Therefore, what gives ethical sanction to the outcomes of a decision, in this instance to withdraw nutrition and hydration, is not solely the objective calculation that the burdens of treatment outweigh any benefits. However necessary that calculation is, for ethical purposes it is not sufficient to meet the demands of the bodily integrity and self-determination of the patient. That will come from the patient's consent to or refusal of treatment informed by a calculation of its burden proportionate to the benefits.

We have seen that in this question of withdrawing nutrition and hydration there is a real and legitimate tension between the rights of the individual and the communal interests of the state. A parallel tension exists between the rights of the patient and the legitimate claims to professional integrity on the part of the treating physician. Arguably, this tension is never as clearly drawn as when decisions to withdraw nutrition and hydration are being considered. The fundamental ethical question is whether physicians should be involved at all. What in the patient-physician relationship could justify such a decision? Is there anything in the nature of this relationship that would sanction, for example, an obligation on the part of physicians to accede to a patient's request to withdraw nutrition and hydration over their better professional judgment?

At stake, from the physician's point of view, are professional obligations to treat the patient in order to further his or her well-being and to avoid doing harm. In this situation, the question for the physician is how, clinically, does withdrawing nutrition and hydration benefit a patient and also avoid doing harm? Far from being an oxymoron, the question is reasonable in itself and has been made answerable, in part, as a result of the argument that nutrition and hydration can be considered an element in a larger medical treatment. As such, they are morally neither good nor bad in themselves, so there can be no presumption that they should or should not be administered. Like the withdrawal of other treatments then, such as chemotherapy in the case of a patient in the terminal stages of cancer, the withdrawal of nutrition and hydration should be subjected, as we have already said, to a calculation of its benefits proportionate to its burdens in order to provide objective medical reasons why withdrawal not only benefits the patient but also does not cause harm.

Is this possible? One answer to this question is empirical and will tell us what physiologically happens to a patient from whom nutrition and hydration have been withdrawn. The other is ethical and tells us what becomes of the moral standing of the patient from whom this treatment has been withdrawn.

Let us consider the empirical answer first. According to Paul C. Rousseau, artificial hydration has long been thought to ease the discomfort of terminal illness.[18] He points out, however, that recent studies suggest something very different:

> As death approaches, dehydration occurs naturally from inadequate oral intake, gastrointestinal and renal losses, and the loss of secretions from the skin and lungs. Transitory thirst, dry mouth and changes in mental status have been found to develop—but the headache, nausea, vomiting or cramps frequently associated with water deprivation rarely occur. The mental changes—while upsetting to relatives—bring relief to patients by lessening their awareness of suffering.[19]

Rousseau adds that although the administration of intravenous fluids can produce a feeling of well-being, the feeling can be of short duration: "In time, artificial hydration is likely to heighten the discomfort of a terminally ill patient, and often exacerbates underlying symptoms."[20] Additional clinical evidence supports the assertion that nutrition and hydration can be harmful to the dying patient. According to Ahronheim and colleagues, "[t]ube feeding itself may produce pain; erosions or hemorrhage of the nasal septum, esophagus, and gastral mucosa have been reported; and nasogastric feeding as well as gastrostomy feeding has been associated with aspiration pneumonia."[21] Ahronheim et al. conclude that "withholding or withdrawing artificial feeding and hydration from debilitated patients does not result in gruesome, cruel, or violent death."[22] Indeed, Rousseau would go further on the basis of his clinical evidence. "Accompanied by comfort measures and emotional support, dehydration is a humane therapeutic response to terminal illness."[23] The Hastings Center guidelines arrive at a similar conclusion: "Patients in their last days before death may spontaneously reduce their intake of nutrition and hydration without experiencing hunger or thirst."[24] As a result, decisions to withhold such treatment can meet the physician's twin obligation to do what is in the patient's best interests and to do no harm to the patient.

As persuasive as this clinical evidence is, are there ethical reasons as persuasive that would justify a physician withdrawing or withholding nutrition and hydration in order to do what is in the patient's best interests and do no harm to the patient? Essentially, this question is asking what effect the withdrawal of nutrition and hydration has on the moral standing of the patient. If, as some assert, "life is 'the first right of the human person' and 'the condition of all the others,'"[25] what circumstances would justify a decision that would inevitably lead to the death of the patient?

Kevin O'Rourke, a medical ethicist, addresses the same issue when he asserts that "one of the basic ethical assumptions upon which medicine and efforts to nurse and feed people is based is that life should be prolonged and because living enables us to pursue the purpose of life."[26] Included in the purpose of life are happiness, fulfillment, and human relationships, which, O'Rourke observes, "imply some ability to function at the cognitive-affective, or spiritual, level."[27]

Despite the theological orientation of these two particular assertions, there is nothing in either of them that is not reaffirmed in the traditional presumption in

clinical practice, which is to favor life. Implicit in the question under consideration in this chapter is the possibility that now there are clinical circumstances in
which the presumption in favor of life is no longer ethically acceptable.

To rephrase the question for purposes of ethical analysis, what becomes of
the obligation to prolong life when, despite the continuation of treatment, the
patient will remain alive but will not recover sufficiently to be him or herself
physically, mentally, and psychologically? Recover, that is, to resume the central purposes of his or her life knowingly, willingly, and emotionally. That
implies at least that, before the obligation to prolong life ceases, there is a
level of purposefulness to which the patient ought to be able to lay claim and
to obtain such that the physician can reasonably continue to treat. However, if
no such level can be hoped for given the patient's prognosis, we place an
impossible burden on the patient by continuing to treat: the expectation of life
without the means to appropriate it in any personal sense through mental,
volitional, or emotional behavior. Considered in those terms, there seems
ample justification to agree with O'Rourke when he concludes that "if efforts
to prolong life are useless or result in a severe burden for the patient insofar
as pursuing the purpose of life is concerned, then the ethical obligation to prolong life is no longer present."[28]

This is an ethical argument for withholding or withdrawing nutrition and
hydration from the patient; it should not be confused with the clinical argument for withholding or withdrawing nutrition and hydration from the
patient on the grounds that their use imposes burdens disproportionate to any
benefits. However, the basis for making this particular ethical argument rests
in part on the clinical calculation that the burdens of treatment will outweigh
its benefits. The clinical calculation is necessary but not sufficient to make the
ethical argument. It is important to draw this distinction if we are to see the
real limitations of the arguments based on clinical data alone and at the same
time to see how unsatisfactory it is to make principled ethical arguments that
are not informed by clinical data.

The distinction illustrates another critical point. Too frequently, we consider medically supportive interventions such as nutrition and hydration as
though they possessed some moral quotient of their own. It would be more
accurate, as suggested earlier, to view them as essentially amoral or ethically
neutral. Therefore, to be realistic, any ethical analysis of nutrition and
hydration begins with the consequences of their use rather than with nutrition and hydration themselves. Here, the important point is that sustaining
life in modern medical practice can and does overreach itself with consequences for which it is directly responsible, but for which it has no professional ability to determine to be ethically acceptable or unacceptable.
Accordingly, from the perspective of the patient receiving such treatment, we
can no longer presume that medicine, whatever the intentions of physicians,
is a benign exercise, at least as far as its outcomes are concerned. As one commentator has put it, "[d]octors now choose from a vast array of interventions
that, when combined with effective therapies for underlying conditions, often
greatly prolong survival."[29] However, as the evidence of one intensive care
unit after another will verify, "the quality of life so skillfully sought can range
from marginally tolerable to positively miserable."[30]

In other words, the distinction between clinical and ethical reasons for with-holding life-sustaining treatment shows that there is a difference between judging a clinically-supportive intervention, such as nutrition and hydration, to be medically successful in the quantitative, technical sense and judging it to be personally acceptable in relation to the qualitative needs and preferences of the patient. Because of this difference, it is necessary when making an ethical argument for withholding nutrition and hydration, to acknowledge that the patient's preferences and underlying values will take precedence.

Any decision, therefore, to withhold life-sustaining treatment, such as nutri-tion and hydration, should be made only after the most careful consideration of the patients' best interests as reflected in their preferences and apart from the clinical outcomes. (Because they do not necessarily coincide, they must always be viewed separately.) The natural hesitation we feel in making a decision to withdraw or withhold life-sustaining treatment cannot, however, justify holding the patient hostage to our hesitation on the grounds that its initiation or contin-uation will be successful in providing the clinical maintenance intended. Rather, armed with the principles laid out in this chapter, we can conclude not only that it is ethically acceptable to withhold or withdraw nutrition and hydration, but that it might be the only ethical thing to do in the circumstances examined here.

SUMMARY

This chapter deals the decision to withhold or withdraw artificial nutrition and/or hydration in end-of-life situations. It is a sensitive ethical issue because food and nutrition are seen as basic to providing care for the patient. Therefore, removing them may seem unethical or even cruel. Hill presents ethical arguments for making the decision to withhold or withdraw artificial nutrition and/or hydration from the patient. He also suggests that such a deci-sion should always be made only after considering the needs of the patient. Further, he posits that this decision may be the only ethical thing to do in cer-tain circumstances.

QUESTIONS FOR DISCUSSION

1. How does the ethical position of the family influence the decision to withhold or withdraw artificial nutrition and hydration?
2. How is nonmaleficience reflected in the decision to withhold or with-draw artificial nutrition and hydration?
3. What is the obligation of the physician in determining whether to with-hold or withdraw artificial nutrition and hydration?
4. When Hill uses the argument of balancing benefits and burdens, which ethical principles or theories is he using?
5. On what ethical grounds would a practitioner "hold the patient hostage" by hesitating to withdraw artificial nutrition and hydration?

NOTES

1. *In re Quinlan*, 70 N.J., 10, 355 A2d 647.

2. *Cruzan v. Director*, DMH 497 US 261 (1990)

3. "Choice in Dying, Background Paper on Artificial Nutrition and Hydration," *Choice in Dying* (New York: September 1990), 1.

4. CNN/USA Today/Gallup Poll, April 1–2, 2005.

5. See www.co.pinellas.fl.us/forensics; "Autopsy report—Medical Examiner's Report of Autopsy," April 1, 2005.

6. R. J. Devine, "The Amicus Curiae Brief: Public Policy versus Personal Freedom," *America* (April 8, 1989): 323–34.

7. Ibid., 324.

8. *Guidelines on the Termination of Life-sustaining Treatment and the Care of the Dying* (Briar Cliff Manor, NY: Hastings Center, 1987), 59–60.

9. Ibid., 60.

10. J. E. Ruark, et al., "Initiating and Withdrawing Life Support," *New England Journal of Medicine* 318 (1988): 25–30.

11. D. C. Maquire, *Death by Choice* (Garden City, NY: Image Books, 1984), 82.

12. R. Wasserstrom, "Rights, Human Rights, and Racial Discrimination," in *Human Rights*, A. I. Melden, ed. (Belmont, CA: Wadsworth, 1970), 99.

13. T. P. Hill, "The Right to Die: Legal and Ethical Consideration," *Southern Medical Journal* 85 (1992): 25–57.

14. J. Ladd, "The Definition of Death and the Right to Die," in *Ethical Issues Relating to Life and Death*, J. Ladd, ed. (New York: Oxford University Press, 1979), 135.

15. Ibid., 139.

16. Hill, op. cit.

17. *In re Quinlan*, 70 N.J., 10, 355 A2d 647, at 37.

18. P. C. Rousseau, "How Fluid Deprivation Affects the Terminally Ill," *R.N.* (January 1991): 73–76.

19. Ibid., 73.

20. Ibid., 74.

21. J. C. Ahronheim and M. R. Gasner, "The Sloganism of Starvation," *Lancet* 335 (1990): 279.

22. Ibid.

23. Rousseau, op. cit., 76.

24. *Guidelines on the Termination of Life-Sustaining Treatment*, 60.

25. U.S. Bishops' Committee for Pro-Life Activities, "Nutrition and Hydration: Moral and Pastoral Reflections," *Origins* 21, 44 (1992): 705–712.

26. K. O'Rourke, "The AMA Statement on Tube Feeding: An Ethical Analysis," *America* (November 22, 1986): 322.

27. Ibid.

28. Ibid.

29. Ruark et al., op. cit., 25.

30. Ibid.

CHAPTER 13

Ethical Issues Concerning Physician-Assisted Death

Barbara Supanich

OVERVIEW

Obviously, the process of dying creates difficult issues for individuals and families, but it also can be challenging for those who support patient care. In this important chapter, Supanich presents a balanced view of the ethics issues surrounding physician-assisted suicide. She presents arguments made by proponents and those in opposition and provides an explanation of why such requests are made. She also provides some practical advice on how to deal with patient requests for such assistance if you encounter them as a healthcare professional.

INTRODUCTION AND KEY DEFINITIONS

Physician-assisted death is a controversial and challenging concept among the many cultures within U.S. society, which are in many ways ambivalent about death and the process of dying. Every day we see movies, TV serials about doctors, and the evening news showing us film footage of wars, ethnic civil wars, and famines. They all sterilize the death experience, at times making it both surreal and unreal. In contrast are the poignant experiences of our own personal and professional lives that teach us the realities of death and dying—patients, relatives, and friends who have died from acquired immune deficiency syndrome (AIDS), heart disease, cancer, or severe traumatic injuries. It is in this societal, professional, and personal milieu that I ask questions about how people die and how they decide the context of their dying process.[1]

Although various faith traditions and ethical guidelines, including the American Medical Association Council on Ethical and Judicial Affairs and the American Academy of Hospice and Palliative Medicine, prohibit and oppose assisted suicide and active euthanasia, public opinion polls show that U.S. society is divided into thirds on the issue of assisted death. One-third support it under a wide variety of circumstances; one-third oppose it under any circumstances; and one-third support it in a few cases, but not all.[2] It is within this rich and complex societal context that physicians and other healthcare professionals need to attain an understanding and an ethical tolerance for these issues and their corresponding controversies and arguments. In this chapter, I will review some of the major ethical arguments, propose clinical strategies for responding to a patient's request for death assistance, and discuss the broader context necessary for a deeper understanding of the challenge of assisted death.

I would like to clarify some basic definitions and distinctions regarding assisted death. First, *assisted suicide* refers to when a patient intentionally and willfully ends his or her own life, with the assistance of a third party. This assistance may include different levels of involvement, from merely providing information about how to commit suicide to providing the means to commit suicide, such as a lethal quantity of pills. It can also include actively participating in the suicide, such as being present at the scene and inserting an intravenous line through which the patient can then administer a lethal dose.[3] The widely-publicized actions of doctors Timothy Quill[4] and Jack Kevorkian[5] provide examples of the second and third levels of involvement, respectively.

In *voluntary active euthanasia*, patients freely choose to have a lethal agent directly administered to them by another individual, with a merciful intent. *Assisted death* is the term I will use in the reminder of the chapter to refer jointly to the practices of voluntary active euthanasia and assisted suicide. Most of the ethics literature has focused on the special problems of the physician's role; and so I will most commonly refer to *physician-assisted death*. However, in intensive care units (ICUs), step-down units, cancer units, hospice settings, and long-term care facilities, as well as in the homes of those who choose to die there, the roles of other healthcare professionals and the family are critically important. In many of these settings, patients may actually request assistance in dying from one or more of these individuals as well as (or instead of) from the physician.

It is also important to be clear about what assisted death is not. It is not an assisted death if a competent person decides not to initiate a specific therapy (e.g., antibiotics for a pneumonia or other septic process, artificial nutrition and hydration, further cardiac interventions). Nor is it assisted death to withdraw any of these options from a patient. The use of high doses of opioids, where the intent is to relieve pain and not to hasten death, is not physician-assisted death. Although many still believe that high-dose opioids pose a serious risk of fatal respiratory depression, palliative specialists know that this very seldom occurs with proper titration of analgesic doses, even when very large doses opioids are administered in terminal illnesses.[6] Even in the rare case in which respiratory depression is a foreseen (but unintended) consequence of adequate analgesia, administering the analgesic is not considered physician-assisted death. (If however, the true intent is to cause or hasten death, and analgesia is merely a ruse or a rationalization, then I would classify the case as assisted death.)[7]

Withholding or withdrawing life-sustaining treatment is widely accepted today both in ethics and law as appropriate and compassionate care, if the competent patient is fully informed and freely chooses that treatment option. Some philosophers, notably Rachels,[8] have argued that there is no morally relevant difference between this practice and the practice of assisted death. In this chapter, without giving detailed arguments, I will dissent from this view. That is, I will leave open the question of whether assisted death is morally justifiable and will discuss the arguments on both sides of the issue. In addition, I will assume that if assisted death can be justified, it must be justified on its own merits, and not merely because it shares some of the same moral features with the relatively uncontroversial practice of withdrawing and withholding life-sustaining treatment.[9]

ETHICAL ARGUMENTS

The following sections present arguments made by those who support and oppose physician-assisted death. Patient autonomy is also considered an important aspect of ethical consideration. In addition, the concept of compassion plays a significant role in formulating an ethics position on this issue. Consideration for safeguards, professional integrity, and the competence level of the patient are also presented in this section.

Patient Integrity and Autonomy

When patients with terminal illnesses come to see their primary physicians, multiple issues are on their minds. These issues might include personal image, the ability to maintain control over treatment decisions (including pain management and other treatment issues), family dynamics, personal values, and potential conflicts with family and/or physicians. There also are deeper reflections about life goals and how to continue living life. Patients want to be able to have conversations about life and the effects that the illness is having in it with their physicians in an open and supportive atmosphere. It is in this type of an atmosphere that patients will be more apt to discuss their concerns and fears about their dying process and options for management of that process, including assisted death.[10]

Those supporting assisted death claim that they are honoring patient integrity by being willing to have conversations with their patients that are open to discussing all treatment options with the patient (and his or her family members, if so desired by the patient), including assisted death. In support of patient integrity and autonomy, proponents argue that only the patient knows what constitutes harm and may decide that continued life with severe interminable suffering is a greater harm than assisted death.[11]

Opponents claim that patient autonomy is not the supreme moral value and is insufficient to justify choosing assisted death. They understand that autonomy is a valid moral value in treatment decisions regarding the withdrawal or withholding of life-sustaining treatments, because in those situations we are respecting personal bodily integrity. However, they do not extend the justification to include a right to demand that others take specific actions to end one's life.

Compassionate Response to Suffering

Proponents of assisted death are supportive of efforts to improve pain and symptom management by physicians and other healthcare professionals; however, they argue that there remain cases in which the best palliative care measures are insufficient to relieve these patients' suffering. They argue along with Quill and others[12] that a willingness to discuss the option of assisted death with the patient may often act as a suicide preventive. This is true because during this open conversation the physician might be able to alleviate the patient's fears and misunderstandings and propose other viable alternatives.[13] Alternatively, if patients do not feel that such a conversation is an option with the physician, they may choose to commit suicide in a manner that is more traumatic for themselves and their families and friends.

In contrast, opponents remind us that suffering is a multifaceted dimension of the human experience. Suffering, in their view, ties intimately to the individual's values, belief system, and sense of meaning. Therefore, at the end of life, suffering relates to one's unique sense of who one is as a person. It also is about how one experiences an illness in the overall context of one's life journey and personal expectations for the future.[14] To relieve suffering, then, by eliminating the sufferer is always unacceptable. Opponents would argue for physicians and others to more competently attend to the issues of loneliness, fear of death, depression, forgiveness, unresolved family and personal conflicts, anger, and hopelessness. This is a challenging endeavor for the healthcare professional, but ultimately allows for a richer personal resolution for the patient. Attending to these issues is important for another reason—a person might make an assisted death request when the physician or family member is suffering from similar inner turmoil. Rather than actively listen to the reasons and concerns behind the patient's request, the physician or family member might project his or her own suffering onto the patient's request and wrongly conclude that a premature death is a merciful choice for the patient.[15]

Safeguards and the Slippery Slope

Persons on both sides of this issue agree that a policy of assisted death would pose a danger to patients and society.[16] Some physicians might abuse this option at the end of life. Table 13–1 lists some safeguards and guidelines commonly proposed by supporters of assisted death.[17]

Table 13–1   Safeguards and Guidelines for a Policy of Assisted Death

---

1. The patient must have a condition that is incurable (not necessarily terminal) and is associated with severe suffering without hope of relief.
2. All reasonable comfort-oriented measures must have been considered or tried.
3. The patient must express a clear and repeated request to die that is not coerced (e.g., emotionally or financially).
4. The physician must ensure that the patient's judgment is not "distorted"; that is, the patient is competent to make rational treatment choices.
5. Physician-assisted death must be carried out only in the context of a meaningful physician-patient relationship.
6. Consultation must be obtained from another physician to ensure that the patient's request is rational and voluntary.
7. There must be clear documentation that the previous six steps have been taken, and a system of reporting, reviewing, and studying such deaths must be established.

Proponents argue that the safeguards and guidelines presented in Table 13–1 create the structure needed for the appropriate conversations between the patient and physician regarding treatment plans for the control of the patient's pain and suffering. These conversations create the rapport and trust necessary for a truly healing relationship. Proponents strongly support recommendations for a consultation from another physician and that there be clear and accurate documentation that all of the guidelines were followed. Adherence to these guidelines, proponents argue, would adequately guard against the slippery slope that opponents fear.

Opponents believe that the slippery slope is a serious and valid concern. Once there is dissolution or weakening of the legal protections against physician-assisted death, society will lose interest in protecting the vulnerable against physicians making inappropriate decisions to hasten death. Given the pressures of cost containment and biases toward vulnerable populations such as the poor, the uninsured, minorities, immigrants, and those living with a disability, there is also concern that once the legal constraints are lifted, physicians might feel obligated to provide assisted death.[18]

Opponents view guidelines and safeguards as, at best, a well-intentioned but inadequate protection against these powerful social forces leading to inevitable abuse. At worst, they are a hypocritical façade erected by proponents to win over public opinion. Those in opposition are concerned that when physicians start providing the means of death for their patients that the patient-physician relationship will be eroded. Because physicians would be tempted to choose a like-minded physician to serve as a consultant, second opinions would provide dubious safety. Documentation systems could not ensure that physicians are consistent and compassionate and that patients would be truly safeguarded.[19]

The debate over safeguards and the slippery slope comes into sharp focus by examining differing interpretations of the Dutch experience. Proponents point to the Netherlands' history of legally-permitted assisted death to support their claim that abuses are minimal and are identified and contained when they occur.[20] Opponents view the Dutch experience as confirming our worst fears of the slippery slope.[21]

Professional Integrity

Opponents of physician-assisted death equate professional integrity with the physician's role as a healer, and thus view physician-assisted death as antithetical to the physician's basic role and moral integrity. Physicians, in their view, are to use their knowledge and skills for healing, restoring, and relieving suffering when possible and to offer comfort always, but never to kill.[22] Similar arguments of integrity are in the literature for other healthcare professionals, including nurses and pharmacists.[23]

Many proponents would argue that opponents have narrowly restricted the definition of *physician integrity* to a very traditional understanding of "healing." They would also argue for an expanded understanding of professional integrity to include relief of suffering, respect for the patient's voluntary choices, and aiding patients to achieve a dignified and peaceful death. For proponents, an exception to the general prohibition against physician-assisted death would be a patient who, despite excellent palliative measures, is still having unremitting suffering. This patient also is making repeated voluntary requests to his or her physician for death assistance. In such a narrowly defined case, a physician of integrity could respond affirmatively to the patient's request, if such an action was not in conflict with his or her personal moral or religious convictions.[24]

Substituted Judgment

The slippery slope argument also raises concerns about extending physician-assisted death to incompetent patients. Presently, proposals for physician-assisted death specifically exclude the option of choosing physician-assisted death by an advance directive. Opponents, however, fear that if a legal right to assisted death were ever accepted, death assistance for now-incompetent patients by advance directive would be a logical and unavoidable extension of any such right.[25] A 1996 United States Court of Appeals ruling stated that patients have a constitutional right to physician-assisted death and left open the possibility that a surrogate on behalf of an incompetent patient might exercise such a right. The final decision by the United States Supreme Court has been issued: A patient does not have a "right to die."[26]

CLINICAL MANAGEMENT OF REQUESTS FOR ASSISTED DEATH

As outlined in the previous section, the ethical debate over assisted death seems as intractable as the abortion debate. One might conclude that proponents and opponents would disagree radically about the actual management of individual patients and could not possibly work cooperatively in team settings. However, this is not entirely true.

In my opinion, the apparent irresolvability of the debate masks a broad area of practical convergence. Opponents do not favor merely abandoning the terminally ill to whatever pain and suffering befalls them. Nor do proponents favor assisted death as the first choice for any terminally ill patient. Both share a strong commitment to trying as hard as possible to relieve the patient's distress to the extent that the patient no longer wishes to die. Proponents are committed to this effort so that they can be sure that assisted death is truly a last resort. Opponents are committed to this effort because they believe that such efforts will ultimately remove any serious demands for assisted death. Moreover, neither believes that health professionals should be required to participate in any activity that is against their personal moral or religious convictions.

Table 13–2 outlines suggested steps for the clinical management of a request for assisted death. Some scrutiny of these steps will show that most can be followed equally well by physicians who support and who oppose the assisted death option.

Table 13–2   Suggested Steps for the Clinical Management of a Request for Assisted Death

---

- The provider should listen to the request for assisted death in an open and sympathetic manner and evaluate the issues underlying the request.
- Providers should share their personal stance with patients in an open and professional manner, always assuring patients that they will be supported throughout this personal decision-making process.
- All providers should take appropriate steps to process their personal emotional reactions to the patient's request (e.g., hospice team meetings).
- The provider should have a continuing dialogue with the patient and appropriate family members or support persons concerning the development and implementation of the therapeutic treatment plans, including a request for assisted death, in a manner that is consistent with the provider's moral values and belief system.

Listen Openly and Evaluate Underlying Issues

Patients demonstrate both courage and trust when they express a request for assisted death to their primary physician. Such a request might trigger strong feelings in the physician. However, the physician should not allow those feelings to derail the necessary conversations with the patient over the ensuing days, weeks, or months. The physician is encouraged to have multiple supportive conversations with the patient that identify the patient's crucial issues. It is important to let the patient know that he or she is not alone, among those facing a terminal illness, to consider assisted death as a personal option. It is also important for the physician to convey to the patient that the fact that the patient chooses to confide in him or her is an honor, and that he or she is be prepared for honest discussions about the option of assisted death.

Both the physician and the patient need to seek out support for themselves as they ponder such a significant decision. The patient might want to discuss the request with family members, other members of the healthcare team, clergy, or a close friend. Physicians should not isolate themselves when they are presented with such a request. They should seek out supportive persons in their personal and professional lives to assist them as they reflect on the implications.

Physicians need to make every effort to understand the reasons that motivate such a patient request and respond appropriately with the information and support that the patient needs. For some patients, this might mean addressing issues of loss of dignity, depression, and feelings of intense loneliness. For these patients, psychological counseling would be an appropriate intervention. Others might have a desire for more information about their disease or specific issues related to the "how" of their dying process. Still others might have concerns about how their illness affects their family and friends, and a social-work consult might be an appropriate intervention. Some might have deep spiritual issues that their terminal illness has brought into sharper focus and an appropriate referral to their religious or spiritual mentor would be a critical next step.

As one can see from these brief examples, an initial request for assisted death, when approached with active listening and sensitivity to the patient's underlying issues, is always more complex that one initially anticipates. It requires repeated conversations to ensure that the request is both enduring and consistent with the patient's life values and goals.

Share Personal Stance with the Patient

It is premature to allow the physician's personal stance on assisted death to disrupt the deep and careful inquiry into the patient's issues and needs. Physicians are obliged to be sincere and candid with patients regarding all aspects of their treatment options, and therefore the next step is for the physician to be transparent regarding her or his stance on assisted death.

Physicians who morally oppose physician-assisted death should couple refusal to provide it with an assurance that they will stand with the patient until the moment of death and will exhaustively search out all appropriate treatment options to ameliorate the patient's suffering. The physician should stress the importance of continuing the dialogue about the patient's perceptions of his or her suffering, so that they can explore mutually acceptable solutions together. Finally, it is important to let the patient know that although the idea of assisted death is morally objectionable to the physician, the person making the request is not.

The physician who is morally willing to be actively involved in assisted death needs to inform the patient of the required procedure for confirming that the patient is making a voluntary and thoughtful choice; and that the patient's suffering cannot be relieved by other any accepted means. The actual amount of time to make such determinations varies and needs to be negotiated with the patient. The physician should also inform the patient that in most cases of this sort, other interventions could improve a person's quality of life that might remove the need for death assistance. These interventions should be identified and considered before proceeding with a request for assisted death.

At this stage, an occasional patient will break off the dialogue—either because the patient demands death assistance and the physician is not willing to provide it, or because the patient feels entitled to this assistance without going through a long process of exploring alternatives. A few patients might choose to commit suicide without the physician's assistance, perhaps in a way that causes great suffering for both the patient and the survivors. Although such outcomes are very tragic, they do not, in my view, count as an argument against the stepwise approach. Safeguards will count for nothing if patients are allowed, in effect, to use a threat of suicide by other means as emotional blackmail to force the physician to circumvent the process. In such cases, the physician's obligation to act out of professional integrity takes priority over any rights or wishes of the patient.

Assure Adequate Comfort Care

Several reports in the literature document physicians' and other healthcare providers' poor knowledge about appropriate pain management and other comfort measures at the end of life.[27] When a patient makes a request for death assistance, it behooves the physician to ensure that all reasonable comfort measures have been discussed and a trial offered to the patient.

Most patients have concerns and fears regarding suffering. Primarily the fear is that they will have unremitting pain with no hope for adequate relief. Frequent discussions about the multiple technologies and techniques available for easing suffering and increasing comfort will help to alleviate their fears. Patients also have concerns about loneliness, abandonment, unresolved family or other personal conflicts, changes to body image, and/or personal identity issues. Spiritual counseling can help to restore a sense of meaning and hope for patients in the context of their hopes, values, and lifeview. Many persons have found that the use of narrative, as a form of life review, is very comforting and can facilitate the restoration of meaning and hope for the patient. I, as well as many other colleagues in palliative medicine, encourage patients to engage in telling or writing stories about their illness, their hopes for survival or their legacy, and the life events and relationships that have enriched their lives and are an expression of their most sacred personal values.

Ensure the Voluntary Nature and Reasonableness of Request

Using transparent conversations with their patients, physicians should seek a deeper appreciation of the nature of the patient's request and ensure that it is a clear, uncoerced, and voluntary decision. The compassionate and responsible physician will want to ensure that the patient made the request after serious consideration of other treatment alternatives. The physician needs to verify that the patient rationally rejected the alternatives and that he or she was not depressed at the time of the decision for assisted death. Quill et al.[28] appropriately emphasized that any sign of ambivalence or uncertainty on the part of the patient should stop the process. The patient's desire for death assistance must be strong, continuous, clear, and convincing.

Just as important, the physician must seek assurance that the patient's judgment is based on a clear and accurate understanding of the facts of his or her case. Further, the patient must understand the implications of his or her decision for assisted death. Frequent and compassionate discussions with the patient will facilitate a better understanding of the reasons for the request and ascertain the perseverance of the request. The physician must be especially alert for signs of depression, which could interfere with executive functions, as well as add to the patient's suffering. Consultation with a skilled psychiatrist is imperative if there is any suspicion of depression. In some cases, a trial of antidepressant therapy with a rapid-acting drug might be essential before acceding to a request for death assistance.

Patients should be strongly encouraged to share their decision for death assistance with family members. The decision to share should not be forced, and they should be able to choose whom to involve and inform, as well as when to share the decision with family members. The primary physician can often function as a facilitator in the discussions between the patient and family members when there are conflicting concerns and opinions.

PLACING THE DEBATE IN CONTEXT

The apparent intractability if the assisted-death debate has done more than obscure the broad area of consensus around optimal patient care at the end of life. Reducing the debate to the technical level of "should we or shouldn't we?" distracts us from broader social and spiritual questions. Unless we address those questions, we will be unable to comprehend why our society and our healthcare system are having this particular debate now and why it has assumed the appearance of intractability.

A critical question is whether physicians view their professional obligation as primarily biomedical or whether they include in that obligation the importance of understanding the narrative life journey of the patient. If they choose the latter, then they would describe their profession as one of promoting health and wellness, and of sojourning with their patients through all of life, including the dying process—our final journey. Persons who have this viewpoint do not describe death as the enemy, but rather as a part of life's journey. Medicine would finally accept death as a limit that cannot be overcome and use that limit as an indispensable focal point in thinking about illness and disease.[29] Medicine would change its focus from fighting death at all costs to helping each person live his or her life to its fullest potential.

A key issue often lost in the current intellectual and legal debate is the critical need to improve the quality of care and support for dying patients throughout our healthcare system. My own estimate from the current debate is that only about three percent of patients who might request assisted death have symptoms that are not remediable by current therapeutic options. This means that proponents and opponents of assisted death agree fully on what should be done to help 97 percent of all patients. Yet, the best available evidence is that far too many of that 97 percent are poorly served within our present system. Healthcare professionals in particular have an obligation to provide leadership in reforming the culture of the health system to be more responsive to the needs of terminally ill patients and their families, including better pain and symptom management and coordination of care for the dying.

Many perceive the assisted-death debate as rooted in unrealistic expectations of what technology can offer in the management of disease and the belief that there is a technological cure available for everyone somewhere in the United States. It is a moral obligation of healthcare providers to help all of our patients seek a balance between the technological imperative and the "pursuit of a peaceful death," as described by Daniel Callahan.[30] It is Callahan's observation that the technological imperative for some patients and their physicians becomes oppressive and serves "to make our dying all the more problematic: harder to predict, more difficult to manage, the source of more moral dilemmas and nasty choices, and spiritually more productive of anguish, ambivalence, and uncertainty."[31]

Merely saying that we accept the inevitability of death does not necessarily free us from the seductive power of the technological solution. For some, the "technical fix" might be a "suicide machine." For some, it is the hope that excellent hospice care will allay all suffering and put an end to all requests for death assistance. Both positions represent a failure to grapple with the meaning of suffering and death at the deeper cultural and spiritual levels.

Because physician-assisted death is an issue with serious personal and societal implications, I strongly encourage continuing dialogue on this issue in as many societal arenas as possible. Within this dialogue, the physician-patient relationship and conversations are primary, but not exclusive. Because we, as humans, are communal by our very nature, discussions about life and death demand that we go beyond the individual context and challenge us to contemplate what it means to live together and die well in a compassionate society.

SUMMARY

The chapter begins with definitions that are important in understanding the differences in the types of assisted death. Supanich then presents arguments used by those who oppose and favor this action that include respecting patient integrity and practicing compassion. Suggestions for managing requests for assisted death are given including following steps for clinical management, sharing one's personal view, and assuring that comfort care will be provided. Finally, Supanich suggests that, because of its significance, we continue the dialogue about this issue and even consider a societal view.

QUESTIONS FOR DISCUSSION

1. Do you think that there will be an increase in patient requests for physician-assisted suicides as we move forward in the twenty-first century? Why or why not?

2. What ethical issues does the physician face when he or she receives a request for assisted suicide?

3. What do you think is the underlying cause of patients making requests for ending their lives with support?

4. Why does technology not hold the complete answer to a "good death"?

5. What principles of ethics should you consider in responding to a patient's request for physician-assisted suicide?

NOTES

1. D. E. Meier, C. A. Emmons, A. Litke, S. Wallenstein, and R.S. Morrison, "Characteristics of Patients Requesting and Receiving Physician-Assisted Death," *Archives of Internal Medicine* 163 (2003): 1537-1542; E. Emmanuel, "Whose Right to Die?" *The Atlantic Monthly* 279, no. 3 (March, 1997): 73-79.

2. D. T. Watts and T. Howell, "Assisted Suicide Is Not Voluntary Active Euthanasia," *Journal of the American Geriatric Society* 40 (1992): 1043.

3. Ibid.

4. T. Quill, "Death and Dignity: A Case of Individualized Decision Making," *New England Journal of Medicine* 324 (1991): 691.

5. J. Kevorkian, *Prescription Medicide: The Goodness of Planned Death* (Buffalo, NY: Prometheus Books, 1991); G. Annas, "Physician-Assisted Suicide: Michigan's Temporary Solution," *New England Journal of Medicine* 328 (1993): 1573.

6. W. C. Wilson, et al., "Ordering and Administration of Sedatives and Analgesics during the Withholding and Withdrawal of Life Support from Critically Ill Patients," *Journal of the American Medical Association* 267 (1992): 949.

7. H. Brody, "Commentary on Billings and Block's 'Slow Euthanasia,'" *Journal of Palliative Care* 12 (1996): 38–41.

8. J. Rachels, *The End of Life: Euthanasia and Morality* (New York: Oxford University Press, 1986).

9. G. Annas, "Death by Prescription: The Oregon Initiative," *New England Journal of Medicine* 331 (1994): 1240; D. Callahan, "Pursuing a Peaceful Death," *Hastings Center Report* (July/August 1993): 33; *Euthanasia: California Proposition* 161; New York: Commonweal Foundation (September 1992; Special Supplement): 1–16; E. J. Emmanuel, "The History of Euthanasia Debates in the United States and Britain," *Annals of Internal Medicine* 121 (1994): 793.

10. J. Peteet, "Treating Patients Who Request Assisted Suicide," *Archives of Family Medicine* 3 (1994): 723; B. Ferrel and M. Rhiner, "High-Tech Comfort: Ethical Issues in Cancer Pain Management for the 1990's," *Journal of Clinical Ethics* (Summer 1991): 108; D. Steinmetz, et al., "Family Physician's Involvement with Dying Patients and Their Families," *Archives of Family Medicine* 2 (1993): 753.

11. M. Battin, "Voluntary Euthanasia and the Risks of Abuse: Can We Learn Anything from the Netherlands?" *Law, Med, Healthcare* 20, no. 1–2 (Spring–Summer 1992): 133; J. Davies, "Altruism towards the End of Life," *Journal of Medical Ethics* 19 (1993): 111.

12. T. Quill, et al., "Care of the Hopelessly Ill: Proposed Clinical Criteria for Physician-Assisted Suicide," (Sounding Board), *New England Journal of Medicine* 327 (1992): 1380; H. Brody, "Assisted Death: A Compassionate Response to a Medical Failure," *New England Journal of Medicine* 327 (1992): 1384; T. E. Quill, *Death and Dignity: Making Choices and Taking Charge* (New York: W.W. Norton, 1993).

13. T. Quill, "Doctor, I Want to Die, Will You Help Me?" *Journal of the American Medical Association* 270 (1993): 870.

14. E. J. Cassell, "The Nature of Suffering and the Goals of Medicine," *New England Journal of Medicine* 306 (1982): 639; id., *The Nature of Suffering and the Goals of Medicine* (New York: Oxford University Press, 1991).

15. S. Miles, "Physicians and Their Patients' Suicides," *Journal of the American Medical Association* 27 (1994): 1786.

16. M. Battin, "Voluntary Euthanasia and the Risks of Abuse"; T. Quill, et al., "Care of the Hopelessly Ill"; F. Miller, et al., "Regulating Physician-Assisted Death," *New England Journal of Medicine* 31 (1994): 119; R. F. Weir, "The Morality of Physician-Assisted Suicide," *Law, Med, Healthcare* 20, no. 1–2 (Spring-Summer 1992): 116.

17. T. Quill, et al., "Care of the Hopelessly Ill"; F. Miller et al., op. cit.

18. C. S. Campbell, "'Aid-in-Dying' and the Taking of Human Life," *Journal of Medical Ethics* 18 (1992): 128.

19. D. Callahan and M. White, "The Legalization of Physician-Assisted Suicide: Creating a Regulatory Potemkin Village," *University of Richmond Law Review* 30 (1996): 1-83.

20. G. Van de Wal, et al., "Euthanasia and Assisted Suicide, 1: How Often Is It Practiced by Family Doctors in the Netherlands?" *Family Practice* 9 (1992): 135-140; *Position Statement* (Gainesville, FL: Academy of Hospice Physicians, 1988); *Statement Opposing the Legalization of Euthanasia and Assisted Suicide* (Arlington, VA: National Hospice Organization, 1989).

21. T. Quill, et al., "Care of the Hopelessly Ill"; Miller et al., op. cit.; G. Van der Wal and R.J. Dillmann, "Euthanasia in the Netherlands," *British Medical Journal* 308 (May 1994): 1346; Van der Wal, et.al., "Euthanasia and Assisted Suicide, 1"; id., "Euthanasia and Assisted Suicide, 2."

22. W. Gaylin, et al., "Doctors Must Not Kill," *Journal of the American Medical Association* 259 (1998): 2139; L. R. Kass, "Neither for Love Nor Money: Why Doctors Must Not Kill," *The Public Interest* 94 (Winter 1989): 25.

23. C. S. Campbell et al., "Conflicts of Conscience: Hospice and Assisted Suicide," *Hastings Center Report* 25 (1995): 36; A. Haddad, "'Physician-Assisted Suicide' the Impact on Nursing and Pharmacy," *Of Value* (Society for Health and Human Values Newsletter) (December 1994); M. T. Rupp and H. L. Isenhower, "Pharmacists' Attitudes toward Physician-Assisted Suicide," *American Journal of Hospital Pharmacy* 51 (1994): 69; A. Young and D. Volker, "Oncology Nurses' Attitudes Regarding Voluntary, Physician-Assisted Dying for Competent, Terminally Ill Patients," *Oncology Nurse Forum* 20 (1993): 445; S. Kowalski, "Assisted Suicide: Where Do Nurses Draw the Line?" *Nurse Health Care* 14 (1993): 70.

24. F. G. Miller and H. Brody, "Professional Integrity and Physician-Assisted Death," *Hastings Center Report* 25 (1995): 8.

25. Euthanasia: California Proposition 161; New York: Commonweal Foundation; D. Callahan, "Aid in Dying: The Social Dimensions," *Commonweal* (Supplement, 9 August 1991): 12.

26. Supreme Court, June 1997.

27. "Pain Management: Theological and Ethical Principles Governing the Use of Pain Relief for Dying Patients," *Health Progress* (January/February 1993): 30; Ferrel and Rhiner, "High-Tech Comfort"; *Management of Cancer Pain Guidelines Panel, Management of Cancer Pain, Clinical Practice Guidelines* no. 9 (Rockville, MD: Agency for Health Care Policy and Research, 1994).

28. T. Quill, et al., "Care of the Hopelessly Ill."

29. D. Callahan, "Pursuing a Peaceful Death."

30. Ibid.

31. Ibid., 33.

Critical Issues for Healthcare Organizations

Part III moves away from the individual and concentrates on healthcare institutions. It features examples of issues that will be a part of their future in the twenty-first century. Chapter 14 presents a discussion of the differences between ethical issues in a clinical situation and those faced by an organization. It includes the complexities of organizational ethics in the changing healthcare environment. The chapter also shows how organizations must address clinical situations, legislation, and community responsibility and still make money. The author challenges you to think beyond the clinical arena and to consider the broader view held by institutional ethics.

Chapter 15 includes an overview of the institution's response to ethical challenge—the ethics committee. It provides you with an understanding of the function, membership, and future challenges for these committees. The practitioner's view section discusses some challenges that ethics committees face because of financial concerns, technology demands, and scrutiny in end-of-life situations.

Chapter 16 features managed care, an aspect of health care that is challenging for both clinicians and organizations. It begins with a review of the distinctions between the types of managed care organizations (MCOs). It then presents the ethical challenges that are part of such practices, such as utilization review, capitation, and physician incentives. The author also gives examples of forces that will balance the negatives of MCOs and provides a managed care model that includes ethics. This chapter should evoke much thought and discussion among your fellow professionals.

Chapter 17 examines current and future ethical dilemmas for specific types of healthcare organizations—those that deal with prehospital and emergency care. The chapter suggests that emergency departments (EDs) are struggling to be the safety net for the poor, and they might be losing the struggle. It acquaints you with such controversial areas as the need for paternalism, assisted suicides and emergency room practices, and prehospital DNR orders. In addition, the need for security for those who work in the ED, the practice of teaching on the newly dead, and the ability to conduct research on critical patients are presented as ethical concerns that will continue into the future.

Another specific organization that is included in Part III is the home care industry, which will be discussed in Chapter 18. Technology's almost miraculous ability to prolong life has led to an increasing problem for healthcare organizations and individuals. Some patients require care beyond the ordinary, and home health care tries to provide this care. The chapter provides information on the home health model and its history of dealing with medically fragile, technology-dependent adults and children. Ongoing ethical issues for home health are stressed, and the impact of the aging boomers on its future is included for your consideration.

Chapter 19 introduces a global ethics issue for healthcare organizations. It asks the question, "what is the role of spirituality in a healthcare organization?" The chapter explores the definition of *spirituality* in general, its application to work, and reasons why it will be an issue for healthcare organizations in the twenty-first century. It also includes the effect of the spirit on transition and the ethical theories and principles that support spirituality in the healthcare organization.

Part III does not include every future ethical situation faced by healthcare organizations. However, it does provide a beginning for considering issues that will affect all these organizations. It also gives an overview of some of the quandaries faced by specific healthcare organizations, such as home health and the emergency department. In this part of the text, you will be challenged to "think outside of the clinical box" and consider ethics from the organization's view.

CHAPTER 14

Healthcare Institutional Ethics: Broader than Clinical Ethics

Carrie Zoubul*

OVERVIEW

This chapter provides an examination of the current and future ethics issues that challenge healthcare institutions. They are addressed from several viewpoints, mirroring the model for this text. For example, issues facing individual managers in terms of their need for practicing ethical integrity are presented (individual). Issues involving nonprofit institutions as they struggle with providing care and making payroll and the need for healthcare institutions to provide proactive care are discussed (organizational). Finally, the schizophrenic view of American society about its healthcare system is presented in a matter that fosters understanding of this often complex issue (society). This chapter will greatly increase your understanding of the business side of health care and the ethical issues it faces in its future.

INTRODUCTION

Bioethical problems have dominated the ethical concerns of hospitals and other healthcare institutions for the past 35 years. Clinical issues such as the termination of treatment, patient autonomy, informed consent, confidentiality, advance directives, and other individual case-based issues have occupied center stage. In the late 1980s and early 1990s, the focus of bioethics began to broaden. With the onset of rapid change in the structure of the healthcare delivery system, many institutions began to recognize and address ethical issues inherent in business practices, corporations, and managed care organizations. As managed care took its place as primary mode of healthcare delivery, questions were raised about how to expand bioethics to address institutional structure and the business aspects of health care.

Institutional focus on clinical, business, and ethical matters eventually began to give way to network concerns. Networks comprised of institutions, physician organizations, financing mechanisms, other health businesses, and community organizations began to emerge. This change resulted in new and organizationally complex ethical dilemmas that demanded different analytical frameworks and broader ethical analysis. In the bioethics literature, this area of inquiry has become known as "organizational ethics," applicable to both individual healthcare institutions (e.g., hospitals) and to the other entities

---

* Revised from D. Brodeur, "Health Care Institutional Ethics: Broader then Clinical Ethics," in *Health Care Ethics: Critical Issues for the 21st Century*. Original ed., 1998, edited by John. F. Monagle and David C. Thomasma. Sudbury, MA: Jones and Bartlett, 2005.

that make up the modern healthcare system.[1] Several definitions of organizational ethics have been formulated. Some examples include: it "aims to enhance the overall ethics of an organization with the goal of changing the climate and then the culture of the organization;"[2] it "deals with an organization's positions and behavior relative to individuals (including patients, providers, and employees), groups, communities served by the organization, and other organizations;"[3] it is described as "the intentional use of values to guide the decisions of a system;"[4] and it "focuses on the ethical climate of the entire organization...which encompasses and integrates all other ethics resources and activities within an organization."[5]

Today, healthcare networks and their member institutions constitute complex, interdependent systems of patients, families, professionals, payers, processes, communities, and businesses. These multiple players interact in intricate ways. Their daily activities, missions, institutional values, strategic goals, and their impact on the community and the community's health status are ethically significant. The bioethical principles of autonomy, beneficence, nonmaleficence, and justice as traditionally formulated may not be sufficient to address the ethical issues that arise. Although these principles have their place, questions of distributive justice demand greater attention and the principles of business ethics, such as "honesty, truthfulness, and keeping promises"[6] may also be useful.

Since patient care is still the focus of much of an institution's activity, the need to address clinical bioethical issues remains a priority. These issues are addressed in other chapters of this book. This chapter focuses on the ethical issues that healthcare network and institutional administrators (and sometimes trustees) need to address from a personal, institutional, and communal perspective. These include justice issues (social, distributive, and commutative), the promotion of the common good, the role of the community in the healthcare system, preservation of human resources, the definition of health, the role of law and government regulation, promoting access to quality health care, conflicts of interest, and the allocation of resources, to name a few. This chapter will not outline a comprehensive theory of justice, argue for a process of allocating or rationing resources, or define the concept of health. Rather, it will attempt to outline important considerations and describe potential ethical issues and value conflicts that arise in healthcare networks and institutions at the organizational level.

Healthcare organizations play an important public role in their communities, providing medical care, medical education, and significant employment opportunities. Trustees and managers confront ethical issues that involve clinical matters, corporate and institutional structure, strategic direction, personal and personnel commitments, and the public nature of health care.

MOVING FROM A CLINICAL FOCUS TO INCORPORATE ORGANIZATIONAL CONCERNS

For many years, healthcare institutions have been expected to be attentive to clinical ethics issues that arise in the context of patient care. Some of these expectations are embodied in laws and regulations, for example, the Patient

Self-Determination Act, required education for Medicaid recipients, organ donation request laws, EMTALA (the "anti-patient-dumping" statute), HIPAA (the privacy rule), the Patients' Bill of Rights, and regulations governing human subjects research. However, independent accreditation bodies also play a role in defining the requirements for institutional ethics activities. In the patient-rights section of its accreditation manual for hospitals, the Joint Commission on Accreditation of Healthcare Organizations (JCAHO) requires that "the patient or the patient's designated representative participate in the consideration of ethical issues that arise in the care of the patient."[7] Institutions must develop processes that provide patients (or their representatives) access to ethics consultants, an ethics committee, or other procedural mechanism designed to address ethical questions and concerns.

Clinical issues are typically dealt with using traditional ethical principles such as autonomy, beneficence, nonmaleficence, and justice.[8] The limits of these principles might force healthcare institutions to confront ethical issues that reach beyond the clinical setting (e.g., the limits of the institutional or professional obligation to treat a patient who requests "everything"). Clinical issues often wind up involving questions of community need,[9] accreditation and government regulation,[10] and organizational structure.[11]

New clinical ethical issues arise as medicine and technology continue to develop new financial structures that more intimately link hospitals and physicians to financial concerns. These issues also raise organizational questions as to their effects on the provision of appropriate, quality medical care. Examples of the issues raised include: the nature of advocacy in the patient-physician relationship, when physicians are subject to outside influences that might affect care decisions[12]; the potential for financial conflicts of interest[13]; challenges to the traditional fiduciary nature of the physician-patient relationship[14]; and the provision of preventative or primary healthcare services to the community for which the institution might not be reimbursed.

In 1995, JCAHO introduced a new accreditation standard in its "Patient Rights and Organizational Ethics" chapter of its accreditation manual, requiring hospitals to "operate according to a code of ethical behavior."[15] A hospital's code must address business ethics concerns, including the marketing, billing, admission, transfer, and discharge practices of the hospital and its relationship to "other healthcare providers, educational institutions, and providers."[16] With this standard, JCAHO expects hospitals to approach these issues in an ethical manner that reflects its moral responsibility to patients and the community they serve.[17] Soon after, the American Society for Bioethics and Humanities Task Force on Standards for Bioethics Consultation acknowledged the growing importance of organizational ethics issues and the need to develop institutional capabilities to address these issues as part of its ethics consultation service or ethics infrastructure.[18]

These developments led to a flurry of scholarship in the bioethics literature addressing the emergence of organizational ethics problems, including special journal issues, conferences and symposia, and books on the topic.[19] For example, the American Medical Association's Institute for Ethics formed an organizational ethics-working group,[20] and the American College of Healthcare Executives created a code of ethics setting forth standards to guide the conduct of executives.[21] The discussions focus on questions of what the concept of organizational ethics means for healthcare institutions and how its principles can be successfully implemented and sustained.[22]

The following questions have been addressed in these discussions: Are business ethics and healthcare ethics compatible?[23] Can healthcare organizations or corporations be considered morally responsible for their actions?[24] Who will do the work, the existing clinical ethics committee, a risk management committee, or a new committee focused solely on organizational issues? What additional education or expertise will ethics consultants need to address ethics on the organizational level? What are the differences and similarities between clinical ethics and organizational ethics consultations?[25] What process should be used to address organizational issues?[26] How can an organization build an "ethical culture," and how will the program thrive? How do you ethically negotiate the tension between patient needs and the institution's financial viability?

Stakeholder theory, defined as "an approach to business ethics that takes into account the rights and interests of the broad range of individuals and organizations who interact with it and are affected by business decision making,"[27] is an example of business ethics theory that has been applied in the healthcare arena. Incorporating principles of business ethics into an existing healthcare ethics program implies expertise in an area not traditionally represented on ethics committees. Although some authors suggest that organizational ethics should be viewed as an additional task for the ethics committee, they recognize that new members must be added or existing members must receive additional training.[28] To many, the goal of an organizational ethics initiative should be to arrive at a system of "integrated ethics," one that combines clinical, organizational, and community goals.[29]

It might be easier to achieve consensus when addressing clinical concerns rather than in the group of issues that involve the network or institution's work life, its sense of justice, the concept of health, or the definition of a socially accountable healthcare network. Although certainly a challenge, attention to these issues should lead to better design and implementation of healthcare services that are patient focused and morally sound.

HUMAN RESOURCES AND THE INSTITUTIONAL CLIMATE

Usually there is consensus about the organization's ethical commitments to human resources and personnel issues. An organization's greatest resource is its human resources, and many would agree that the inappropriate or unethical treatment of the workforce can lead to a collapse of the institution's mission and its ability to serve the public. A list of ethical principles and rules could be developed that, prima facie, seem to be normative. These include treating people as an end, not as a means; providing fair compensation; not being deceitful or manipulative; and instituting mechanisms for participatory decision making and consensus building. They also include ensuring that personnel policies are just and nondiscriminatory; treating employees with dignity and respect; implementing fair disciplinary policies; and protecting against physical or sexual harassment in the workplace.

Surveys of human resources professionals reveal an empirical basis for this normative agreement about what is ethical in the workplace.[30] For example, in one survey 22.6 percent of personnel managers indicated that sex discrimination in recruitment and hiring was an ethical issue they confronted. Nearly 31 percent indicated that the hiring, training, or promotion of personnel based on favoritism was an issue.[31]

Clearly, this prima facie agreement on normative principles does not ensure that all people in the workplace act ethically. The temptation might be to dismiss unethical practices as aberrant behaviors of unethical managers or employees, but the root cause might lie in the culture of the organization or its inability to address or control the unethical practices of its employees.

Employees of healthcare organizations have diverse professional backgrounds (e.g., medicine, nursing, social work, administrators, etc.), and each individual has a personal sense of what is just or moral, in addition to those values identified in the workplace. Because of this, organizations must focus on building a strong "ethical climate" by identifying core values and beliefs that are visible to both patients and staff, who can then abide by them and expect the organization to live up to them.[32] Hospital staff might also benefit from educational programs that focus on organizational ethics, helping them to spot issues as they present themselves on the job.[33]

Organizational assistance must be provided to workers to ensure that they are able to assert their rights and act on their values. One way this can be accomplished is providing protection for whistle-blowing actions in the workplace.[34] If this protection is not provided, employees who witness unethical behavior will be less likely to come forward, and, if they do, they may suffer negative consequences for speaking up.[35] Owners/managers need to make a commitment to the assurance of employee rights and to the inclusion of workers in the process of creating, nurturing, and sustaining the workplace environment.

Trustees or administrators who establish ethical parameters for personnel policies and the managers who implement these policies must think about the factors that contribute to unethical behavior. Furthermore, in order to create an ethical climate they need to carefully consider the content of policy manuals, the design of disciplinary procedures, the organization's mission and strategic goals, and other activities that reflect the ethical commitment of the organization. Furthermore, employers must create an environment where the staff feels comfortable expressing ethical concerns without fear of retaliation or other negative consequences. This attention to ethical matters in personnel policies has to be deliberate, ongoing, and public.

Emerging healthcare networks raise additional concerns. Key among them is a change in an institution's commitment to its workforce. In today's healthcare climate, the ethical question is not necessarily about loyalty, but rather about an organization's commitment to its human resources that enables workers to learn new skills and respond to rapidly changing work environments. Conversely, employees need to be open to change and be willing to learn and take on new challenges.

Work is a means through which human beings express significant aspects of personal life, support the development of family, build community, and create a culture. Healthcare institutions employ a great number of individuals who view their work as a vocation, a calling, or a ministry. Even workers who perform more routine tasks often characterize their work activity as contributing to a greater end—the care of those in need. Therefore, the ethical challenge for healthcare administrators is to create a work environment in which all employees are able to express their personal dignity, achieve personal fulfillment, and realize their creative possibilities.

Those authors who focus on the question of work, including management-science authors, describe a number of additional "normative" principles that help to create a meaningful work environment. First is the principle of *subsidiary*; that is, that decisions should be made at the level where they have the most impact and involve the owners of work processes. The second principle is that decisions, whenever possible, should be based on consensus. This suggests that people who work together, examining the root causes of problems, and seeking functional and cross-functional solutions, are more likely to find effective solutions and to create a respectful work environment.

Finally, although perhaps not purely an ethical commitment, managers need to think about what management style, technique, or process best helps to build a positive and respectful work environment. Management style will have a direct impact on the type of managers recruited and hired. Furthermore, high-level management must be supportive of creating and affecting the ethical climate of the workplace.[36] Management style should be seen as a means to achieve an ethical end—a workplace where employees are respected, are able to assert their rights, and are comfortable expressing their own moral views if they conflict with the practices or policies of the institution.

ORGANIZATIONAL IDENTITY AND STRATEGIC DIRECTION

Another area for ethical reflection for trustees and managers is the mission of the healthcare organization and the means it uses to accomplish this mission. In the late 1980s and early 1990s, issues related to organizational mission came to the forefront when many healthcare institutions saw their nonprofit tax status challenged in state and federal courts.[37] The issue was raised to new heights when proprietary organizations, such as Columbia/HCA, questioned the tax status of community nonprofit organizations.

What are the ethical duties owed by a healthcare institution to the community it serves? Potter suggests that the incorporation of organizational and community bioethics "will be a time to recover the social responsibility of healthcare institutions."[38] In part, this responsibility arises out of the commitment to meeting the needs of the community. Ideally, managers lead healthcare organizations in an analysis of community needs and develop and design its strategic directions to meet these needs.

For the purposes of this part of the discussion, the focus will be on nonprofit (voluntary) healthcare organizations. Nonprofit institutions must be financially sound, act as appropriate stewards of resources, and generate excess revenues over expenses. Questions about whether a manager behaves as a responsible steward of these resources or whether the organization acts justly in the "business community" are questions of business ethics. The more specific question to be addressed here is: What are the organizational ethics concerns of nonprofit healthcare institutions as they provide goods and services to the community?

Paul Starr and Rosemary Stevens each trace the growth of the voluntary healthcare sector.[39] According to Stevens' analysis, this growth involved a shift from voluntary hospitals, whose purpose was to mobilize local resources, to a range of disparate institutions that successfully fought government intervention and organized medicine. By the late 1930s, voluntary hospitals exemplified (in ideal cases) "public responsibility without government compulsion" and "private initiatives untainted by selfish gain."[40]

In time, nonprofit institutions lost touch with the principles of that earlier era. Medicine became increasingly more organized, healthcare institutions became more dependent on federal and state funding, and the government had an increasingly larger role in designing healthcare financing and delivery systems. This was especially evident with the growth of Medicare and Medicaid. Healthcare institutions adjusted their practices to survive and grow in the new environment. As a result, some people looking at health care began to see big business rather than public charitable corporations. More recently, the focus has changed again as care has shifted from traditional nonprofit hospitals to community-wide networks that include proprietary insurance companies and physician networks with equity incentives. The values of the "health system," as described by Stevens and Starr, seem to be long gone.

Municipalities, pressed for tax dollars to maintain other community services, began to question the appropriateness of the tax status of healthcare institutions and emerging networks in light of the amount of "charity" care and community benefit they provide. If things have changed so much, and if the organizations look more like businesses, then perhaps they should pay the same taxes and municipal fees that for-profit enterprises are required to pay. Critical focus on the tax-exempt status of nonprofit healthcare organizations and the provision of charity care has only grown over the last 10 years. However, a recent empirical analysis comparing the provision of services by for-profit and nonprofit healthcare organizations finds that, comparatively, nonprofit hospitals provide more "private and public goods in the public interest" and that the focus on tax exemption is misplaced, because it does not constitute a large percentage of overall public spending.[41]

Furthermore, U.S. society has a schizophrenic attitude toward its healthcare institutions. On the one hand, communities expect that healthcare institutions will (1) be close to home; (2) be filled with the latest technology; (3) abound in expertise; (4) be efficient, quality, full-service providers; (5) take care of the poor and uninsured; (6) not be concerned about insurance or payment arrangements; and (7) not be prohibitively expensive. Communities expect the costs of providing these services will be covered by income derived from the overall activities of the institutions, free from overdependence on public money. Healthcare institutions should also provide services as needed, without addressing questions of the national healthcare budget or rationing resources. On the other hand, the community expects that healthcare institutions (1) should not be involved in projects that raise money through non-health-related activities (except for philanthropic fund-raising); (2) should be wary of joint ventures and other business practices; and (3) should compete openly in the marketplace while not looking like a business. Obviously, these conflicting expectations need to be resolved.

This is not to suggest that there are not appropriate limits to a nonprofit institution's use of excess revenue, capitalization of proprietary projects, inurement, or executive compensation. However, at the root of these issues are questions about whether healthcare services are public or private goods, whether competition and the marketplace help or hinder the provision of these goods, and how many tiers of healthcare services society really wants.

No clear policy will resolve every issue. In the absence of a national health plan (and even if there were a national health plan), managers and trustees of voluntary institutions must do their best to create institutions that respond to the needs of the communities they serve. This is not be easy, and strategies differ depending on applicable laws, regulations, and court decisions. Managers and trustees need to develop strategic directions that guide their institutions through the regulatory maze while simultaneously meeting the needs of as many people as possible. This is not only sound business strategy, it is an ethical imperative if one understands health care as a social good.

The ethical components of institutional strategy are definitional and procedural. Definitional concerns include defining *health*: What is health? Is it the optimal functioning of the whole person? Should the definition of health focus on the individual, or should it have a broader community (public health) perspective? What goals is the organization aiming for? Which services benefit individual patients and which address community health? Increasingly, health benefits are measured in terms of both community and individual gain. Consequently, preventive services, community-education programs, primary health care, outreach and advocacy programs, and other activities become part of the institution's mission in the community.[42]

The procedural aspects of strategy require managers to define the process of the allocation and rationing of healthcare resources. Although there may be no ascertainable national healthcare budget to frame spending, each institution or organization has a general sense of an "annual total budget" available to it through implementation of the strategic/financial planning process, its cash reserves, its charitable funds, and its debt capacity. After determining the health needs of the community, managers must allocate the human and fiscal resources necessary to meet these needs. If all health needs cannot be met, the institution must then ration services based on the revenues it has.

Therefore, the institution must devise a procedure for rationing—the denial of possibly beneficial resources to some or all people—that is publicly defensible, socially accountable, quantitative, and clear.[43] Often this is not the case, and rationing is instead surreptitious and secret and not publicly recognized (although managed care organizations can be considered a very public form of rationing).[44] Managed care rationing often is perceived as a "denial" of treatment by healthcare consumers, consequently weakening public trust in the healthcare system. In the hospital setting it is an uncomfortable reality, but failure to ration care appropriately can lead an institution into fiscal difficulty when services are provided beyond its resources or without full reimbursement.

Not all people agree that rationing is necessary, and some believe that the elimination of inefficiencies and waste could go a long way toward ensuring universal access to cost-effective and quality healthcare services. The ethical challenge for those who believe this is to define appropriate outcomes and cost-efficient practices and then to build a system that allows sound steward-ship of available resources.

Other procedural concerns include ensuring that managers exhibit integrity[45] and behave ethically. For example, financial managers must be honest and must establish mechanisms that are not illegal or unscrupulous. Planners must honestly assess the needs of the community when developing healthcare services and match available financial resources with the institu-tion's commitment to serve that community. Operations personnel must make decisions about services and personnel that are aligned with strategic direc-tions and goals, and the chief executive officer must integrate these activities within the institution and, when necessary, revise them accordingly.

THE PUBLIC NATURE OF THE CORPORATION

A healthcare organization's commitment to service is a public statement. Such a statement is ethically significant because it can contribute to the build-ing of a community. Trustees and executives must ask basic questions such as: How will this network or institution make a difference to the community that it serves in the future? The fiduciary responsibility of trustees can be back-ward-looking: What was the financial performance of the organization last month (or last year)? How many goals were achieved last year? However, their ethical responsibility is mainly forward-looking: How will this organization make a difference in the world tomorrow? Planning how the ethical obliga-tions of the organization will be met is the work of the board.[46]

Creating tomorrow's vision demands ethical sensitivity to the public nature and service orientation of the organization. Generally, this includes a special concern for the uninsured, disenfranchised, and the poor. The managers and trustees should respond to community, state, or national demands for social justice, consider the social determinants of health, work to ameliorate factors that contribute to poor health, and use their considerable financial and insti-tutional power to help shape the community's future. These ethical concerns often are addressed through community networking, by building partnerships between community entities (businesses, educators, etc.), as well as working with public and elected officials to promote positive changes that will improve the health status of the community.

The preferential tax treatment of most healthcare organizations, their pub-lic trust, and their service mission obligates trustees and managers to work for the public good, At times, this obligation requires an institution to chal-lenge the medicalization of social problems and help eradicate the social deter-minants of health. For example, an organization must take on the causes of lead poisoning (poor housing conditions); the prevalence of malnutrition; abu-sive treatment of children, the elderly, and other vulnerable populations; the lack of vaccinations; and access to healthcare services and insurance. If healthcare organizational leadership does not address these issues, costs will rise, people will continue to be harmed, and the health status of the community will deteriorate.

Often, healthcare organizations, whether alone in smaller communities or in groups in larger communities, constitute a leading economic and political force. Leveraging an institution's powerful economic position for community gain is an ethical requirement flowing from the mission of the institution. Moral persuasion might be the tool most often employed in these situations, but a community's trust in and dependence on healthcare institutions or networks gives tremendous ethical power to trustees and managers.

The ethical commitment to the common good has implications for other institutional practices as well. Why would a healthcare institution not be sensitive to environmental issues? In the wake of the increasing costs of cure and care, can healthcare organizations be indifferent to returning people to a polluted or harmful environment? Environmental awareness will lead institutions to consider more closely the appropriate disposal of their wastes and toxins and promote the use of environmentally-friendly products.

Healthcare organizations also need to be self-critical when making strategic decisions. When deciding where to place the newest clinic or professional office building, they need to consider how the location might affect access to care for the poor and uninsured or contribute to the geographic isolation of the sick. What policies or regulations should institutions advocate to increase access, equitable reimbursement, and community support? Sometimes it seems there is a tendency in healthcare organizations to advocate for policies that will ensure their own continued existence, rather than those that benefit patients or the community. With ever-increasing external stresses on the healthcare system, the ethical concern for tomorrow is whether healthcare institutions will advocate for changes that are consonant with patient needs, such as increased outpatient services. Can there be a redistribution of public dollar commitments to address preventive health needs and decrease institutional and technological use? What social structure improvements will prevent illness and increase the health status of the community? There will always be a need for healthcare institutions, but perhaps the most equitable healthcare structure will consist of a new and different alignment of institutions, payers, and providers.

CONCLUSION

Healthcare networks, organizations, and institutions are powerful forces in public and political life. The ethical concerns of health care are broader than those that arise in the clinical context, and they are still being defined. Managers and trustees of healthcare organizations, if faithful to their mission, identity, and public commitment, must systematically address their role in promoting public welfare, protecting employees, creating a better environment for healthy living, influencing the politics and economics of the community, and helping to develop a just public order. Trustees and managers should focus on distinct, but complementary, objectives to achieve these general goals. To accomplish this, there must be a deliberate and systematic approach to address, implement, and monitor the ethical commitments of healthcare organizations.

SUMMARY

Issues in healthcare ethics are not restricted to clinical situations; they are also increasingly difficult for the institutions that address healthcare needs. This chapter presents some of the areas of concern for these institutions and systems including their role in clinical concerns, issues surrounding personnel, and the nature of the work itself. Because of healthcare organizations' unique mission, a discussion concerning organizational identity and obligation to the community is included. Finally, the reader is reminded of the need to be aware of ethical issues and to continue to address them, now and in the future.

QUESTIONS FOR DISCUSSION

1. Why do you think there has been an interest in ethics with respect to the institutional part of health care by organizations such as JCAHO and others?
2. What is the role of the administrator or manager in institutional ethics?
3. Why are healthcare businesses interested in being proactive in meeting the community's healthcare needs?
4. Why do you think Americans are so schizophrenic about their attitude toward health care?
5. What principles of ethics would be most important to institutions as they consider their ethics actions in the future?

NOTES

1. R. L. Potter, "On Our Way to Integrated Bioethics: Clinical, Organizational, Communal," *Journal of Clinical Ethics* 10, no. 3 (Fall 1999): 172.
2. C. F. Thurber, "Assessing Quality in HCO's: A Paradigm for Organizational Ethics," *HEC Forum* 11, no. 4 (1999): 358–363.
3. R. M. Arnold, et al., "Society for Health and Human Values—Society for Bioethics Consultation, Task Force on Standards for Bioethics Consultation," *Core Competencies for Health Care Ethics Consultation: The Report of the American Society for Bioethics and Humanities* (American Society for Bioethics and Humanities, Glenview, IL, 1998), 24.
4. R. L. Potter, "From Clinical Ethics to Organizational Ethics: The Second Stage of the Evolution of Bioethics," *Bioethics Forum* 12, no. 2 (1996): 3–26.
5. E. Spencer and A. Mills, "Ethics in Healthcare Organizations," *HEC Forum* 11, no. 4 (1999); 323–332.
6. W. Mariner, "Business versus Medical Ethics: Conflicting Standards for Managed Care," *Journal of Law, Medicine and Ethics* 23 (1995): 237.
7. Joint Commission on Accreditation of Healthcare Organizations, *Accreditation Manual for Hospitals, vol. 1* (Oakbrook Terrace, IL; Joint Commission on Accreditation of Healthcare Organizations, 1996).

8. See T. L. Beauchamp and J. Childress, *Principles of Biomedical Ethics*, 5th ed. (New York: Oxford University Press, 2001), 59–220.

9. See D. Seay and R. Sigmond, "The Future of Tax Exempt Status for Hospitals," *Frontiers of Health Services Management* 5, no. 3 (1989): 3–39.

10. C. Mackelvie and B. Sandborn, "Mooring in Safe Harbours," *Health Progress* 70 (1989): 32–36; J. Inglehart, "The Recommendations of the Physician Payment Review Committee," *New England Journal of Medicine* 320 (1989): 1156–1160; D. Kinzer, "The Decline and Fall of Deregulation," *New England Journal of Medicine* 318 (1988): 112–116.

11. See, for example, A. Enthoven and R. Kronick, "A Consumer-Choice Health Plan for the 1990s," *New England Journal of Medicine* 320 (1989): 29–37; U. Reinhardt, "Whither Private Health Insurance? Self Destruction or Rebirth?" *Frontiers of Health Services Management* 9, no. 1 (1992): 5–31.

12. A. Regan, "Regulating the Business of Medicine: Models for Integrating Ethics and Managed Care," *Columbia Journal of Law & Social Problems* 30 (1997): 635.

13. M. Rorty, "Ethics and Economics in Healthcare: The Role of Organizational Ethics," *HEC Forum* 12, no. 1 (2000); 65.

14. G. J. Agich and H. Forster, "Conflicts of Interest and Management in Managed Care," *Cambridge Quarterly of Healthcare Ethics* 9 (2000): 189; S. Wolf, "Toward a Systemic Theory of Informed Consent in Managed Care," *Houston Law Review* 35 (1999): 1660–1662.

15. Joint Commission on Accreditation of Healthcare Organizations, *Accreditation Manual for Hospitals, vol. 1* (Oakbrook Terrace, IL: Joint Commission on Accreditation of Healthcare Organizations, 1996), 44–45.

16. Ibid.

17. Ibid.

18. R. M. Arnold, et al., "Society for Health and Human Values—Society for Bioethics Consultation, Task Force on Standards for Bioethics Consultation," *Core Competencies for Health Care Ethics Consultation: The Report of the American Society for Bioethics and Humanities* (Glenview, IL: American Society for Bioethics and Humanities, 1998), 24–26.

19. See, for example, *Bioethics Forum*, 12, no. 2 (Summer 1996); *HEC Forum* 10, no. 2 (June 1998): 127–229 (the *HEC Forum* regularly features articles in a special section covering organizational ethics); *Journal of Clinical Ethics* 10, no. 3 (Fall 1999); and *Cambridge Quarterly of Healthcare Ethics* 9, no. 2 (Spring 2000); 145–298 (the papers in this issue were generated at a 1998 conference on healthcare organizational ethics, sponsored by the University of Virginia's Center for Biomedical Ethics and the Olson Center for Applied Ethics at the business school). For books on the topic, See P. J. Boyle, et al., *Organizational Ethics in Healthcare: Principles, Cases, and Practical Solutions* (San Francisco, CA; Jossey-Bass, 2001); The Kennedy Institute of Ethics, *Organizational Ethics and Healthcare: Expanding Bioethics into the Institutional Arena* (Washington, DC: Kennedy Institute of Ethics, 1999); R. T. Hall, *An Introduction to Healthcare Organizational Ethics* (New York: Oxford University Press, 2000); M. L. Pava and P. Primeaux, eds., Symposium on Health Care Ethics (*Research in Ethical Issues in Organizations*, 2 (New York: JAI Press, 2000); E. Spencer, et al., *Organization Ethics in Health Care* (New York: Oxford University Press, 2000); J. Blustein, L. Farber Post, and N. Dubler, *Ethics for Health Care Organizations: Theory, Case Studies, and Tools* (New York: United Hospital Fund, 2002); S. D. Pearson, et al., *No Margin, No Mission: Health Care Organizations and the Quest for Ethical Excellence* (New York: Oxford University Press, 2003); A. S. Iltis, *Institutional Integrity in Health Care* (New York: Springer, 2003).

20. American Medical Association, Institute for Ethics, *Organizational Ethics in Healthcare: Toward a Model for Ethical Decision-making by Provider Organizations* (Chicago, IL: American Medical Association, 2000).

21. American College of Healthcare Executives, *Code of Ethics*, November 10, 2003. Available at www.ache.org/ABT_ACHE/CodeofEthics.pdf.

22. G. Khushf, "Struggling to Understand the Nature of Organizational Ethics," *HEC Forum* 11, no. 4 (1999): 285–287.

23. J. Andre, "The Alleged Incompatibility of Business and Medical Ethics," *HEC Forum* 11, no. 4 (1999): 288-293.

24. L. L. Emanuel, "Ethics and the Structures of Healthcare," *Cambridge Quarterly of Healthcare Ethics* 9 (2000): 152.

25. N. J. Hirsch, "All in the Family—Siblings but Not Twins: The Relationship of Clinical and Organizational Ethics Analysis," *The Journal of Clinical Ethics* 10, no. 3 (Fall 1999): 210–215.

26. S. Dorr Goold, et al., "Outline of a Process for Organizational Ethics Consultation," *HEC Forum* 12, no. 1 (2000): 69–77.

27. P. H. Werhane, "Business Ethics, Stakeholder Theory, and the Ethics of Healthcare Organizations," *Cambridge Quarterly of Healthcare Ethics* 9 (2000): 172.

28. E. M. Spencer, "A New Role for Institutional Ethics Committees: Organizational Ethics," *Journal of Clinical Ethics* 8, no. 4 (Winter 1997): 374.

29. R. L. Potter, "On Our Way to Integrated Bioethics: Clinical, Organizational, Communal," *Journal of Clinical Ethics* 10, no. 3 (Fall 1999): 171; C. R. Seeley and S. L. Goldberger, "Integrated Ethics: Synecdoche in Healthcare," *Journal of Clinical Ethics* 10, no. 3 (Fall 1999): 202.

30. Surveys of human resource professionals reveal that there are issues underneath this normative agreement about what is ethical in the workplace. A survey of human resource management personnel indicates that the 10 most serious ethical situations are as follows: (1) hiring, training, or promotion based on favoritism; (2) allowing differences in pay, discipline, promotion, and so on, because of friendships with top management; (3) permitting sexual harassment; (4) yielding to sexual discrimination in promotion; (4) using discipline for managerial and nonmanagerial personnel inconsistently; (5) not maintaining confidentiality; (6) tolerating sex discrimination in compensation; (7) using nonperformance factors in appraisals; (8) arranging with vendors or consulting agencies; (9) situations leading to personal gain; and (10) acquiescing to sex discrimination in recruitment and hiring. See *Human Resources Management: 1991 SRHM-CCH Survey* (Commerce Clearing House, Chicago, June 26, 1991), 1–12.

31. Ibid.

32. J. Fletcher, J. Sorrell, M. Cipriano Silva, "Whistle-blowing as a Failure of Organizational Ethics," *Online Journal of Issues in Nursing*, December 31, 1998, p. 10. Available at www.nursingworld.org/ojin/topic8/topic8_.htm.

33. C. R. Seeley and S. L. Goldberger, op. cit., 206.

34. J. Fletcher, J. Sorrell, M. Cipriano Silva, op. cit.

35. Ibid.

36. A. E. Mills and E. M. Spencer, "Organization Ethics or Compliance: Which Will Articulate Values for the United States Healthcare System?" *HEC Forum* 13, no. 4 (December 2001): 329.

37. Seay and Sigmond, op. cit.; D. Pellegrini, "Hospital Tax Exemption: A Municipal Perspective," *Frontiers of Health Services Management* 5, no. 2 (1989): 44–46.

38. R. L. Potter, 1999, op. cit., 171–177.

39. P. Starr, *The Social Transformation of American Medicine* (New York: Basic Books, 1982); R. Stevens, *In Sickness and in Wealth: American Hospital in the Twentieth Century* (New York: Basic Books, 1989).

40. Stevens, op. cit., 141.

41. J. R. Horwitz, "Why We Need the Independent Sector: The Behavior, Law, and Ethics of Not-for-Profit Hospitals," *UCLA Law Review* 50 (2003): 1345–1347.

42. See the American Hospital Association, *Community Benefit and Tax Exempt Status: A Self-Assessment Guide for Hospitals* (Chicago: American Hospital Association, 1988); Catholic Health Association, *Social Accountability Budget: A Process for Planning and Reporting Community Service in a Time of Fiscal Constraint* (St. Louis: Catholic Health Association, 1989).

43. One suggested approach is presented in Catholic Health Association, *With Justice for All? The Ethics of Health Care Rationing* (St. Louis: Catholic Health Association, 1991).

44. S. Wolf. "Toward a Systemic Theory of Informed Consent in Managed Care," *Houston Law Review* 35 (1999): 1631.

45. For a discussion of integrity in today's healthcare market, see R. Dell'Oro, "The Market Ethos and the Integrity of Health Care," *Journal of Contemporary Health Law and Policy* 18 (2002): 641–647.

46. J. Carver, *Boards That Make a Difference: A New Design for Leadership in Non-Profit and Public Organizations* (San Francisco: Jossey-Bass, 1991), 1–23, 40–55.

CHAPTER 15

Hospital Ethics Committees: Roles, Memberships, Structure, and Difficulties

John F. Monagle and Michael P. West

OVERVIEW

Monagle reviewed this chapter from the first version of the text for inclusion in this new edition. His conclusion was that although the material is from older sources, the issues are substantially the same. They will remain significant for ethics committees into the twenty-first century. As a practitioner, West researched current issues facing hospital ethics committees and his findings have been added to this chapter.

Note that ethics committees are not just "window dressing" in today's healthcare world. Even with their limitations, they provide much needed guidance for healthcare professionals in dealing with the significant issues faced within healthcare facilities. Surely, they will face issues that are even more complex as health care becomes more technologically complicated and has its resources challenged by ever-increasing numbers of patients.

INTRODUCTION

It has become commonplace for technological growth to outstrip society's methods of dealing with it.* Nowhere is this more true than in medical care. At times, life-saving equipment and techniques work only to preserve a semblance of life. These tragic results are becoming increasingly common. Physicians, when unable to predict what treatment will achieve in an individual case, must apply the best treatment available in emergencies.

However, after a patient is stabilized and the prognosis becomes clear, the patient's family and physician might have to confront difficult questions: Is it ethical to discontinue treatment? Is it ethical to continue? Having to make hard decisions is becoming more frequent, producing in recent years a number of highly-publicized, emotionally-charged court actions over the ethical approach to withdrawal of treatment.

Two California physicians agreed with a patient's family that they should remove life-support systems, including medical feeding and hydration, from a hopelessly brain-damaged patient. The physicians were accused of murder, although the charges were eventually dismissed.[1]

---

*The following material is reprinted from *CHA Insight* 8, no. 26, (June 1984): 1–4, with permission of California Hospital Association, © June 1984.

Baby Doe cases are proliferating, with some families and physicians deciding to treat, and others refusing to treat, children born with serious birth defects. What is society's ethical position? Is there any consensus toward resolution?

BASIC ROLES OF THE ETHICS COMMITTEE*

The idea that ethics committees can form a consensus toward resolution and assist in bioethical decision making has now become widespread. Enough has been written about the ideal scope of such committees to allow their intended roles to be summarized as follows:

- *Education.* Educating hospital staff about issues in ethical decision making and about how to use the hospital ethics committee[2]
- *Multidisciplinary discussion.* Providing a locus for interdisciplinary participation in value clarification and prioritization, leading to conflict resolution[3]
- *Resource allocation.* Recommending in-hospital allocation policies to maintain quality of care in the face of cost-containment measures[4]
- *Institutional commitments.* Expressing the spirit of the hospital regarding its stated mission, philosophy, image, and identity (most often applicable to religious or private hospitals)[5]
- *Policy formulation.* Developing policies and guidelines regarding ethical issues
- *Consultation.* Assisting attending physicians regarding difficult decisions

Education

Even if a hospital ethics committee cannot function, because of its large membership, as the ethical decision maker or directly in a consulting or policy-formulating capacity, it nevertheless can become the backbone of an institution's effort to educate its staff about ethics, ethical principles, and ethical issues. Initially, a process for conducting interdisciplinary discussions about specific ethical issues is needed. Later, as issues become more clearly defined, a process should be established whereby ideas and guidelines about specific hospital policies can be directed to the hospital's ethical policy subcommittees for their consideration and for policy formulation. Although it may function mainly to recommend guideline policies for further review and formulation, the hospital ethics committee remains deeply involved in ethical issues and is never cut off from the clashes of fundamental values experienced by clinical staff and administration.

What kinds of educational activities are appropriate? Many hospital staff members are interested in discussing ethical issues but feel that their train-

---

*The following material is from the © *Quality Review Bulletin*. Oakbrook Terrace, IL: Joint Commission on Accreditation of Healthcare Organizations, 1985, pp. 204–208. Reprinted with permission.

ing in ethics is inadequate. They may also see formal education in ethics as too esoteric and remote from real-life problems. Given this common intimidation about ethics education, it is best to concentrate on case discussions in the context of a formal plan and under the leadership of an educator or medical ethicist. Most university medical centers employ such professionals,[6] as do many other hospitals and hospital systems.[7] Also, as existing hospital ethics committees have discovered, the faculty of nearby colleges might include professionals interested in discussing ethical problems in health care.

A necessary activity for the hospital ethics committee is to provide bioethical education for patients, their families, and the larger community in order to promote an understanding of ethical problems and an awareness of the desire and responsibility of physicians and hospitals to respond in an ethical manner. Hospital ethics committees, given the specific charge to analyze the community's ethical concerns, issues, and dilemmas and the authority to develop (through ethical policy subcommittees) policies for the care of severely handicapped infants and terminally ill patients, can be a source of great help to families and physicians directly involved in difficult decisions. Properly structured, an ethics committee thereby demonstrates the hospital's and the medical staff's commitment to protecting patients' rights and community values.

Multidisciplinary Discussion

An interdisciplinary approach both to the makeup of hospital ethics committees and to proposed ethics discussions in hospitals is essential for several reasons. Ethical dilemmas are not confined to the physician-patient relationship; they occur with respect to many other healthcare professionals, institutional demands, and social factors. The increased specialization of health care demands "defragmentation" of staff during attempts to resolve ethical issues. Communication across disciplines regarding difficult emotional issues (often involved in ethically-complex cases) tends to minimize disruptions that could damage healthcare delivery.

For example, when a patient's wife and children request that the father be taken off a respirator, does the request represent the wishes of the father or of the family? Sometimes the nurses or the significant attending nurse know the answer better than the attending physicians, who in many hospital situations might not know the family well. In such cases, a sound decision cannot be reached without involving the nursing staff (or the significant nurse) and other relatives who know the patient's lifestyle, desires, and requests.

A second consideration is the effect that the decision will have on the caregivers. Staff members often form emotional bonds with patients, especially when the patient is so helpless as to need ventilator support. A physician's order to "wean" the patient off the respirator when this action may result in death requires at the very least some discussion with the attending nurses and respiratory specialists who have been providing the care (see the section "Consultation: Ethics Advisory Groups" later in this chapter). Nurses often ask hospital ethicists to approach physicians about such determinations—not in a spirit of rebellion, but with a simple request that the decision be discussed with them. Any attempt to avoid such interdisciplinary discussion at the specific case level not only ignores the emotional dimensions of ethical issues, but also causes new ethical issues to arise for those who must carry out the orders. As one nurse stated privately years ago, the most fundamental ethical issue for nurses concerns the expectations that they will remain silent and "get used to" being excluded from the decision-making process.

Multidisciplinary discussion does not merely address the emotional aspects of ethical issues; it is required by the inherently multidisciplinary nature of the ethical dilemmas that occur today. The federal government is directly involved in promulgating guidelines on research and on the care of defective newborns. State authorities are involved in executing prospective payment policies that might cause some persons not to receive the care they need. Insurance companies are involved, especially through preferred provider organizations (PPOs) and health maintenance organizations (HMOs), because they reward physicians who keep their patients away from expensive care. Hospital administrators are involved in determining who will receive expensive care that will not be reimbursed. In addition, physicians and consultants are involved in day-to-day decisions to which they bring legal, moral, and professional standards. It becomes impossible to resolve some clinical ethical problems without considering the involvement of all these participants.

Resource Allocation

One of the least discussed of the possible functions of a hospital ethics committee is assisting the hospital governing body to develop policies for resource allocation.[8] As the trend toward cost containment continues, more difficult allocation issues will arise in every institution. For example, can the hospital ethically limit the number of certain types of expensive cases it accepts should reimbursement fail to meet its actual costs? Should certain services no longer be offered at the hospital? Has the community been represented in these decisions?

A study at Rush-Presbyterian-St. Luke's Medical Center in Chicago revealed the loss of approximately $20,000 per elderly patient receiving care in an intensive care unit, despite reimbursement under Medicare's prospective payment system. The researchers expressed a concern that if costs cannot be recovered elsewhere, critical care for the aged will dwindle, and patients will not receive the quality of care to which they have become accustomed.[9] Their concern rests on a profound ethical principle of medicine: Physicians must act in the best interests of their patients, no matter the cost. Fortunately, at Rush, as elsewhere, costs for some services have been recovered through reimbursement for other more cost-effective services. However, this momentary respite from hard choices is just that—momentary. The national plan, of course, is to equalize the payment for each procedure throughout the country. When this is fully accomplished, cost shifting will no longer be possible, and resource allocation decisions will become all the more difficult.

The luxury of individual cases for which payments can be received will almost completely cease, replaced by the hardship of being no longer able to provide expensive services for which little or no payment will be received. Cost will become an essential ingredient in the ethical decisions regarding allocation of scarce resources unless the necessary funds are made available. The claim to necessary but expensive health care is to be weighed in the balance (of resource allocation).

As outside entities establish even greater control over reimbursement for specific diseases, each institution will face a major ethical question: How can cost containment and institutional survival be balanced with quality of care? If it is the responsibility of a hospital to fulfill its stated mission, philosophy, identity, and image, then particular judgments regarding allocation should be appropriate discussion matter for relevant administrators, staff, and community members.

Each hospital employee ostensibly commits himself or herself to the aims of the institution, and individual determinations and actions should further these aims. When the achievement of these aims is in jeopardy, consensus should be sought on how to maintain the best possible balance of values. This balance can then be conveyed to the community that the hospital serves. The hospital ethics committee can be central to this effort to renew and communicate the hospital's aims and the community's values and choices.

Institutional Commitment

The hospital ethics committee can begin to develop (or, in private and religious facilities, continue to develop) an ethical tradition for the hospital. Hospital ethics subcommittees need to consider such issues as the care of newborns, cardiopulmonary resuscitation, do not resuscitate (DNR) orders, resource allocation, and procedures that will not be performed. The hospital ethics committee should then recommend policies. Through this process, the ethics committee itself in effect becomes the conscience of the institution, linking the institutional philosophy with practical judgments about how to proceed in the best interests of the patient and the larger community.

Because of the extraordinary pressures currently brought to bear on hospitals as social institutions, they face the same kind of crisis regarding goals that universities faced in the 1960s. The social good traditionally offered—the highest quality of care—is called into question not only by "bureaucratic parsimony"[10] but also by alternative forms of delivery, ranging from HMOs to surgical, emergency, and ambulatory care centers. Hospitals are responding to the challenge by altering their characters, becoming less like social institutions and more like businesses. Departments become product lines, and services become ciphers in computer printouts of cost analyses.

However, one fact that often becomes lost in the jumble remains essential: Hospitals provide a good that people cannot obtain on their own using their own resources.[11] This good is not like most consumer products, which in some sense are luxuries. To reduce it to mathematical or economic analysis alone is to diminish its vast importance.

To preserve its aims in the thicket of economics and bureaucracy, the hospital must have at its disposal a realistic but firm vision of its nature and purpose. Siegler has suggested that if we are to ration health care, perhaps we should begin by withholding it from the wealthy and articulate and giving it to the poor and downtrodden.[12] Less dramatic, a hospital ethics committee might suggest a policy that would involve donating several hours a week to care for the poor. Further, it might consider practical measures to foster cooperation among competing hospitals so that needed care can be provided to all who seek it. Philanthropy, charitable giving, marketing, and fund-raising must be encouraged to ensure survival. Diversified business endeavors should be explored and implemented.

Policy Formulation: Ethical Policy Subcommittees[13]

Every hospital governing body has the duty to ensure that the institution reflects the mission and philosophy stated in its charter and developed in its traditions.[14] Staff turnover and a natural tendency, especially in institutions, for ideals to decay over time make it desirable to establish perdurable policies regarding ethical decision making. In effect, such policies are a form of prescriptive or directive ethics.

Yet one of the most astonishing features of hospitals to outsiders is precisely the lack of such directive ethics. Although most hospitals have numerous policies directing healthcare practice within their walls, few have attempted, until recently, to establish ethics guidelines. Religious hospitals have long had "mission and philosophy" committees, which have offered guidelines about procedures such as abortion and elective sterilization. Many other hospitals have developed guidelines for DNR orders as well. Apart from these exceptions, however, little attention has been given to policies regarding the significant ethical problems that challenge daily practice in the hospital (e.g., stopping certain forms of therapy for terminally ill patients, interprofessional conflicts, informed consent, and decision making for incompetent patients).

Resistance to policies governing such ethical problems stems from several sources. Inertia is certainly one; distractions and the pressures of time are two others. Some people think decisions by committee do not represent a sufficient advancement over individual decisions to warrant the effort. Still others are concerned that guidelines about care will adversely affect physician-patient relationships. Resistance also almost certainly results from the wrongheaded philosophy of medicine that views the one-on-one relationship of the physician and patient as sacred and exempt from outside interference.[15] Evidence exists that traditional Hippocratic ethics have been welded to an entrepreneurial concept of health care.[16]

In a traditional fee-for-service system, emphasis on the almost "sacred" quality of the physician-patient relationship is not entirely altruistic. Keeping other interests out of the relationship could be seen, at least in part, as a protectionist rather than a beneficent action. Traditional ethics and entrepreneurship can be decoupled without damage to the important ethical dimensions of the physician-patient relationship.

The hospital ethics committee's preliminary work serves as a starting point for more detailed analysis by ethical policy subcommittees appointed to study and recommend policy on specific areas of ethical uncertainty. The subcommittees, composed of physicians, some members of the hospital's ethics committee, and other health professionals with expertise in the subject area, forward the results of their analyses to the hospital ethics committee, which then can send them on to the appropriate authority for adoption as hospital policy.

Consultation: Ethics Advisory Groups*

These hospital policies are then available as guidance for ethics advisory groups, which are formed ad hoc when a specific case involving ethical issues arises. At this level, there is direct involvement of the attending physician and the patient and/or family.

The composition and membership of an ethics advisory group might include the following:

- Attending physician
- Patient and/or family members
- Significant nurse in the case
- Clergy or bioethicist
- Physician or other member of the ethical policy subcommittee of the subject area

In cases where there seem to be unresolved civil or criminal liabilities, an attorney for the hospital should be included. In certain cases, upon request of the patient or family, the attorney for the patient can also be invited to participate.

Perhaps the most important and most problematic role of the ethics advisory group is consultation.** Should the consultation on cases be, strictly speaking, an offering of advice to the physician or, alternatively, an actual decision-making process? Physicians often resist interpolations of decision-making bodies between themselves and their patients.[17] In part, this resistance stems from the view that the physician-patient relationship is the moral center of medicine.[18] It might also derive from a failure to recognize that medical ethics is no longer the private domain of physicians, if it ever was. The issues almost always involve public perceptions, social and political presuppositions, legal standards, and ethical traditions.[19]

It is not yet clear which of the two options should predominate. At present, the group should function at least as an advisory body. Successful optional consultation by the ethics advisory group requires support from the board members, administrators, and medical executive committee, along with continuing educational activities for the staff. Because ethically and legally society has placed the burden of medical decisions on the attending physician, the final treatment decision remains with the physician and the patient or family.

The bioethics committee at High Desert Hospital, Lancaster, California, operated by the Department of Health Services, County of Los Angeles, was

---

*The following material is reprinted from *CHA Insight* 8, no. 26, (June 1984): 1–4, with permission of California Hospital Association, © June 1984.

**The following material is from the © *Quality Review Bulletin*. Oakbrook Terrace, IL: Joint Commission on Accreditation of Healthcare Organizations, 1985, pp. 204–208. Reprinted with permission.

the first to be named in a malpractice suit. The plaintiff was 30-year-old Elizabeth Bouvia, and her attorney was Richard S. Scott. Bouvia had suffered since birth from cerebral palsy, and she was a spastic quadriplegic, immobile, and entirely dependent on others. She alleged that a nasogastric tube for forced feeding was inserted against her will and without her consent on January 16, 1986. On April 16, 1986, the Court of Appeals, Second Appellate District, Division Two, ordered the tube removed. In an amended complaint filed on July 23, 1986, in the Superior Court of the State of California for the County of Los Angeles, Bouvia named the hospital's bioethics committee and individual members as defendants. (Case No. C583828). Bouvia's attending physicians were free to disregard the advice of the bioethics committee.

In this case, the physicians were legally responsible for their actions. However, was the bioethics committee? The suit against the bioethics committee and its individual members should not chill or intimidate members of bioethics committees who act in good faith in the interest of the patient. Bioethics committees reduce, not increase, legal exposure.

Ethics Committees: Membership*

The membership of hospital ethics committees should represent a broad range of value perspectives, professional expertise, and community representation. The committee should include:[20]

- ***Medical staff.*** Staff from specialty areas such as obstetrics, neurosurgery, neurology, nephrology, oncology, psychiatry, and so forth
- ***Nursing staff.*** The director of nursing, operating room supervising nurse, emergency department supervising nurse, etc.
- ***An administrator.*** A high-level qualified administrative person who is interested in ethical issues, sensitive to medical staff responsibilities, patient and employee rights, financial realities, and community concerns
- ***A social services representative.*** A person knowledgeable about what the hospital, as well as the larger community, can provide in the way of care for patients
- ***Clergy or bioethicist.*** Having at least one such person is essential for multidisciplinary discussions. Candidates should have training not only in moral theology, but also in the formal discipline of philosophical ethics in order to present the ethical theories and principles that can be applied to the individual case. Some clergy do not have these credentials. Although they can bring important and essential insight to the committee, it cannot replace the formal discipline in ethics that also is needed.
- ***A member of the hospital board.*** Because the hospital board represents the community, the person selected should be knowledgeable about the larger community's concerns as to the kinds of medical procedures and treatments that are needed in the demographic area that the hospi-

---

*The following material is reprinted from *CHA Insight* 8, no. 26, (June 1984): 1–4, with permission of California Hospital Association, © June 1984.

tal serves. In addition, because all of the hospital's services are ultimately the responsibility of the hospital board, the governing-body representative should participate in and have knowledge of the hospital ethics committee's discussions and decisions.

STRUCTURES: THREE MODELS*

Three structures are possible for an ethics committee. The structure of the committee is determined by the part of the hospital that has authority over its operations. The three organizational designs to be considered include an ethics committee as a committee of the hospital's governing board, as a committee reporting to the hospital's chief executive officer, and as a committee responsible to the hospital medical staff executive committee.

Each structure has its advantages and disadvantages. The committee's structure and membership, its authority and responsibility, its charge and scope of activity, and its limits of purpose and authority should be clearly defined according to the particular needs of each hospital.

Under the governing-board model, the ethics committee uncovers, discusses, and clarifies ethical concerns or problems and, in consultation with the medical staff executive committee and the hospital administration, forms an ethical policy subcommittee to analyze the available information on the subject.

The subcommittee's policy recommendations are reviewed by the ethics committee and forwarded for adoption by the governing board as hospital policy. When a case involving those issues arises, those policies serve as guidelines to ethics advisory groups formed to help the family and physician understand the ethical choices involved. The flow of information and development of hospital policies is similar in the other two models, but in those models the hospital's administration or the medical staff executive committee has more or less direct authority for final review and approval of the policies.

One of the differences among the governing board, administration, and medical staff organizational models is the level of public disclosure each affords. Because the ethics committee's primary focus is on patients' rights and hospital and community education in bioethical issues, it might not be advisable to seek the protection from discovery in legal action that state law gives to the deliberations of medical staff quality-care review committees.[21]

To the extent that the discussions and recommendations about or solutions to ethical concerns, issues, and dilemmas are shared openly, the medical staff's and the institution's assumption of ethical responsibility for policies and actions will be visible and recognized. Furthermore, if a hospital's ethical practices are challenged through civil or criminal suit, summary documentation of the ethics committee's proceedings may well serve as a defense for the physicians and the hospital.

---

*The following material is reprinted from *CHA Insight* 8, no. 26, (June 1984): 1–4, with permission of California Hospital Association, © June 1984.

Under the medical staff organizational model, the ethics committee might seek protection from discovery for the records and proceedings of its ethical policy subcommittees, because these committees report to the ethics committee of the medical staff. Likewise, protection from discovery might be sought for the ethics advisory groups under either the medical staff or governing board organizational models. The governing board structure might be the most amenable to openness of information, discussion, and recommendations, while at the same time protecting records and proceedings related to individual case discussions of the ethics advisory groups.

The administration model, although unable to seek protection from discovery under quality-assurance confidentiality statutes, might be more responsive to management control of cost-effectiveness and to evaluating risk management and professional liability implications of hospital ethical policies. The medical staff model, although fully protected from disclosure of discussions, has to guard against domination by physicians and lack of interaction with the community.

DIFFICULTIES AND NEEDS: ETHICS COMMITTEES AND ETHICISTS

The following ten areas represent areas of difficulty for most ethics committees and ethicists. They exist in a variety of current healthcare environments. They also promise to be problems for committees into the twenty-first century.

1. The necessary money by which we can fund and allocate time in order to discuss and resolve present and evolving ethical issues, "soft money," is difficult to acquire.[22] It takes time and expert personnel to develop and implement a single ethical policy. If a committee has only one or two hours a month to discuss, formulate, and prepare to implement an ethical policy, only one or two policies can be produced in a year. The issues are many, but the policies are few.[23] A national network of healthcare committees that have formulated and are willing to share policies does not exist. One unified national organization of bioethicists, to educate and share, is necessary, yet it still does not exist.[24]

2. At present, bioethicists are not recognized as "certified" in their discipline, profession, or field.[25] A certification standard needs to be developed and implemented so that bioethics can be recognized in academic and clinical arenas. The Society for Bioethics Consultation has a panel that will make recommendations in the future.

3. Some money-strapped healthcare institutions find it difficult to justify expenditures on "ethicists" or ethics committees because they are not considered necessary for direct patient care.

4. Issues such as abortion, sterilization, surrogate motherhood, transplantations, euthanasia, assisted suicide, and other issues regarding death and dying[26] have not been resolved successfully by any universally applicable solutions to benefit the care of patients. Furthermore, ethicists and ethics committees in general are not able to offer practical discussion and resolution of evolving issues, such as the relationship of high technology to possibilities for

cloning and all other forms of genetic manipulation and engineering. The academic discussions are presented, but clinical resolutions to the problems are not discussed.

5. Pass-through costs for academic or clinical services are under scrutiny. Managed care, curtailed by cost, has led to severe limitations on the consultative care offered. Physician survival has forced professionals into managed care organizations. Less money spent by managing care is the dominant goal of these organizations. In fact, because of these organizations' rules and regulations, the quality of patient care is a secondary consideration. The prime directive is reduction of managed care costs. This is the reality.[27]

6. Most ethicists and ethics committees are not trained in business or managed care ethics. Ethicists come more readily from the humanities background and are not corporate business practitioners. They do not easily deal with enforced government rationing, as demonstrated by Medicare and Medicaid. Not all demands can or will be met by a corporate business mentality into which healthcare institutions and professionals have been forced. In general, ethicists are not financially experienced in the cost of personnel staffing requirements. They have not been trained in business marketing and health service plans. In addition, most ethicists are not able to contribute to the ethical and financial issues involved in healthcare mergers, joint ventures, corporate restructuring, and the financial limitations of institutions in providing uncompensated care. Consequently, ethical demands are not fully understood in the context of financially-based insurance policies limiting or denying certain options of coverage.

7. Comparatively few ethicists have entered into public discussion and initial proposals reflecting public desires related to the financial problems of the healthcare industry. Only recently have several states conducted educational public inquiries addressing public demands and preferences for healthcare treatments and procedures. Examples include the Health Care Decision Making Surveys conducted in California, Colorado, Oregon, and Massachusetts.[28] Ethicists need to establish and participate in similar statewide activities involving decision making and policy planning related to bioethical and financial interests. Furthermore, they should increasingly become part of the organizations that raise the "soft money" that finances public studies of patients' viewpoints, priorities, preferences, and desires regarding health care. Eventually, state legislatures might modify and mandate publicly-acceptable solutions, based on the activities of these statewide organizations.

8. Bioethics has reached a crisis in its young adulthood. It needs to identify (a) who its practitioners are, what their qualifications are, and what their training and experience should be and (b) what problems and issues they can professionally and skillfully handle. In addition, it must address (c) in what areas ethicists need to educate themselves and contextualize their views; and (d) to what extent they need to adopt a financial or "Wall Street" approach to managed care.

9. Most of the bioethicists who will survive and progress in the new millennium will be those who become involved in the administrative, financial, and clinical functions of managed care organizations, healthcare facilities, and socially responsible entities. These organizations will deal with comprehensive

ethical issues, which may include environmental concerns, including hazardous waste, and issues involving the homeless, the disabled, home care, and hospice efforts. A focus on these efforts will be necessary if bioethicists are to be considered necessary and valued to the administrative and public views of the healthcare system.

10. There has been reluctance in the past, as there undoubtedly will be in the future, by some bioethicists to become involved in "the dirty business of finance." Unless so fortunate as to have an endowed academic or clinical chair, an ethicist will quickly realize the necessity for knowledge of healthcare financing as he or becomes involved in the financial concerns pervading the healthcare industry, because these concerns influence ethical issues and decisions constantly. Otherwise, some might come to consider bioethicists and ethics committees as parasitic to the financial efficiency of healthcare entities. They cannot afford to be marginalized in this way.

CONCLUSION*

Hospitals interested in ethics committees can select from the roles discussed in this chapter. The needs of each institution are different, as is each institution's capacity to establish such committees. Some of the roles are more problematic than others are. In many hospitals, several of the roles are already carried out by other committees—allocation decisions by the quality assurance committee, institutional commitments by the mission and philosophy committee, and so on. None of these functions, however, will be successfully integrated within the hospital unless the ethics committee is part of an educational effort that involves both the primary disciplines responsible for patient care and the personnel responsible for hospital governance.

Ethical issues are not going to diminish in frequency or complexity.* The individual treatment dilemmas raised by new technology are difficult enough. However, dilemmas that are even more agonizing have surfaced, with the introduction of PPOs, HMOs, diagnosis-related groups, and the other responses to limited resources.

In Securing Access to Health Care,[29] the President's Commission for the Study of Ethical Problems in Medicine and Biomedical and Behavioral Research concluded that society is obligated to provide "equitable" access to "adequate" health care.[30] But as new technology redefines what care is adequate, its cost restricts access to its benefits. The inequity of limited access, first to the poor, but eventually to everyone, might become society's thorniest bioethical dilemma—one that will necessitate more hospitals to establish and support ethics committees.

*The following material is from the © Quality Review Bulletin. Oakbrook Terrace, IL: Joint Commission on Accreditation of Healthcare Organizations, 1985, pp. 204–208. Reprinted with permission.

UPDATE FROM A PRACTITIONER'S VIEW

The following section presents the results of West's research with hospital ethics committees. It introduces the issues of current concern and suggests those that will be part of the future. There appears to be a struggle with social justice or balancing the benefits of care with the burdens of financing that care. It is important that ethics not be forgotten in this struggle.

Healthcare costs continue to increase by double digits despite managed care's promise to control costs and provide high-quality preventive healthcare services. Medicare and Medicaid pay as little as seven percent of billed charges to many of the country's hospitals. The cost of patient care technology has been rising, with the added conundrum that the technology often is outdated before it is even delivered and installed.

This financial crisis has forced hospital ethics committees to not only consider quality-of-life and quality-of-death issues, but also the financial implications of treatment alternatives. Committees are now being scrutinized for their high-profile decisions regarding value-of-life issues in futile situations and the costs that arise from those decisions. The case of Tirhas Habtegiris, a poor black woman in Plano, Texas, clearly demonstrates the impact of these decisions. Habtegiris, a terminally ill 27-year-old cancer patient, was removed from a ventilator while she was conscious and died within a few minutes. Her prognosis was hopeless, and her future cost of care was considered in the decision to cease all treatment. Compare this to the case of Mickey Mantle. The famous 63-year-old baseball celebrity was a lifelong alcohol abuser. He received a liver transplant after being on the transplant list for only two days and died shortly after receiving his transplant. These two cases demonstrate the disparity in the selection process, whereby treatment considerations were made based on the individual's social status and ability to pay, not on the patient's clinical presentation. Because financial considerations are included in the decision-making process, celebrity, wealth, and/or high levels of insurance coverage seem to be weighted more heavily than clinical status.

Advances in technology and patient care bring increased expectations for positive outcomes from patients and their families. These sometimes unrealistic hopes can cloud decisions made in emotionally charged situations. Hospital ethics committees must be an integral part of the patient care decision-making process in futile cases, but the committee must make decisions based on what is ethically best for a patient's situation and not just consideration for the institution's bottom line. This requires that committees have knowledge of the technologies involved and their benefits and limitations. It also requires time to deliberate from an ethical stance without undue pressure concerning facility financial concerns. The need to make ethics-based decisions also makes a case for the involvement of nonhospital members from the community, including ethicists.

To meet this societal demand for the use of technology and appropriate end-of-life decisions, hospitals must adequately fund and support ethics committees. Making ethics committees a viable part of the organization's decision making by seriously considering their recommendations should go a long way to assure fair and equitable distribution of medical treatment to those who will benefit. As health care becomes even more complex in the twenty-first century, the work of the ethics committee will have even greater importance for providing care that is both clinically sound and just.

SUMMARY

Ethics committees are the primary way that healthcare institutions address increasingly difficult institutional and patient ethical issues. This chapter reviews the roles of these committees and details the duties of ethics subcommittees. In addition, current and future issues for these committees are presented. Finally, through his research on practicing hospital ethics committees, West suggests that they may face even more difficult issues in the future including the challenge of providing clinically-sound, cost-effective care that is also socially just.

QUESTIONS FOR DISCUSSION

1. How do you think ethics committees can contribute to the organization's commitment to ethics-based practice?
2. Do you think that patient advocates or community members should be included on ethics committees?
3. What effect will the continuing progress of technology have on the job of the ethics committee?
4. If you were an ethics committee member, how would you address the following question: "At what point should treatment cease in futile cases?"
5. If you were an ethics committee member, how would you address the following comment: "Futile care policies are a humane action."
6. If you were an ethics committee member, how would you address the following statement: "Futile care policies are institutionalized murder."

NOTES

1. 47 Cal. App. 3d 1006 (1983). See J. F. Monagle, "A Question of Ethics on Murder," *CHA Insight* 13 (April 1984): 1–4.
2. A. R. Fleischman and T. H. Murray, "Ethics Committees for Infants Doe?" *Hastings Center Report* 13 (December 1983): 5–9; J. A. Robertson, "Ethics Committees in Hospitals: Alternative Structures and Responsibilities," *Quality Review Bulletin* 10 (January 1984): 6–10; R. J. Rooney, "Ethics from the Bottom Up: A Participative Approach to Health Care Ethics," *Bioethics Reporter* 3 (1984): 970.
3. J. Curtis, "Multidisciplinary Input on Institutional Ethics Committees: A Nursing Perspective," *Quality Review Bulletin* 10 (July 1984): 199–208; D. Ozar, "The Challenge of Multiple Professional Perspectives in Institutional Ethics Committees," *Bioethics Reporter* 1 (1984): 153.

4. A. Griffin and D. Thomasma, "Health Care Distribution and Hospital Impartial Panels," *Bioethics Reporter* 1 (1984): 124.

5. B. Bader, "Medical Moral Committees: Guarding Values in an Ambivalent Society," *Hospital Progress* 63 (October 1982): 80; E. Lisson, "Active Medical Morals Committee: Valuable Resource for Health Care," Hospital Progress 63 (October 1982): 36.

6. T. K. McElhenny and E. D. Pellegrino, *Teaching Ethics, the Humanities, and Human Values in Medical Schools: A Ten-Year Overview* (Washington, DC: Institute on Human Values in Medicine, Society for Health and Human Values, 1981).

7. M. M. McDonnell, "Holy Cross Health System: Medical Ethics Program," *Bioethics Reporter* 3 (1984): 960; G. Graber, "One Philosopher's History in His Work with Hospital Ethics Committees," *Bioethics Reporter* 3 (1984): 956.

8. Griffin and Thomasma, op. cit.

9. P. W. Butler, et al., "Technology Under Medicare Diagnosis-Related Group Prospective Payment: Implications for Medical Intensive Care," *Chest* 87 (February 1985): 229–234.

10. M. Siegler, "Should Age Be a Criterion in Health Care?" *Hastings Center Report* 14 (October 1984): 24–27.

11. D. Ozar, "Justice and a Universal Right to Basic Health Care," *Social Science and Medicine (Ethics)* 15 F (March 1981): 135–141.

12. Siegler, op. cit.

13. J. F. Monagle, "Blueprints for Hospital Ethics Committees," *CHA Insight* 8, no. 20 (26 June 1984), see note 23.

14. D. Thomasma, "Hospitals' Ethical Responsibilities as Technology, Regulation Grow," *Hospital Progress* 63 (December 1982): 74–79.

15. D. Ozar, "Social Ethics in the Philosophy of Medicine, and Professional Responsibility," *Theoretical Medicine* 6 (1985): 281–294.

16. W. B. Schwartz and H. J. Aaron, "Rationing Hospital Care: Lessons from Britain," *New England Journal of Medicine* 310 (1984): 52–56.

17. Robertson, op. cit.

18. E. D. Pellegrino and D. C. Thomasma, *A Philosophical Basis of Medical Practice* (New York: Oxford University Press, 1981).

19. D. Thomasma, "Medical Ethics Committees Find New Roles," *Quality Assurance—Risk Management Bulletin* 5 (January–February 1985): 1–3; D. Callahan, "Shattuck Lecture: Contemporary Biomedical Ethic," *New England Journal of Medicine* 302 (1980): 1228–33.

20. Monagle, 26 June 1984, op. cit.

21. Forty-five states protect medical staff committee records under the state's evidence code or peer-review statute.

22. *Hospital Ethics* 11, no. 5 (1995): 1.

23. J. F. Monagle and D. C. Thomasma, eds., *Medical Ethics: Policies, Procedures, Guidelines, and Programs* (Gaithersburg, MD: Aspen, 1997).

24. *Hospital Ethics*, 5

25. *Hospital Ethics*, 4.

26. *Hospital Ethics*, 6, 11, 13.

27. "To Confess Role in Man's Death," *San Francisco Chronicle*, April 15, 1997, pp. A13, A15. A Kentucky physician for the Humana HMO allegedly saved $500,000 for the HMO, an allegation that the HMO denies.

28. *Hospital Ethics*, 15ff.

29. *President's Commission for the Study of Ethical Problems in Medicine and Biomedical and Behavioral Research, Securing Access to Health Care, vol. 1* (Washington, DC: U.S. Government Printing Office, 1983). For a review of its conclusions, see Allen Toon, "Equitable Access to Adequate Care," *CHA Insight*, (October, 19 1983): 9.

30. Bader, op. cit.

ADDITIONAL RESOURCES

American Hospital Association, *Hospital Committees on Biomedical Ethics* (Chicago: American Hospital Association, 1984).

P. L. Chinn, *Ethical Issues in Nursing* (Rockville, MD: Aspen, 1986).

R. P. Craig, *Ethics Committees: A Practical Approach* (St. Louis: The Catholic Health Association, 1986).

B. Hosford, *Bioethics Committees* (Rockville, MD: Aspen, 1986).

CHAPTER 16

Ethically-Important Distinctions Among Managed Care Organizations

*Jessica Moore**

OVERVIEW

Managed care is a major influence on healthcare delivery and is here to stay in one form or another. This chapter provides an excellent overview of the types of managed care options currently in use, and more importantly, the ethics issues they face. The author stresses the impact of managed care business practices on ethical problems for providers, those who are covered by such plans, and for society as a whole. These issues and others that new managed care options might create, will continue to be part of the ethical dilemmas for the twenty-first century.

INTRODUCTION

The term *managed care* describes a diverse set of organizational forms. Wide variations in approach, financing, physician involvement, and philosophy exist among the different types of managed care organizations (MCOs). Although many articles on the ethics of managed care acknowledge this variety, most analyses focus on for-profit entities, paying less attention to the ethical distinctions among the different forms of managed care.[1] This chapter discusses the key distinctions among MCO types, in particular the difference between for-profit and nonprofit plans. It also examines the relationship of the physician to the MCO, incentives used to control costs, incentives to improve patient care, and the organizational features that nurture the principled practice of medicine.

THE IMPACT OF MANAGED CARE

Throughout the literature on managed care, certain themes predominate. First, there is a great concern that MCOs are not fulfilling the goals for which they were initially designed. Second, there is overwhelming agreement that managed care has the potential to compromise the doctor-patient relationship. Some of the dangers to the physician-patient relationship take the form of financial incentives for physicians, putting the physician in the role of gatekeeper and implementer of gag clauses. However, much of the literature also refers to several positive aspects of managed care.

---

*Revised from K. T. Christensen, "Ethically Important Distinctions Among Managed Care Organizations," in *Health Care Ethics: Critical Issues for the 21st Century*. Original ed., 1998, edited by John F. Monagle and David C. Thomasma. Sudbury, MA: Jones and Bartlett, 2005.

Initially, managed care was conceived as a way to manage the skyrocketing cost of health care. The need for cost controls was the result of several factors. Private employers could no longer afford to subsidize healthcare costs for their employees under the third-party fee-for-service system. The government visualized managed care as a way to reduce costs in the Medicare and Medicaid systems. Managed care was also seen as a means to increase access to health care, because making health insurance more affordable would surely make it financially accessible for more people. In theory, managed care offers purchasers of health care competitively priced insurance, institutes quality-control measures to determine and encourage cost-effective care, and provides enrollees fair access to quality health care from credentialed providers within a budget. At the beginning of the new century, these goals have not been fully realized. Somewhere between theory and implementation, the system has fallen short in many ways, engendering public discontent and a struggle among stakeholders.[2]

Unfortunately, managed care has fulfilled few of its expectations:

1. Fewer Americans have access to health care, and there are more underinsured than ever before. The number of people with health insurance coverage increased by 1.4 million, to 247.3 million, between 2004 and 2005. However, the number of people without health insurance coverage also rose by 1.3 million, to 46.6 million, in 2005.[3]

2. Healthcare costs continue to rise. According to the American Medical Association's (AMA) Private Sector Advocacy Unit, health insurance premiums increased by more than 42 percent from 1998 to 2002, more than double the overall increase in medical inflation (17%) and triple the increase in overall inflation (10%) during the same period.[4]

3. MCOs have a financial responsibility to their stockholders, thus profits from cost savings are passed on to stockholders, instead of being realized in the form of rate reductions for plan participants.

4. Returning profits to stockholders reduces the amount of resources that can be directed toward the poor and uninsured.

5. The competition between MCOs is so fierce that few can afford to provide discounted or free access for the uninsured and underinsured. This competition has led to mergers that have created larger organizations with greater control over the market and the cost of care. According to the AMA, over 384 managed care mergers and acquisitions occurred between 1995 and 2002, with the top 10 largest national health plans covering at least 50 percent of commercially insured persons as of March 2004.[5]

A number of effects of managed care that compromise the physician-patient relationship have been discussed in the literature. These include conflicts between financial incentives and the patient's best interest, conflicts between individual patient interests and other patient's interests and society's interests, and gag clauses versus informed consent and patient autonomy. Additional concerns have been expressed about the physician's fiduciary responsibility to the patient versus financial responsibility to self, partners, company, and family. Some are concerned about the effects of the continuous pursuit of the cheapest managed care rates forcing frequent changes in providers on the quality of patient care received and questions of distributive justice to the group versus commutative justice in interpersonal relationships. Finally, the effect of cost containment on patient care is of major concern.

It also is important to note the consistently mentioned positive aspects of managed care. Managed care places a greater emphasis on preventive care. It tends to pay for preventive and maintenance (chronic) care more often than fee-for-service plans. This practice has led to more effective early detection and better chronic disease management. Managed care also places an emphasis on stewardship and community by attempting to balance the needs of both individual patients and the community in which they live. Another benefit is the inclusion of payment for medications in plan coverage. When properly administrated, managed care also reduces the amount of paperwork required for medical coverage. According to Kassirer, managed care has produced a number of benefits:

- In-hospital stays are shorter.
- Surgical procedures that previously required hospitalization are now safely performed in same-day surgery.
- Many medical practices have been standardized, producing better outcomes.
- Patient satisfaction has become an explicit goal.[6]

KEY DISTINCTIONS AMONG MCOs

In order to understand the ethics issues associated with managed care, it is necessary to grasp the critical distinctions between managed care organizations. This section presents information about the differences between for-profit and nonprofit managed care operations and the relationship between physicians and MCOs. In addition, there is an explanation of how capitation works and the ethics strain it produces for physicians.

For-Profit Versus Nonprofit Managed Care

Although MCOs come in a bewildering array of structures, three crucial distinctions can be made among them: profit status, the relationship of physicians to the organization, and the nature of the capitation arrangement. The most important difference is between for-profit and nonprofit health plans. For-profit plans make up the fastest-growing segment of the managed care market, are growing at a much faster rate than the nonprofits, and receive most of the attention in the business press.[7] For-profit healthcare conglomerates now dominate the healthcare system as a whole.[8] Although all MCOs must generate surplus revenue to continue to operate, for-profit plans differ from nonprofit ones in that they trade their shares publicly and are not governed by the rules of charitable organizations.[9] As a result, their administrative costs, as a percentage of total income, tend to be much higher.

For-profit administrative costs often include extraordinarily large chief executive officer (CEO) salaries and bonuses, dividends to shareholders, and cash reserves for acquisition of competitors.[10] In California, where 85 percent of the insured population belongs to a managed care plan, a 1994 survey revealed a wide range between the total administrative expenses of MCOs. These expenses ran as high as 30.9 percent of total revenue in the for-profit MCOs, but only 3.1 percent in the nonprofit organizations, such as the Kaiser Foundation Health Plan.[11] Nonprofit healthcare plans also tend to have a larger share of income devoted to health services and a smaller profit/income ratio.[12] A 1996 study by the California Medical Association of that state's health maintenance organizations (HMOs) demonstrated a similar trend: The largest portion of revenue spent on medical care was found in the nonprofit plans.[13]

This difference becomes ethically relevant when we consider the pressure on physicians to limit healthcare costs. Subscriber premiums or dues are set by the marketplace, and, because of direct competition between plans, the costs of the different plans tend to lie within a narrow range. Therefore, in order to create more profit for shareholders, the surplus is generated elsewhere.

Part of the surplus comes from reducing the amount spent on physicians, tests, treatments, and hospitalization.[14] Corner cutting, or erring on the side of doing less instead of more, is the feature of managed care that engenders the most concern. All MCOs keep costs down by decreasing the amount of money spent on unnecessary treatment or visits, making healthcare delivery more efficient. However, between the area of clearly unnecessary treatment and the clearly necessary there is a margin of uncertainty. It makes sense that physicians in an MCO that has both less to spend on patient care and stock-holders to please will be under more pressure to keep this margin as narrow as possible.[15]

In one major review published in *Consumer Reports* in August 1996, the public came down solidly in favor of the nonprofit MCOs.[16] *Consumer Reports* polled more than 30,000 readers who were members of health maintenance organizations (HMOs) and preferred provider organizations (PPOs) for their opinions of their health plans and examined the data available comparing quality of care. *Consumer Reports* compared how tightly the various MCOs restricted physician discretion in patient care decisions. The top 11 plans were all nonprofit MCOs, and the bottom of the list was made up of for-profit MCOs. Only future research will tell us whether such practices also are having a negative impact on clinical outcomes in patient care, such as rehospitalization rates and asthma mortality.[17] Even into the first decade of the twenty-first century, research indicates that patients are not happy, providers are not happy, and purchasers are not happy.[18]

Physicians and the MCO

The relationship between physicians and MCOs is clarified in this section. The type and scope of incentives are discussed because they create different ethics issues for practicing physicians. The idea of utilization reviews and practice guidelines as ways to control physician practice patterns are also included as ethics issues. Finally, issues of physician autonomy versus administration control are discussed.

Incentives

The second relevant distinction between MCO types is the relationship of the physician to the organization,[19] which manifests itself in the various incentives used to control patient care costs.[20] For physicians, incentives can influence professional autonomy, as well as practice stability and the quality of professional work life, which in turn impacts the quality of patient care in a variety of ways.[21] According to the AMA, "[t]he foundation of the physician-patient relationship is the trust that physicians are dedicated first and foremost to serving the needs of their patients."[22] These incentives have the potential to affect this trust as well as patient care.

All healthcare delivery systems have financial incentives that can influence physician behavior. Under the traditional fee-for-service (FFS) model, physicians are rewarded financially for overtreating patients.[23] Because many patients still believe that more health care is better health care, physicians have a further incentive to keep patients happy by doing more. This system (along with technological advances and increased public expectations) has led to spiraling healthcare costs and, at times, iatrogenic harm to patients. Few tests or procedures are entirely risk-free, and incidental findings can cause unnecessary anxiety as well as further tests or procedures. Although FFS allows physicians more practice and administrative autonomy than any other system does, it is rapidly withering in the face of the massive growth and consolidation of MCOs, as well as the cost-containment measures to limit Medicare and Medicaid reimbursements. Many FFS physicians are now contracting with a variety of MCOs.[24]

For many years, Kaiser Permanente was the only large-scale private alternative to FFS in the United States. Now MCOs include a growing array of reimbursement and healthcare delivery systems. Many MCOs offer a number of different products to enrollees and employers, giving each a choice from a menu of managed care and traditional indemnity plans. The basic forms currently are the independent practice associations (IPAs), PPOs, the group model HMOs (such as Kaiser Permanente), and the staff model HMOs.

PPO physicians contract with the MCO and are usually paid on a FFS basis (see Table 16–1).[25] Fees are usually discounted deeply by the health plan, and, as a result, many FFS physicians have experienced declining incomes.[26] Physicians in PPOs typically have contracts with a number of different MCOs and some indemnity plans. Because these physicians are still paid per service rendered, an inherent incentive arises to generate more healthcare costs by seeing patients more often and/or by ordering more tests and interventions (see Table 16–2).[27]

PPO physicians also are exposed to sudden changes in their relationships with the health plan, such as contract termination and the subsequent loss of covered patients. Therefore, income security is lowest for this group of physicians, in particular for the subspecialists. Physicians in IPAs also contract

Table 16–1   The Financial Relationship of the Physician and the MCO

Practice Type	Relationship of the Physician to the MCO	Physician Payment	Physician Involvement in Quality Assurance/ Utilization Review
PPO	Physicians contract with MCO	Discounted FFS	High
IPA/network	Physicians contract with MCOs through IPA	Usually capitation	High
Group model HMO	Group contracts with MCO	Capitation to group; salary with various incentives	High
Staff model HMO	Physician is employee of MCO	Salary with various incentives	Low

with one or more MCOs, but are given organizational coherence and negotiating power by the IPA. They are usually reimbursed on a capitated basis.[28]

The earliest forms of MCOs were group or staff model HMOs, such as Kaiser Permanente and the Group Health Cooperative of Puget Sound.[29] These two organizations had their foundations in benevolent aid societies set up for working immigrants in urban and rural communities across the country between the 1880s and the 1930s.[30] As healthcare costs rose in the 1960s and 1970s, policymakers and employers began to consider these prepayment arrangements as an attractive alternative to FFS plans.[31] In the group model HMO, the physician is part of a group that contracts with the health plan.[32]

Table 16–2   Spectrum of Physician Incentives*

	Traditional Fee for Service	Managed Care
Compensation	Fee per service rendered	Fee per person enrolled (capitation)
General incentive	Do more, get more	Do less, get more
Examples of specific financial incentive	Direct reimbursement for patient care; income from laboratory or radiology services, partnerships in hospital	Withhold part of income; capitation, direct or diffused; bonuses; threat of deselection

*This table is abstract in that it does not take into account the many variations on these basic themes among MCOs.

Instead of receiving a fee for each service rendered, the group is paid a capitated amount by the health plan in advance of providing patient care services. The physicians are typically paid a basic salary plus a variety of financial incentives, such as bonuses.

In contrast, physicians in staff model HMOs are employees of the MCO. They are salaried and are paid a variety of incentives—similar to group model physicians—that are designed to promote cost-effective medical care. Job security is often low because of the physicians' employee status. Some predict that in the future the majority of physicians will be working for staff model HMOs.[33] Some insurers offer "multitiered" plans. By combining features of HMOs, PPOs, and point-of-service (POS) plans, this approach offers patient choice and allows the patient to weigh the trade-offs between the options at the time of illness rather than during the annual enrollment period.[34] Such plans implement selected parts of the managed care toolkit.[35]

Financial incentives offered by many MCOs include the payment of bonuses from any unspent funds and the withholding income that is then paid out at the end of the year if certain cost-containment targets are met. Such targets might include keeping hospital utilization below a certain rate or limiting referrals to specialists. The larger the amount of the withheld income, the stronger the incentive to toe the line.[36] Laboratory and radiology costs are frequently deducted from the pooled funds as well.[37] In all but the group model HMOs, the threat of job loss or loss of one's patients also serves as a potent incentive to adhere to the MCO's rules.

Control over Clinical Practice: Utilization Review and Practice Guidelines

Another significant aspect of the relationship of physicians to MCOs is the degree of control physicians have over the administrative and clinical aspects of their practices. In IPAs and PPOs, income security may be low, but physician autonomy over medical practice is high because physicians retain much of the traditional FFS prerogatives and practice format. Although practice autonomy is more restricted in the group model HMOs than in IPAs or PPOs, physicians in all models typically manage their own utilization review, quality assurance, and cost controls. Practice autonomy is usually lowest in the staff model HMOs, where utilization review and cost controls are usually managed and implemented by health plan administrators. When control over the clinical aspects of practice rests with nonphysician administrators, the quality of patient care is threatened and physician morale plummets.[38]

Many physicians are happy to relinquish administrative responsibility for their medical practices but are uncomfortable with losing control over the clinical aspects, such as utilization and quality management. Physicians in MCOs know that utilization review can be benign or malignant, depending on who is doing it and to what end. This is the nightmare of utilization review: A stranger in another city, who has no clinical experience, calls the doctor and tells her to discharge a patient or denies approval for a test the physician deems necessary. When used in this way, utilization review can function as a barrier to patient care.[39] Negotiating these hurdles on behalf of their patients can greatly increase physicians' job stress.[40] That situation also raises a direct conflict of interest between physicians' duty to provide good patient care and their own financial well-being.[41]

However, when managed and implemented by physicians, utilization review can both promote better patient care (by minimizing unnecessary treatments or hospital stays) and save money. Utilization review should not put up barriers to good patient care, and in the hands of physicians, it is less likely to do so.[42]

Similarly, practice guidelines can be imposed on physicians, as in many staff model MCOs, or developed and implemented by physicians, as in group model MCOs.[43] When used inappropriately, such guidelines are applied as standards to measure, reward, and punish physician behavior.[44] However, with physician involvement this process serves as a useful extension of peer review and helps to maintain a high quality of care. When physicians are involved in the development and implementation of the guidelines, it is less likely that they will mistake guidelines for standards (which require more stringent outcomes studies and stricter enforcement)[45] and inappropriately use the guidelines to reward and punish.

Capitation

Another useful distinction among MCOs is the way members' premiums are distributed to the physicians.[46] Capitation forms the core financial process in all of the systems previously discussed. In a capitated system, the pool of funds for the provision of services is collected by the health plan and then distributed in various ways, which often is called *risk sharing*. Some plans give a physician group the money (reducing administrative costs and, if applicable, profit), and the money is kept in a central pool to pay for healthcare services. Other plans give the funds to the physicians or to small physician groups, and the physicians then keep whatever is left at the end of the period (monthly, quarterly, or yearly).

The more individualized the capitation arrangement is in relation to the physician, the greater the ethical strain on the physician's relationship with the patient.[47] For example, if a physician in a large group with a centralized fund orders an MRI to evaluate a young woman for multiple sclerosis, cost will not be a primary concern, because it is spread out over the group. If that same physician orders the MRI and the money comes out of the physician's own capitated fund, it directly affects that physician's income. The temptation to assign a heart murmur a benign status or to forgo a cardiology consult is greater if every penny spent comes out of the physician's own pocket. Most conscientious physicians will resist this temptation, but it injects an unnecessary "ethical stress" into the clinical encounter and might influence treatment decisions to the detriment of good patient care. Many HMOs now shy away from such direct capitation and instead capitate physicians as a group.

CONSEQUENCES OF MANAGED CARE FINANCIAL INCENTIVES

What are the possible consequences of capitation and other financial inducements to physicians to control costs? The most widely discussed is the temptation to withhold needed services.[48] Whether this really happens is hard to prove and has not been supported in the few studies that have examined it.[49] However, anecdotes about harm to patients from undertreatment abound, and this issue remains a primary concern of those who study managed care.[50] It might also be that a disincentive arises to retain ill patients in one's health plan or patient panel, because they will tend to cost more than they (or their employers) pay into the plan. This could endanger the care of patients with complex chronic illnesses.[51]

The beneficial impact of managed care incentives includes the reduction of wasteful treatments and less iatrogenic harm to patients because of the avoidance of unnecessary tests and procedures. Managed care also creates more emphasis on preventive care, the potential for better case management of very ill patients in an integrated setting,[52] and cost savings.[53] All of these benefits result in improvements in the quality of the care provided under managed care.[54] Although the degree of cost savings under managed care also has been contested,[55] it is this aspect of managed care that has propelled it to the forefront of healthcare delivery systems.

However, the moral test of a managed care system is not in the balance sheet of the HMO. Nor is it in the dividend reports of the investor, in the bonus to the "provider," or even in the costs saved, bed days reduced, efficiency gained, or productivity improved. The moral test of any system of care is its impact on the patient for whom the system is presumably designed and on the physician from whom the patient seeks help.[56]

So far, this chapter has focused primarily on the financial relationships that are intended to influence physician behavior and to decrease healthcare costs. However, physicians are influenced by nonfinancial considerations as well.[57] What kinds of incentives exist that might balance or buffer the temptation to limit treatment for the physician's own pecuniary benefit?

The strongest forces that balance the temptation to undertreat are those principles that most physicians acquired in medical school.[58] The most important and pervasive principle is the physician's professional duty to benefit, and not to harm, his or her patients. Applying this principle in traditional FFS would counteract the temptation to overtreat. Under managed care, physicians will be less likely to withhold necessary treatments if their primary allegiance is to the patient's well-being.[59]

Next in importance is the maintenance of the physician's professional and personal integrity, which again requires that the physician prevent harm to his or her patients. The approval of one's colleagues also exerts a strong effect on the behavior of many physicians, which is why peer review is such a powerful tool in changing physician behavior. If the philosophy and practice of the physician group reflect the primacy of good patient care over all other considerations, it is less likely that patients will suffer under managed care.[60] Reinforcing these principles in medical school and residency will be an important factor in maintaining good patient care as practiced in the managed care setting.

Health systems have mechanisms for reinforcing the principle of beneficence and for maintaining high-quality patient care, such as peer review and practice guidelines. These mechanisms offer the physician feedback if the physician is not providing the quality of care that colleagues expect or lets they physician know, for example, if he or she is not ordering enough mammograms or vaccinations.

Table 16–3   Forces that Balance the Negative Consequences of Managed Care Incentives

Principle Benefits
- Desire to prevent harm from undertreatment (beneficence)
- Professionalism/self-respect (integrity)
- Desire for the respect of one's peers

External Forces
- Treatment guidelines
- Peer review
- Fear of malpractice
- Patient/member involvement
- Regulation and legislation

The threat of malpractice is a reality in all treatment settings, and it can both promote overtreatment in FFS and deter undertreatment in managed care (see Table 16–3). State and federal regulations also are having an impact on MCO incentives and policies.[61] Finally, if health plan subscribers are educated and involved in their health care, they may be less likely to accept inadequate care and more likely to understand the financial trade-offs involved in every health-care decision.

THE ETHICAL HMO

Many authors suggest that the traditional clinical ethics framework is not sufficient for the organizational situations created by the managed care system.[62] Managed care controls healthcare access for both groups and individuals. Because of this power it has a duty to use resources appropriately, protect the community's interests, and assure the quality of clinical practice.[63] The Ethical Force Program (EFP) identified five core qualities that mark an ethically sensitive "benefits package." Such a package must be transparent, participatory, equitable and consistent, sensitive to value, and compassionate. Using these issues as a starting point, The Harvard Community Health Plan's LORAN Commission conducted additional research on improving fairness in coverage decisions.[64] Similarly, Allen Buchanan discusses the core elements of procedural justice within the context of managed care that must utilize methods of rationing to best serve the interests of the enrolled population and society while avoiding harm or injustices to individuals. These core elements include nondiscrimination; impartiality; publicity of rules; publicity of justifications for those rules; and accessible, fair, and timely procedures for appeals of denials of coverage.[65]

Enumerating ethical principles and good practices is not enough to help us identify those organizations that are best suited to promote the provision of health care in an atmosphere relatively untainted by financial conflicts of interest. Many authors have developed important and useful guidelines and principles for MCOs.[66] Let's summarize from the previous discussion on the structural features of healthcare organizations that nurture and reinforce the best principles of medical practice. MCO structure determines in large part the nature of the conflicts providers within it have to face, and it can also impact the quality of the care delivered.[67] For example, preauthorization requirements for hospitalization or emergency care are a structural barrier to good patient care.[68] A direct financial incentive to reduce hospital admissions is an ethical hurdle the physician must overcome to keep the patient's welfare foremost.

What would an MCO look like if it were structured to buffer or neutralize the incentive to undertreat patients and to maximize the incentives to provide quality medical care? What features should we look for in evaluating the degree of ethical stress a physician experiences in providing health care in different practice settings?

- The organization should be nonprofit.[69] This removes the shareholder and profit maximization as the bottom line, which theoretically puts less pressure on the physician to meet financial goals (as opposed to patient-outcome goals).

- To remove the cash register from the examination room—physician income should primarily come from a salary.[70] Divorcing the individual patient encounter from the physician's immediate income helps to focus the encounter on meeting the patient's needs and frees the physician to practice according to his or her professional principles. Group model and staff model HMOs both meet this ideal.

- Sharing the risk of capitation among a large group of physicians dilutes the temptation to cut corners inappropriately.[71] The manner in which capitated funds are distributed varies and influences the degree of conflict of interest that the physician experiences. Direct or individual capitation and linking financial incentives directly to cost-containment targets should be avoided.

- Clinical practice should be managed by physicians. Physicians should be centrally involved with utilization review, quality management, and the development and implementation of clinical practice guidelines. Utilization review should not serve as a barrier to providing healthcare services, and it should focus on undertreatment as well as overtreatment.

- The patients or members of the MCO should have a role in the operations of the organization at a number of levels.[72] First, subscribers should receive full disclosure from the health plan about any incentives to limit treatment and any restrictions on coverage. Second, MCOs need a mechanism to include health plan members in discussions of benefit coverage and conflict-resolution procedures. Third, community members should be involved in the ethics committees of managed care hospitals and organizational ethics committees of the health plans, where these committees exist.[73] Fourth, vigorous efforts at patient/member health education should be ongoing, both to improve the health of members and to improve their understanding of the financial trade-offs involved in treatment and benefit decisions. An educated member might be more likely to challenge unfair limits to treatment. Many other authors similarly suggest that public education and open communication are key elements of both an ethical framework and an increase in patient understanding, satisfaction, and participation in a beneficial managed healthcare system.[74]

CONCLUSION

Managed care is not one entity, but a broad category that includes a variety of healthcare delivery structures and practices, relationships with physicians, and physician incentives. Although all managed care forms face the challenge of avoiding conflicts of interest leading to undertreatment, some are more challenged than others. Whether an MCO minimizes conflict of interest for physicians depends on the way it is organized and financed, the degree of physician involvement in managing patient care quality, and the nature of the incentives used to control costs. The form of managed care that currently works best to prevent undertreatment is one that is nonprofit and has a large salaried physician group that manages the clinical aspects of the provision of healthcare services.

Having drawn these distinctions, it is clear that managed care, as a subject of study, is a rapidly moving target. Nonprofit HMOs are sorely challenged to compete with the for-profit entities.[75] All nonprofit HMOs are taking measures to cut costs, and in many instances, are adopting the methods of the for-profit HMOs.[76] If this trend continues, it is possible that the distinction between for-profit and nonprofit MCOs will blur. Moreover, for-profit organizations are rearranging themselves into new and unique forms at a rapid rate. Thus, as these new structures evolve, we must encourage the growth of those that foster the highest quality of patient care and physician satisfaction.

SUMMARY

The need to control healthcare costs will continue to be a fiscal and ethical issue into the twenty-first century. This chapter discusses managed care, which has evolved into the predominant method for attempting to control these costs. In addition to featuring the key distinctions among MCOs, it presents the ethical consequences of its use of financial incentives. The chapter also describes an MCO organizational model that reduces the ethical stress placed on physicians as they struggle to provide beneficent, high quality care within the structure of a MCO.

QUESTIONS FOR DISCUSSION

1. If John Stuart Mill analyzed the ethics of the managed care, as it currently exists, would he think it was a good idea? Why or why not?
2. Physicians have many ethical duties in their practice of medicine and healing. What is the impact of managed care on their duty to benefit patients?
3. What ethical temptations does the reimbursement scheme present for the physician?

4. What is the impact of managed care on the patient's autonomy?
5. Some have said that ethical managed care is an oxymoron. Do you think this is true? Why?

NOTES

1. A. Relman, "The Impact of Market Forces on the Physician–Patient Relationship," *Journal of the Royal Society of Medicine* 87 (supp. 22) (1994): 22–25; A. Relman, "Medical Insurance and Health: What about Managed Care?" *New England Journal of Medicine* 331, no. 7 (1994): 471–472; E. Pellegrino, "'Ethics," *Journal of the American Medical Association* 271, no. 21 (1994): 1668–1670.

2. K. G. Gervais, "Managed Care," in Stephan J. Post, ed. *Encyclopedia of Bioethics* 3rd (Cleveland, OH: Thompson and Gale, 2004): 1463–1467.

3. Public Information Office, U.S. Census Bureau, *U.S. Department of Commerce, U.S. Census Press Release No. CB06-136, Income, Poverty, and Health Insurance Coverage in the United States: 2005* (Washington, D.C.: Public Information Office, 2006).

4. A. D. Hoven, *Impact of the Health Maintenance Organization Act of 1973.* Report of the Council on Medical Service no. 4-A-04. (Chicago: American Medical Association, 2004).

5. Ibid.

6. J. P. Kassirer, "Managed Care and the Morality of the Marketplace." *The New England Journal of Medicine* 333, no. 1 (July 6, 1995): 50–52.

7. J. Johnsson, "Mega-merger of Two Public Plans Spurs New Interest in Stock Offering," *American Medical News* (April 24, 1995): 1; M. Freudenheim, "Penny-Pinching H.M.O.s Showed Their Generosity in Executive Paychecks," *New York Times* (April 11, 1995): C1.

8. K. G. Gervais, op. cit.

9. California Code for Non-Profit Corporations, section 5130-B.

10. See Freudenheim, supra note 7; M. Rodwin, "Conflicts in Managed Care," *New England Journal of Medicine* 332, no. 9 (1995): 604–607; J. Kassirer, "Mergers and Acquisitions—Who Benefits? Who Loses?" *New England Journal of Medicine* 334, no. 11 (1996): 722–723.

11. S. Thompson and Z. Valentine, "The Profiteering of HMOs," *California Physician* (July 1994): 28–32, based on a California Department of Corporations report for 1992.

12. Alameda-Contra Costa Medical Association, "Latest CMA Study Shows Rise in HMO Costs and Profits," *ACCMA Bulletin* (February 1995): 14; M. Freudenheim, "A Bitter Pill for the HMOs," *New York Times* (April 28, 1995): C1.

13. L. Kreiger, "Study Finds HMOs Less Efficient If For-Profit," *San Francisco Examiner* (February 13, 1996): A8.

14. M. Freudenheim, "Penny-Pinching H.M.O.'s Showed Their Generosity in Executive Paychecks"; M. Hiltzik and D. Olmos, "Are Executives at HMOs Paid Too Much Money?" *Los Angeles Times* (August 30, 1995): A13.

15. J. Fletcher and C. Engelhard, "Ethical Issues in Managed Care," *Virginia Medicine Quarterly*, 122, no. 3 (1995): 162–167.

16. "How Good Is Your Health Plan?" *Consumer Reports* (August 1996): 28–42.

17. For an interesting discussion of the pros and cons of for-profit HMOs, see M. Hasan, "Let's End the Nonprofit Charade," *New England Journal of Medicine* 334, no. 16 (1996): 1055–1057, and P. Nudelman and L. Andrews, "The 'Value Added' of Not-for-Profit Health Plans," *New England Journal of Medicine* no. 16 (1996): 1057–1059.

18. K. G. Gervais, op. cit.

19. J. M. Eisenberg, "Economics," *Journal of the American Medical Association* 273, no. 21 (1995): 1670–1671.

20. A. Hillman, "Financial Incentives for Physicians in HMOs: Is There a Conflict of Interest?" *New England Journal of Medicine* 317, no. 27 (1987): 1743–1748; see Rodwin, supra note 10, pp. 152–156.

21. L. Prager, "State Licensing Boards Consider Curbing Financial Incentives," *American Medical News* (October 16, 1995): 1, 74.

22. D. Orentlicher, *Council on Ethical and Judicial Affairs, American Medical Association, Ethical Issues in Managed Care* (January 25, 1995): 330–335.

23. E. Emanuel, "Preserving the Physician–Patient Relationship in the Era of Managed Care," *JAMA* 273, no. 4 (1995): 323–329; M. A. Rodwin, *Medicine, Money & Morals: Physicians' Conflicts of Interest* (New York: Oxford, 1993), 98.

24. L. Kreiger, "Family Doctors Are Disappearing," *San Francisco Examiner* (June 18, 1995): A1.

25. M. Gold, et al., "A National Survey of the Arrangements Managed Care Plans Make with Physicians," *New England Journal of Medicine* 333, no. 25 (1996): 1678–1683.

26. D. Olmos, "Some Doctors Head to Idaho, a State Without Managed Care," *Los Angeles Times* (August 29, 1995): A11.

27. S. Herschberg, "Potential Conflicts of Interest in the Delivery of Medical Services: An Analysis of the Situation and a Proposal," *Quality Assurance and Utilization Review* 7, no. 2 (1992): 54–58.

28. B. Shenkin, "The Independent Practice Association in Theory and Practice," *JAMA* 273, no. 24 (1995): 1937–1442.

29. R. A. Dudley, R. and H. S. Luft. "Health Policy 2001: Managed Care in Transition." *The New England Journal of Medicine* 344, no. 14 (April 5, 2001): 1087–1092.

30. W. Knight, *Managed Care: What It Is and How It Works* (Gaithersburg, MD: Aspen Publishers, 1998).

31. R. A. Dudley and H. S. Luft, op. cit.; W. Knight, op. cit.

32. J. Robinson and L. Casalino, "The Growth of Medical Groups Paid Through Capitation in California," *New England Journal of Medicine* 333, no. 25 (1995): 1684–1687.

33. E. Friedman, "Changing the System: Implications for Physicians," *Journal of the American Medical Association* 269, no. 18 (1993): 2437–2442.

34. R. A. Dudley and H. S. Luft, op. cit.

35. K. G. Gervais, op. cit.

36. Council on Ethical and Judicial Affairs, American Medical Association, "Ethical Issues in Managed Care," *Journal of the American Medical Association* 273, no. 4 (1995): 330–335.

37. M. A. Rodwin, *Medicine, Money & Morals: Physicians' Conflicts of Interest* (New York: Oxford University Press, 1993), 138–144.

38. A. S. Relman, "Medical Practice under the Clinton Reforms—Avoiding Domination by Business," *New England Journal of Medicine* 329, no. 21 (1993): 1574–1576.; Vincent Cangello, "The Real Issue," *ACCMA Bulletin* (January 1995): 18; M. C. Beach, et al. "Physician Conceptions of Responsibility to Individual Patients and Distributive Justice in Health Care," *Annals of Family Medicine* 3, no. 1 (January–February 2005): 53–59; James F. Childress, "Conscience and Conscientious Actions in the Context of MCOs," *Kennedy Institute of Ethics Journal* 7, no. 4 (1997): 403–411.

39. M. Hiltzik, "Emergency Rooms, HMOs Clash over Treatments and Payments," *Los Angeles Times* (August 30, 1995): A12.

40. W. Phillips, "Hassle Hypertension: A Risk of Managed Care," *Journal of the American Medical Association* 274, no. 10 (1995) (letter to editor): 795–796.

41. M. A. Rodwin, op. cit., 135.

42. One study of IPAs and physician groups with capitated contracts showed that physicians tended to employ the same type of barriers to care, such as preauthorization requirements, as health plans. The study did not include the largest group practice HMO in California, Kaiser Permanente, which does not use preauthorization requirements to control costs. E. Kerr et al., "Managed Care and Capitation in California: How Do Physicians at Financial Risk Control Their Own Utilization?" *Annals of Internal Medicine* 123, no. 7 (1995): 500–504.

43. F. J. Crosson, "Why Outcomes Measurement Must Be the Basis for the Development of Clinical Guidelines," *Managed Care Quarterly* 3, no. 2 (1995): 6–11; D. Eddy, "Broadening the

Responsibilities of Practitioners: The Team Approach," *Journal of the American Medical Association* 268, no. 14 (1993): 1849–1855; L. Zendle, "Controlling Costs: The Case of Kaiser," *Journal of the American Medical Association* 274, no. 14 (1995): 1135; J. LaPuma, D. Schiedermayer, M. Siegler, "Ethical Issues in Managed Care," *Trends in Health Care, Law & Ethics* 10, no. 1/2 (1995): 73–77.

44. E. Friedman, op. cit.

45. F. J. Crosson, op. cit.

46. A. Hillman, "Health Maintenance Organizations, Financial Incentives, and Physicians' Judgments," *Annals of Internal Medicine* 112, no. 12 (1990): 891–893.

47. M. A. Rodwin, op. cit., 139–141.

48. N. S. Jecker, "Managed Competition and Managed Care," *Clinics in Geriatric Medicine* 10, no. 3 (1994): 527–540; E. Emanuel, op. cit.; Council on Ethical and Judicial Affairs, American Medical Association, op. cit.

49. D. Clement, et al., "Access and Outcomes for Elderly Patients Enrolled in Managed Care," *Journal of the American Medical Association* 271, no. 19 (1994): 1487–1492.

50. Council on Ethical and Judicial Affairs, American Medical Association, op. cit.; D. Sulmasy, "Managed Care and Managed Death," *Archives of Internal Medicine* 155 (1995): 133–136; M. Hiltzik and D. Olmos, "A Mixed Diagnosis for HMOs," *Los Angeles Times* (August 27, 1995): A1.

51. J. Richmond, "The Health Care Mess," *Journal of the American Medical Association* 273, no. 1 (1995): 69–71; E. Rosenthal, "Managed Care Has Trouble Treating AIDS, Patients Say," *New York Times* (January 15, 1996): A1.

52. S. Miles, "End-of-Life Treatment in Managed Care: The Potential and the Peril," *Western Journal of Medicine* 163, no. 3 (1995): 302–305.

53. J. M. Eisenberg, op. cit.; "Study: Managed Care Lowers Hospital Costs, Improves Quality," *American Medical News* (June 19, 1995): 6.

54. J. Meisel, "Quality of Care in HMOs: A Review of the Literature," September 1994, *CAHMO*, Sacramento, California; California Cooperative HEDIS Reporting Initiative, Report on Quality of Care Measures (San Francisco: CCHRI, February 1995); National Committee for Quality Assurance, *Report Card Pilot Project / Technical Report* (New York: NCQA, 1994).

55. J. Somerville, "CMA Study: High HMO Administrative Costs for Medicaid," *American Medical News* (May 15, 1995): 12.

56. E. D. Pellegrino, "Managed Care at the Bedside: How Do We Look in the Moral Mirror?" *Kennedy Institute of Ethics Journal* 7, no. 4 (1997): 321–330.

57. A. Hillman, op. cit.

58. Woodstock Theological Center, *Ethical Considerations in the Business Aspects of Health Care* (Washington, D.C.: Georgetown University Press, 1995), 9–14.

59. Woodstock Theological Center, supra note 46, 20–22.

60. Board of Directors of Kaiser Foundation Hospitals and Kaiser Foundation Health Plan, "Principles of Responsibility," 1984.

61. Forces external to managed care are exerting a growing pressure against under treatment; for example, the 1990 Medicare amendment restricts prepaid plans contracting with the Health Care Financing Administration (HCFA) from creating an "incentive plan as an inducement to reduce or limit medically necessary services to a specific individual"; see Medicare law in 42 USC § 1395 mm (1)(8)(A); legislation pending in several states would put limits on the type of cost-control measures that MCOs can employ: E. Ogrod, "The Many Faces of Managed Care," *California Physician* (August 1995): 10; J. Johnsson, "State Laws on Managed Care Spur New Battles," *American Medical News* (July 24, 1995): 3, 51.

62. K. G. Gervais, op. cit.; L. Randel, et al., "How Managed Care Can Be Ethical," *Health Affairs* 20, no. 4 (July–August 2001): 43–56; E. D. Pellegrino, op. cit.; A. Allen, "Trust in Managed Care Organizations," *Kennedy Institute of Ethics Journal* 10, no. 3 (2000): 189–212.

63. K. G. Gervais, op. cit.; E. D. Pellegrino, op. cit.; A. Buchanan, "Trust in Managed Care Organizations," *Kennedy Institute of Ethics Journal* 10, no. 3 (2000): 189–212.

64. J. J. Paris, *Improving Fairness in Coverage Decisions: Insights from the Harvard Community Health Plan's LORAN Commission Report* (Boston: The Center for Strategic and International Studies, Massachusetts Institute of Technology, 2004). See also Ethical Force Program, *Ensuring Fairness in Health Care Coverage Decisions: A Consensus Report on the Ethical Design and Administration of Health Care Benefits Packages* (Chicago: The American Medical Association, 2004).

65. A. Buchanan, op. cit.

66. J. D. Biblo, et al., *Ethical Issues in Managed Care: Guidelines for Clinicians and Recommendations to Accrediting Organizations* (Kansas City. MO: Midwest Bioethics Center, 1995); S. M. Wolf, "Health Care Reform and the Future of Physician Ethics," *Hastings Center Report* (March–April 1994): 28–41; Council on Ethical and Judicial Affairs, American Medical Association, op. cit.; H. T. Engelhardt and M. A. Rie, "Morality for Medical-Industrial Complex: A Code of Ethics for the Mass Marketing of Health Care," *New England Journal of Medicine* 319, no. 16 (1988): 1086–1089.

67. D. Barr, "The Effects of Organizational Structure on Primary Care Outcomes under Managed Care," *Annals of Internal Medicine* 122, no. 5 (1995): 353–359.

68. L. Johnson and R. Derlet, "Conflicts between Managed Care Organizations and Emergency Departments in California," *Western Journal of Medicine* 164 (1996): 137–142.

69. A. S. Relman, op. cit.; M. Angell, "The Beginning of Health Care Reform: The Clinton Plan," *New England Journal of Medicine* 329, no. 21 (1993): 1569–1570; Cardinal J. Bernadin, "Making the Case for Not-for-Profit Healthcare" (speech by Cardinal Joseph Bernadin, The Harvard Business School Club of Chicago, 12 January 1995).

70. M. A. Rodwin, op. cit., 136.

71. Council on Ethical and Judicial Affairs, American Medical Association, op. cit.

72. E. Emanuel, "Managed Competition and the Patient–Physician Relationship."

73. J. Harding, "The Role of Organizational Ethics Committees," *Physician Executive* 20, no. 2 (1994): 19–24; E. Emanuel, "Preserving the Physician–Patient Relationship in the Era of Managed Care."

74. K. G. Gervais, op. cit.; L. Randel, et al., op. cit.

75. D. Azevedo, "Can the World's Largest Integrated Health System Learn to Feel Small?" *Medical Economics* 23 (January 1995): 82–103.

76. D. Azevedo, "What You Can Bargain for When HMO's Compete," *Business & Health* (June 1995): 44–56.

CHAPTER 17

Bioethical Dilemmas in Emergency Medicine and Prehospital Care

Kenneth V. Iserson

OVERVIEW

In this chapter, Iserson presents ethics dilemmas for an area of medicine that potentially affects all Americans—emergency medical services. His 10 ethical issues provide an outline for an in-depth discussion of current and future critical areas for medical service systems and practitioners. Note how often aspects of autonomy play a role in these dilemmas. Concerns about who is able to provide informed consent, the right of patients to refuse life-sustaining treatment, and even the autonomy of the dead contribute to ethical decisions that must be made in the fast-paced, critical care environment of the emergency department. As the health-care system becomes more and more troubled, the issues discussed in this chapter will be exacerbated and lead to even greater concerns for those who practice in this vital area of medicine.

INTRODUCTION

Emergency medicine is at once the oldest and the newest of medical specialties. Stemming from the aid given to injured comrades, the modern domain of emergency medicine includes care provided in hospital emergency departments (EDs), urgent-care centers, and areas outside of medical facilities via ambulance and medically-trained flight crews (i.e., prehospital care). Emergency medical practitioners, physicians, nurses, and prehospital personnel face not only the traditional ethical dilemmas common to all healthcare providers, but also new ethical challenges arising from their added responsibilities in the health treatment system and the unique demands of emergency medical care.

These relatively new ethical dilemmas stem from the changing nature of the health treatment system and the technical practice of medicine. The U.S. health system increasingly fails to meet the needs of the medically indigent, and EDs have attempted to take up this slack; however, they often lack the resources to perform both this task and their primary duty to treat the acutely ill and injured. Emergency medical practitioners face 10 key ethical issues.[1] These issues are as follows:

1. How to continue to care for the critically ill and injured while also acting as a medical safety net for the medically indigent

2. How to aggressively treat critical patients and yet avoid paternalism toward those who can participate in their own healthcare decisions

3. How to preserve patient autonomy while implementing prehospital advance directives

4. How to respond to failed physician-assisted suicides (PAS)

5. How to best break bad news and provide end-of-life care

6. How to evaluate patients' decision-making capacity and work with surrogate decision makers

7. How to keep emergency medical providers safe while caring for patients

8. How to approach triage/disasters ethics

9. How to respect both the living and the dead while staying current in necessary lifesaving skills

10. How to ethically perform research to advance the field of emergency care while safeguarding patients

Each of these topics will be discussed in the chapter.

SAFETY NET AND OVERCROWDING

The U.S. health treatment system is in need of resuscitation. EDs, which have been described as the system's safety net, are losing their ability to provide this service.[2] Medically indigent patients often access health care through EDs, because they often cannot access the health treatment system in any other way.[3] EDs have taken up the slack, but they often lack the resources to perform both this task and their primary role of treating the acutely ill and injured. Serious ED overcrowding has been a national problem for more than 20 years and is a result of decreasing hospital capacities, the closure of many EDs, increased numbers of patients, and decreasing reimbursement as the number of uninsured seeking treatment in EDs has proportionately increased.[4] Additionally, hospital EDs and trauma centers are "the only providers required by federal law to accept, evaluate, and stabilize all who present for care, regardless of their ability to pay. An unintended but predictable consequence of this legal duty is a system that is overloaded and under funded to carry out its mission."[5] This last situation poses a significant dilemma: whether to focus on emergency medicine's primary duty to treat the acutely ill and injured or to provide a major source of care to medically indigent patients.

Paradoxically, as EDs see increasing numbers of patients for a wider spectrum of problems (many of which are nonemergent), they also are being targeted as a convenient site to access socially underserved populations. Emergency medical personnel find themselves castigated for not providing general medical screenings, preventive care, and public medical education programs. Social problems are being "medicalized," putting the onus of the remedy for multifactorial problems on medicine—and, increasingly, on emergency medicine. In part, this is due to crumbling social supports as well as the confusion about how to solve serious social ills. The ethical dilemma facing emergency medicine is whether to assume these various social roles and dilute (or change) its primary mission or to take a hard line and ignore these ills—as have most others in our society.

Unfortunately, studies now show that as an ED becomes overwhelmed with patients and the waiting times increase, ED patient mortality increases.[6] Thus, the results of ED overcrowding are not simply a matter of longer wait times or even increased illness, but sometime a matter of life and death. What are emergency medicine providers to do?

PATERNALISM

Paternalism, in the medical context, denotes the belief that "the doctor knows best." A physician with a paternalistic attitude intervenes to do what he or she believes will be beneficial, whether or not the patient desires an intervention.[7] Although paternalistic behavior has long characterized physicians in cultures around the world, it is beginning to be replaced in many Western settings by increased patient autonomy.

In the emergency medical care setting, paternalism often results from a constant pressure to optimally use time and resources to aid critically ill or injured patients who often lack decision-making capacity. Time pressures to make critical decisions are nowhere as intense or as constant as in emergency medicine. Simply doing without asking often saves time, which is the major resource in emergency medical systems (EMS). However, this paternalistic attitude may put practitioners' values and their patients' desire to exercise autonomy in direct conflict.

Emergency medicine, in its most basic form, as practiced during wars and disasters, is the immediate decision of one provider regarding who receives treatment and who is allowed to die. In the common hospital and prehospital scenario, this translates into rapid unilateral decisions to intervene to save lives or limbs with tubes, fluids, medications, electric shocks, and surgery. Such actions are generally desired and are considered beneficial, rather than paternalistic. Patients want and expect aggressive and immediate action by emergency medical teams. Too easily, however, this aggressive behavior can become paternalistic when applied toward the patient who is not critically ill. ED and prehospital patients commonly complain that "things are done to them" without prior discussion or acquiescence once they enter the emergency medical system. Significantly, these "things" often commit patients to large expenses for tests or procedures. In cases where patients lack decision-making capacity and patient benefit can be expected from the medical team's actions, aggressive intervention is not only reasonable, but essential. Transferring this attitude to other patients who maintain decision-making capacity, however, is problematic.

Paternalism can also arise in the guise of "futility." In emergency medicine and prehospital care, two questions are closely linked: What constitutes futility for the emergency patient? When should life-sustaining measures be withheld or withdrawn? Even as advanced cardiopulmonary life support and other techniques in trauma resuscitation increase practitioners' capacity to extend biological life, the patient benefits remain uncertain. Few guidelines exist to aid either prehospital or ED practitioners in the decision to abandon therapeutic interventions other than their lack of success in a "reasonable" amount of time. Prehospital advance directive orders are, unfortunately, still rarely seen. Clinicians in these situations are, therefore, forced to make unilateral decisions regarding further care—and often choose unwanted treatments.

PREHOSPITAL ADVANCE DIRECTIVES VERSUS DNR ORDERS

Most EMS systems still mandate that ambulance personnel called to the scene of a patient in cardiac arrest must attempt resuscitation unless it is physiologically futile (generally meaning rigor mortis, decomposition, burned beyond recognition, or other situations incompatible with life). Over the past decade, an increasing number of systems have adopted rules or state laws whereby patients (or their surrogates) can opt out of resuscitation if an ambulance is erroneously requested. Ethicists and emergency medical personnel have jointly helped to address the tragedy of unwanted resuscitations through the development of prehospital advance directives (PHAD). A danger, however, has arisen.

Although some states have successfully maintained patient autonomy by using patient- or surrogate-initiated PHADs, others have rigidly attempted to preserve physician prerogatives by changing the nature of these laws and rules to mimic in-hospital DNR orders.[8] Prehospital DNR (PHDNR) orders, although requested by (or at least discussed with) patients or their surrogate decision makers, must be approved and signed by physicians.[9] This eliminates patients' autonomous decisions regarding what is perhaps the most important decision of their lives—deciding how they will die. Occasionally, patients try to use their own forms of PHAD, such as tattoos or jewelry, but physicians or EMS personnel risk incorrectly interpreting the messages, so they are rarely followed.[10]

Although, initially, the laws and EMS rules governing PHDNR orders stemmed from concerns about the misuse of and possible criminal activity associated with using patient-initiated forms, experience with patient-initiated PHADs has shown that these concerns are unwarranted. Although physicians espouse patient autonomy, the widespread continued use of physician-initiated PHDNR rules belies this attitude.

Emergency medicine has three significant challenges regarding prehospital directives: (1) increasing the locales where these programs are available, (2) increasing patient awareness of how to best use these programs, and (2) ensuring that patient autonomy is preserved. The American College of Emergency Physicians, among other groups, is attempting to correct this situation.[11]

ASSISTED SUICIDES AND EMERGENCY DEPARTMENT RESUSCITATIONS

As assisted suicide laws spread throughout the United States over the next decades, experience shows that the number of failed suicides will increase—perhaps dramatically. Will this change the role of the entire emergency medical services system and that of emergency physicians in particular?

At present, all emergency medical personnel operate under the general rule of when in doubt, preserve life. This rule stems from their frequent lack of information about the patient, the circumstances surrounding the incident bringing the patient to the ED, and any wishes or values the patient might have. The rule includes committing to psychiatric hospitals those patients who pose a danger to themselves. Although this is, in fact, at odds with patient autonomy, both legal and ethical theorists agree that protecting suicidal patients is a necessary medical function.

In situations in which physicians (and sometimes EMS personnel through a PHAD or PHDNR order) know that a patient does not want resuscitation, the patient's wishes are generally followed.[12] Yet, when the need for resuscitation arises from a failed assisted-suicide attempt, how will ED physicians respond? What if there is an underlying condition that also precipitated signing a PHAD? (Patients without a serious medical illness generally will not fall under current assisted-suicide statutes, although it may be difficult for EMS or ED personnel to initially determine whether they have such a condition.) Such cases of failed assisted suicides have already appeared in the bioethics literature.[13] These cases indicate that another complicating factor might be interference (perhaps self-motivated) from the physician who prescribed the almost-lethal drugs.

Emergency medical personnel may well be caught between several very unacceptable options—maximal resuscitative efforts, no resuscitative efforts, or providing temporizing measures while gathering information. The only indication of how emergency physicians will respond is an Oregon study that suggests that many emergency physicians will abstain from aggressively resuscitating such patients only if they have clear proof that the patient desired and tried to die.[14] This result suggests the need to increase the use of PHADs by terminally ill patients.

An ethical analysis of the issue suggested that, whenever possible, emergency physicians should gather as much relevant information as they can and originate life-sustaining treatment to buy time to gather the information. If valid information indicates that physician-assisted suicide is the patient's competent and informed choice in response to a terminal illness, life-sustaining treatments can be withdrawn or not instituted. If such circumstances are not clear, treatment should continue. However, the authors concluded that emergency physicians should not provide direct assistance to patients who have attempted physician-assisted suicide by giving them a lethal drug to ingest or by administering a lethal injection.[15]

BREAKING BAD NEWS AND END-OF-LIFE CARE

One of the most difficult tasks emergency physicians perform is to deliver the news of sudden, unexpected deaths. Similarly, they often must break bad news to patients and families about critical conditions and devastating illnesses. How to do this with sensitivity and professionalism are two of the ethical issues in which emergency medicine residents and emergency department nurses feel they need the most education.[16]

Coupled with end-of-life care, which is often difficult in a stressful ED environment with relatively few appropriate resources, emergency medicine personnel often feel overwhelmed by the need to communicate bad news. The key element is to respect and understand recipients' feelings, which can be more difficult if they speak a different language, are from a different culture, or often both. Sudden-death notification is rarely taught, because teaching physicians often fear that they are mishandling the process, and thus are reluctant to have trainees observe them, an attitude that is passed down through generations of physicians. The key to performing this task with survivors, who are now considered patients, is to prepare in advance to deliver the news; inform them using nontechnical language, appropriate phrases, and active listening; be ready to answer their questions, especially about organ and tissue donation and autopsies;[17] and to provide support however possible.[18]

The delivery of bad news in the ED is made much more difficult when the primary physician has not provided adequate information to the patient or family prior to a critical illness. Even though impending death might be a difficult topic, resources are available to make that discussion easier.[19] No doubt, newer generations of physicians will become more comfortable with performing these tasks as emphasis on these educational topics becomes more common.

DECISION-MAKING CAPACITY AND SURROGATE DECISION MAKERS

Frequently troublesome to ED and EMS providers is the question of whether an individual has the capacity to consent to (or refuse) medical treatment, how to assess that capacity, and who makes the decision if the individual cannot. People often assume, incorrectly, that minors and inebriated or psychiatric patients lack decision-making capacity. Minors can be emancipated (treated as adults) under numerous conditions or may simply fall under the "emergency treatment" category, such as when they present alone or with a nonguardian adult for treatment and then assent to sutures, radiographs, or intravenous hydration. The principle for minors is that they should not be denied because of their age what would otherwise be the standard of care for emergencies.

Inebriated and psychiatric patients, unless they have no contact with reality, usually retain some elements of decision-making capacity, although possibly not enough to make important medical decisions. The rule is that the more serious the decision, the higher level of capacity a person must have. For example, the person might be able to decide what he wants to eat, but not have the capacity to decide whether he needs (or can refuse) a chest tube for a collapsed lung.

In the ED setting, to have decision-making capacity for a particular decision, patients must show an understanding of (1) the treatment options that have been described to them, (2) the risks and benefits to them of each option, and (3) how their decision relates to their normal value system.[20] This last question can be put as simply as, "Why did you make that decision?" If patients retain decision-making capacity, not only can they select treatments, but they can also refuse them, even if to do so might be life-threatening.[21] This often causes consternation among ED and EMS providers who are, by nature, "rescuers."

If adult patients lack decision-making capacity, both their advance directives and any surrogate list in state law come into play. Generally, if a patient has a durable power of attorney for health care (DPAH), it names a surrogate decision maker, who then takes precedence over anyone other than a court-appointed guardian.[22] If no DPAH exists, decisions can be made by individuals named in the state's surrogate list.[23] In all cases, if a surrogate declines to assume the decision-making position, the next person can assume the role. Having an excellent advance directive law and a substantive surrogate list in state law is an example of proactive ethics, which greatly assists ED and EMS patients and practitioners.

PROVIDER SAFETY AND SECURITY

Increasingly, EMS and ED healthcare providers must concern themselves with safety issues. Gang-related and other violent individuals no longer think of the EMS and ED as sanctuaries or "neutral zones," but rather as sources of additional victims. Ethical dilemmas arise when the provider's desire to be beneficent conflicts with the innate need to be safe. This safety concern starts with access to the system. Should EMS personnel enter unsecured (no police) scenes to provide aid to victims of violence or wait and possibly jeopardize their patients' well-being?[24] Similarly, but not as obvious, are the restrictions on ED entry (or entry to patient-care areas) that have become much more common. Self-preservation can be justified both because it is a natural instinct that professionalism does not abolish and because the ED health provider is a valuable societal resource that should not be frivolously endangered.

The underlying theme is that EMS personnel must guard their own safety first. This includes refusing to "play cop" in the ED with violent patients. (Such behavior also distorts physicians' roles, so that patients see them as security guards and may no longer willingly trust them as physicians.) Next, emergency medical practitioners must, whenever possible, safeguard their coworkers' well-being by ensuring that they are not put in harm's way. Only once that is accomplished can emergency medical providers protect their patients.[25] Ideally, this situation rarely arises, but in a crisis, the ethics of resource conservation, if nothing else, dictates this order of priorities.

TRIAGE/DISASTER ETHICS

In an age of devastating natural and human-caused disasters, EDs and EMS systems represent the frontline defenses, the primary medical responders, and those initially called upon to make difficult moral choices. In situations with scarce resources available to treat a multitude of patients, a sorting system—*triage*—must be employed to determine which patients receive the resources that do exist, including time, which equates to priority for treatment.

In modern, overcrowded EDs, triage is the norm, with many patients who seem to have less-acute illnesses or injuries waiting many hours to be seen. In a catastrophic setting, some patients might be considered to be too ill or injured to have resources expended on them. This uilitarian outlook takes a different tack than either the Hippocratic Oath or physicians' normal behavior of prioritizing each patient.[26] In scarce-resource situations, however, it is this outlook that must prevail to save the greatest number of lives and reduce residual morbidity to a minimum. Because these morally, psychologically, and technically difficult decisions often must be made in seconds, they are the responsibility of senior emergency physicians or, in the EMS, senior medics. (In the holding area for the operating room, the senior surgeon makes triage decisions.)

The challenge for ED and EMS providers is how to switch quickly into that role when required. In the prehospital setting, crucial triage decisions are relatively common, such as when a single medic is the first to arrive at a multiple casualty incident or the rural medic is alone in the back of an ambulance with two critical patients.

Numerous distributive justice (fair resource allocation) theories abound. But, in the practical sense, as long as resources exist, experienced emergency medicine personnel, both in the ED and the EMS, will continue to use the utilitarian concept of providing the most good for the most people to determine who receives limited resources.[27] In situations of widespread severe resource scarcity, bioethics committees must work in advance with their entire communities to provide ED and EMS personnel with triage guidance policies or protocols.[28]

PRACTICING AND TEACHING ON THE NEWLY DEAD

The public demands and expects all emergency practitioners to be skilled in critical lifesaving procedures and to teach these procedures to new practitioners. The most efficient and practical way for them to remain proficient in these sometimes little-used, technically difficult skills is for them to practice and teach on the newly dead.

For many years, physicians learned technical skills such as intubation and central-line placement on patients who had recently died. Recently, however, it has been suggested that postmortem procedures are only permissible if prior consent has been obtained from relatives. This position, however, ignores the nature of and purpose for informed consent, contravenes patient altruism, and disregards society's interest in having an optimal number of medical care providers experienced in lifesaving techniques.[29]

The process of obtaining informed consent stems from the concepts of patient autonomy and, ultimately, a respect for others. In theory, the process increases communication between the physician and patient prior to dangerous, disfiguring, or seriously invasive procedures. Requiring prior consent by emergency medical personnel to practice or teach lifesaving procedures on the newly dead, however, misapplies informed consent and misrepresents the concept of patient autonomy.

The dead, of course, have no autonomy claim. Autonomy, based on the principles of freedom and liberty, is a function of personhood. But the dead are no longer persons, although by societal consent they can still implement their wishes for the disposition of their bodies through advance directives or a legal will—neither of which are normally available in the ED. Nevertheless, the former patients' wishes should be respected, which generally means respecting an altruism not found as readily in their relatives.[30] The relatives' "quasiproperty rights" to a corpse are strictly limited and do not give them either moral or legal authority to counteract stronger competing claims.

Society also has a substantial interest in these procedures. That interest is the need to maintain an optimal number of ED and EMS personnel proficient in lifesaving procedures. The medical professions recognize that both primary instruction and continued practice is necessary for proficiency in lifesaving skills. This instruction and practice is best done on fresh cadavers, because the available alternatives are not adequate. But, although they recognize that unreasonable barriers to this training should not exist, limits are equally important. These limits should include the respectful treatment of the body, limiting the training to those who must use these procedures, and eliminating from use any corpses where the person had an available document declining use as an organ or tissue donor or was from a culture that does not permit this. One academic emergency medicine organization suggests that hospitals develop a policy on such practices and recommends asking for consent from next of kin.[31] (Interestingly, the same organization firmly supports resuscitation research on living patients without consent. See next section.)

Alternatives to using fresh cadavers are inadequate—or dangerous. Although models, animals, and donated embalmed cadavers are useful ways to learn or practice some aspects of critical-care techniques, they poorly simulate the critical patient. The use of animals, aside from being logistically ever more difficult, is itself ethically problematic. Donated, preserved cadavers and models are less realistic, are expensive, and have limited availability. (Eventually, we will use virtual reality models for this training at larger training centers, and this discussion will be moot.) The commonly used alternatives to cadavers are to use patients who are undergoing anesthesia for this teaching or to prolong resuscitations beyond the point where the clinicians know it to be futile so that procedures can be done.[32]

If a legal or ethical requirement for consent exists prior to postmortem ED instruction, it decreases the number of clinical personnel trained in lifesaving procedures. A need to request this permission from distraught relatives raises significant emotional barriers for clinicians to overcome in order to practice and teach the procedures. In a survey of medical personnel involved in organ harvesting, a dislike of "adding to relatives' distress by asking permission for donation" was the single greatest barrier to organ procurement.[33] This barrier is unlikely to be breached, especially for the seemingly more trivial request to teach or practice procedures. Any impediment is further compounded by the stringent time limitations imposed by the onset of rigor mortis, by the rapid transport of bodies to the morgue, and by the press of duties for the ED staff once a resuscitation attempt has ended.

In summary, patient autonomy plays an appropriate and vital role in keeping modern medicine from overstepping individual interests. However, its inappropriate extension to requiring consent for ED postmortem practice and teaching cannot be justified. The concept of autonomy would not be advanced, and future patients, the medical profession, and society would be harmed.[34]

RESUSCITATION RESEARCH WITHOUT CONSENT

Lastly, emergency medicine cannot remain static. Research on the treatment of critical patients in the prehospital arena and the ED is essential if the field is to progress. Despite the benefit to society, societal strictures on informed consent increasingly have prohibited much of this research in the United States.[35]

Research in acute care is a troubling area for institutional review board (IRB) approval and informed consent. Confusion about ethical and legal requirements has hampered research efforts and subsequent patient benefits. The acute care patients commonly seen in EDs and prehospital care are the relatively few patients who have suffered unexpected events that carry a high probability of mortality or severe morbidity unless immediate medical intervention is provided. Due to the lack of substantive research on their medical and surgical problems and the difficulty in implementing research protocols, thousands of individuals receive, at best, untested, and, at worst, inappropriate, care each day in the United States. They deserve better. Acute care research can be implemented more widely and still satisfy both bureaucratic mandates and the ethical requirements to protect patients and research subjects.

It has been argued that acute-care research is justified if the usual ethical requirements for research are modified to reflect the uniqueness of the situation. The recommendations are (1) to use an explicit definition of *acute care* as distinct from other modes of critical care, (2) to eliminate the requirement for informed consent (as usually understood), and (3) to require stringent IRB oversight regarding the unique ethical problems raised by this research. It has been further suggested that IRB oversight include review of the protocol by a panel of individuals who represent possible enrollees in the proposed study.[36]

Yet, in 1993 the Food and Drug Administration (FDA), the governing body for individual institutional review boards (IRBs), placed a moratorium on resuscitation research.[37] The Office of Protection from Research Risks (now called the Office for Human Research Protection) halted all human resuscitation research, including studies using alternative consenting mechanisms, such as deferred consent, implied consent, and two-tiered consent.[38]

Toward the end of 1996, the National Institutes of Health (NIH), the FDA, and other government agencies loosened a few of their restrictions on critical care research, publishing the "Final Rule" that permitted limited critical care research without prior informed consent. The restrictions have resulted in a significant decrease in the number of published clinical cardiac arrest trials—and, by implication, other resuscitation research. In contrast, the European Union has significantly increased the number of studies published since 1993.[39]

In part, this led to a 2005 consensus conference held by the Society for Academic Emergency Medicine. Not only was there consensus that this research was vital, but also that systematically excluding any subgroups from such studies would be inappropriate. The group also recommended that a risk-benefit determination for inclusion of vulnerable populations in research without consent should be added to standard IRB deliberations, and that various methods for the difficult, but required, IRB consultation with representative members of the community be tested.[40] One participant summarized the issue as "the societal value of minimizing future morbidity and mortality may conflict with individuals' right of self-determination. In allowing research to take place without informed consent, the current regulations resolve this conflict in favor of the societal benefit."[41]

In sum, despite regulation changes and widespread professional approval, our society remains conflicted about proceeding with unconsented research in critical situations when consent cannot be obtained. How our society will resolve this is still an open question.

OTHER TROUBLESOME AREAS

Although the dilemmas described in this chapter epitomize some of emergency medicine's unique ethical conundrums, many other ethical dilemmas exist. In the ED, the basic beneficent value of alleviating pain runs up against two other values—to patients' detriment. The physicians' stricture against doing harm keeps adequate analgesia from many patients who are suspected of "drug-seeking" behavior. This includes many patients with migraines and back pain, and some with kidney stones (all classic complaints of drug seekers). The majority of patients with these complaints are simply seeking relief for an acute problem. Inadequate treatment also is accorded, although for different reasons, to patients who need pain relief before they are taken to operating or procedure rooms. Many physicians want the patient to be coherent rather than comfortable when they sign an operative or procedure permit. Therefore, they may wait hours without adequate analgesia, especially those with fractures and abdominal catastrophes requiring surgery, due to an ethical (or more likely legal) requirement for the patient's signature on an operative permit.

Emergency physicians commonly face another dilemma, for which there does not seem to be an adequate answer. In most clinical situations, a patient's decision-making capacity is easily determined. If there is a question, clinicians test the patient's understanding. There is a significant question about decision-making capacity under the severe stress of an acute and unexpected illness, compounded by the strange surroundings of the ED. Patient autonomy governs much of modern U.S. biomedical ethics. It is unclear, however, what it takes to be autonomous in a crisis. The patient gasping for breath who refuses intubation, the acquired immune deficiency syndrome (AIDS) patient who at the last moment verbally changes a well-thought-out advance directive, or the patient agreeing to take a risky medication or undergo a major operative procedure under these circumstances might be exhibiting panic behavior rather than autonomy in any accepted sense. Even in these scenarios, many patients continue to want to make their own healthcare decisions. Is this appropriate? We just do not know.

SUMMARY

Emergency medicine also faces ethics challenges as it enters into the twenty-first century and struggles to meet its mission in a changing health-care system. In this chapter, Iserson presents ten dilemmas that are critical for those who provide prehospital or emergency care. Practitioners must be prepared to address such issues as their status as the safety net, paternalism versus patient autonomy, prehospital advanced directives, and failed PAS while maintaining the emotionally and physically grueling pace of emergency care. In addition, the challenges end-of-life care, disaster ethics, and research and training on the newly dead pose additional ethical problems. Finally, these practitioners must be aware of their own safety as they provide quality care to all who enter their systems.

QUESTIONS FOR DISCUSSION

1. How does decreased funding for public health and other community out-patient clinics affect ethical issues faced by emergency medicine (EM) practitioners?

2. How will the aging of the baby boomers increase ethical issues for the EM system?

3. What ethical issues does the lack of implementation of PHADs create for EM staff? What about for the healthcare system itself?

4. What ethical issues are caused by failing to adequately train EM physicians to deliver bad news?

5. How does the theory of utilitarianism relate to the safety of EM practitioners?

6. What is the relationship between autonomy and the ethical dilemmas faced by EM practitioners?

NOTES

1. K. V. Iserson, "Bioethics," in J. A. Marx, R. S. Hockberger, R. M. Walls, et al. (eds.), *Rosen's Emergency Medicine: Concepts and Clinical Practice*, 6th ed. (Philadelphia: Mosby, 2006): 3127–3338.

2. G. D. Velianoff, "Overcrowding and Diversion in the Emergency Department: The Health Care Safety Net Unravels," *Nursing Clinics of North America* 37, no. 1 (March 2002): 59–66, vi.

3. K. V. Iserson and T. Kastre, "Are Emergency Departments a 'Safety Net' for the Medically Indigent?" *American Journal of Emergency Medicine* 14, no. 1 (1996): 1–5; Committee on the Future of Emergency Care in the United States Health System, Institute of Medicine of the National Academies, *Future of Emergency Care Series—Emergency Medical Services At the Crossroads* (Washington, D.C.: National Academy Press, 2006), xii.

4. J. S. Olshaker and N. K. Rathlev, "Emergency Department Overcrowding and Ambulance Diversion: The Impact and Potential Solutions of Extended Boarding of Admitted Patients in the Emergency Department," *Journal of Emergency Medicine* 3 (April 2006): 351–356.

5. Committee on the Future of Emergency Care in the United States Health System, Institute of Medicine of the National Academies, op. cit.

6. P. C. Sprivulis, J. A. DaSilva, I. G. Jacobs, et al., "The Association Between Hospital Overcrowding and Mortality Among Patients Admitted via Western Australian Emergency Departments," *Medical Journal of Australia* 184, no. 5 (2006): 208–212; D. B. Richardson, "Increase in Patient Mortality at 10 days Associated with Emergency Department Overcrowding," *Medical Journal of Australia* 184, no. 5 (2006): 213–216.

7. P. T. Hershey, "A Definition for Paternalism," *Journal of Medical Philosophy* 10, no. 2 (1985): 171–182.

8. K. V. Iserson, "A Simplified Prehospital Advance Directive Law: Arizona's Approach," *Annals of Emergency. Medicine* 22, no. 11 (1993): 1703–1710.

9. K. V. Iserson, "Prehospital Advance Directives—A Better Way," *Journal of Emergency Medicine* 23, no. 11 (2002): 419–420.

10. K. V. Iserson, "Nonstandard Advance Directives: A Pseudoethical Dilemma," *Journal of Trauma* 44, no.1 (1998): 139–142; K. V. Iserson, "The 'No Code' Tattoo: An Ethical Dilemma," *Western Journal of Medicine* 156, no. 3 (1992): 309–312.

11. R. M. Schears, C. A. Marco, and K. V. Iserson, "'Do-not-attempt Resuscitation' (DNAR) Policy in the Out-of-hospital Setting," *Annals of Emergency Medicine* 44, no. 1 (2004): 68–70.

12. R. Byock, "A Slight Postmortem Disagreement," in *Ethics in Emergency Medicine*, 2d ed., K. V. Iserson, et al., eds. (Tucson, AZ: Galen Press, 1995), 80–87.

13. K. V. Iserson, et al., "Willful Death and Painful Decisions: A Failed Assisted Suicide," *Cambridge Quarterly of Healthcare Ethics* 1, no. 2 (1992): 147–158.

14. T. A Schmidt, "Oregon Emergency Physicians' Experiences, Attitudes, and Concerns about Physician-Assisted Suicide," abstract in *Academy of Emergency Medicine* 3, no. 5 (1996): 490.

15. J. Moskop and K. V. Iserson, "Emergency Physicians and Physician-Assisted Suicide, Part I: A Review of the Physician-Assisted Suicide Debate," *Annals of Emergency Medicine* 38, no. 5 (2001): 570–575; J. Moskop and K. V. Iserson, "Emergency Physicians and Physician-Assisted Suicide, Part II: Emergency Care for Patients Who Have Attempted Physician-Assisted Suicide," *Annals of Emergency Medicine* 38, no. 5 (2001): 576–582.

16. M. A. Pauls and S. Ackroyd-Stolarz, "Identifying Bioethics Learning Needs: A Survey of Canadian Emergency Medicine Residents," *Academy of Emergency Medicine* 13, no. 6 (2006): 645–652.

17. K. V. Iserson, *Death to Dust: What Happens to Dead Bodies?* 2nd ed. (Tucson, AZ: Galen Press, 2001).

18. K. V. Iserson, *Grave Words: Notifying Survivors About Sudden Unexpected Deaths* (Tucson, AZ: Galen Press, 1999); American College of Emergency Physicians, "Ethical Issues in Emergency Department Care at the End of Life," *Annals of Emergency Medicine* 47, no. 3 (2006): 303; K. V. Iserson, "Bereavement and Grief Reactions" (Chapter 125), in *Harwood-Nuss' Clinical Practice of Emergency Medicine*, 4th ed., A. B. Wolfson, G. W. Hendey, P. L. Henry, et al. (eds) (Philadelphia: Lippincott Williams & Wilkins, 2005), 649–653.

19. K. V. Iserson, *After-Death Planner*, 2nd ed. (Tucson, AZ: Galen Press, 2001).

20. A. E. Buchanan, "The Question of Competence," in *Ethics in Emergency Medicine*, 2nd ed., K. V. Iserson, et al., eds. (Tucson, AZ: Galen Press, 1995), 61–65.

21. A. R. Derse, "What Part of 'No' Don't You Understand? Patient Refusal of Recommended Treatment in the Emergency Department," *Mount Sinai Journal of Medicine* 72, no. 4 (2005), 221–227.

22. See www.galenpress.com/extras/extra1.htm for Arizona's extremely useable and often-copied advance directives.

23. Arizona's list, one of the most extensive in the nation, lists, in order: spouse, adult children, parents (of an adult), domestic partner, adult sibling, close friend, attending physician in consultation with a bioethics committee.

24. R. A. Lazar, "Prehospital Personnel's Safety versus A Duty to Treat," in *Ethics in Emergency Medicine*, 2nd ed., K. V. Iserson, et al., eds. (Tucson, AZ: Galen Press, 1995), 412–416.

25. K. V. Iserson and B. Morenz, "Ethics of Wilderness Medicine," in P. Auerbach (ed), *Wilderness Medicine: Management of Wilderness and Environmental Emergencies*, 5th Edition (St. Louis: C.V. Mosby, in press).

26. R. M. Veatch, "Disaster Preparedness and Triage: Justice and the Common Good," *Mount Sinai Journal of Medicine* 72, no. 4 (2005): 236–241.

27. K. V. Iserson and J. C. Moskop, "Triage in Medicine—Part I: Concept, History, and Types," *Annals of Emergency Medicine*, in press; J. C. Moskop and K. V. Iserson, "Triage in Medicine—Part II: Underlying Values and Principles," *Annals of Emergency Medicine*, in press.

28. N. Pesik, M. E. Keim, and K. V. Iserson, "Terrorism and the Ethics of Emergency Medical Care," *Annals of Emergency Medicine* 37, no. 6 (2001): 642–646; K. V. Iserson and N. Pesik, "Ethical Resource Distribution After Biological, Chemical, or Radiological Terrorism," *Cambridge Quarterly of Healthcare Ethics* 12, no. 4 (2003) 455–465.

29. K. V. Iserson, "Teaching Without Harming the Living: Performing Minimally Invasive Procedures on the Newly Dead," *Journal of Health Care Law & Policy* 8, no. 2 (2005): 216–231.

30. R. M. Oswalt, "A Review of Blood Donor Motivation and Recruitment," *Transfusion* 17 (1977): 123–135.

31. T. A. Schmidt, J. T. Abbott, and J. M. Geiderman, et al., "Ethics Seminars: The Ethical Debate on Practicing Procedures on the Newly Dead," *Academy of Emergency Medicine* 11, no. 9 (2004): 962–966.

32. K. V. Iserson, *Death to Dust: What Happens to Dead Bodies?*

33. K. V. Iserson, "Teaching Without Harming the Living: Performing Minimally Invasive Procedures on the Newly Dead," *Journal of Health Care Law & Policy* 8, no. 2 (2005): 216–231.

34. K. V. Iserson and D. L. Lindsey, "Research on Critically Ill and Injured Patients: Rules, Reality, and Ethics," *Journal of Emergency Medicine* 13, no. 4 (1995): 563–567.

35. K. V. Iserson and M. Mahowald, "Acute Care Research: Is It Ethical?" *Critical Care Medicine* 20 (1992): 1032–1037.

36. G. B. Ellis, "Dear Colleague" letter: human subjects' protection. *OPRR Report* 93, no. 3 (August 12, 1993).

37. U.S. Department of Health and Human Services. Protection of Human Subjects: Informed Consent and Waiver of Informed Consent Requirements in Certain Emergency Circumstances. In: 21 CFR 50; 45 CFR 46; 1996.

38. K. M. Hiller, J. S. Haukoos, and K. Heard, et al., "Impact of the Final Rule on the Rate of Clinical Cardiac Arrest Research in the United States," *Academy of Emergency Medicine* 12, no. 11 (2005): 1091–1098.

39. J. M. Baren and S. S. Fish, "Resuscitation Research Involving Vulnerable Populations: Are Additional Protections Needed for Emergency Exception from Informed Consent?" *Academy of Emergency Medicine* 12, no. 11 (2005): 1071–1077.

40. M. C. Morris, "An Ethical Analysis of Exception from Informed Consent Regulations," *Academy of Emergency Medicine* 12, no. 11 (2005): 1113–1119.

41. Ibid.

CHAPTER 18

High-Technology Home Care: Critical Issues and Ethical Choices

*Melissa Brandon**

OVERVIEW

This chapter is concerned with the significant issue of the impact of high technology on the quality and ethics of healthcare delivery. Specifically, the chapter focuses on critical issues surrounding the use of technology in home care for medically fragile, technology-dependent patients. Notice how important the principles of autonomy, beneficence, and justice become when addressing the ethics involved in these issues. Notice also that the principles apply not only to the individual, but also to the patient's family, friends, caretakers, and medical staff.

INTRODUCTION

Critical issues and ethical choices facing those concerned about high-technology home care (HTHC) are explored in this chapter. The discussion focuses on medically fragile, technology-dependent (MF/TD) children. This chapter is structured to accomplish the following:

1. *Assess the past*. This section presents the history of those issues resulting from the creation of the initial and subsequent populations of MF/TD children who required HTHC.

2. *Analyze the present*. This section describes the complexity of the present concerns of parents, professionals, and organizations involved in providing services to meet the health care, psychosocial, educational, and developmental requirements of these children with special needs.

3. *Apply for the future*. This section allows you to consider ethical issues and choices so that you can plan future strategies for developing and managing comprehensive/integrated approaches for children/families who require HTHC. It will consider ethical choices within the framework of managed care.

BACKGROUND ON THE ISSUE

Around the world, people are facing rapidly growing healthcare expenditures. Health care must compete with other political, social, and economic pri-

---

*Revised from A. I. Goldberg, E. A. M. Faure, and J. J. O'Callaghan, "High Technology Home Care: Critical Issues and Ethical Choices," in *Health Care Ethics: Critical Issues for the 21st Century*. Original ed., 1998, edited by John F. Monagle and David C. Thomasma. Sudbury, MA: Jones and Bartlett, 2005.

orities for restricted resources. This demand for increasing health finance confronts industrial nations responding to global market pressures and changing societal forces, as well as developing countries and former communist nations undergoing economic transformation. Rapid discovery and application of life-sustaining diagnostic and therapeutic technologies provide one major explanation for this cost escalation.[1]

Countries must also meet the challenge of adapting traditional healthcare delivery to demands arising from unanticipated needs. Specifically, growing numbers of elderly, persons with disabilities, and those with previously unforeseen health issues (drug-addicted infants, people with acquired immune deficiency syndrome [AIDS], and technology-dependent persons) require care for chronic conditions. In addition, the health systems in place are based on an industrial-era model that focuses on acute care, which might not be appropriate for meeting these challenges. These systemic challenges are the outcomes of progress, the successes of modern medical science, and advancing medical technology.

In light of these concerns, a global search has begun for innovative, nontraditional approaches to health systems. In November 1990, the Max Planck Institute held a healthcare summit to analyze alternative delivery models suitable for the elderly and persons with chronic conditions. Participants reviewed the evolution of different community-based models—including home care—in national health systems, national health insurance systems, and evolving market-oriented systems.[2] In addition to analyzing healthcare finance systems, invited health service research experts analyzed national delivery systems to determine differences between countries using the same health finance approach. Among the concerns raised were: (1) What are suitable models for persons with long-term requirements for health care and medical technology? (2) What can other nations' experiences tell us about optimal economic/finance systems to avoid limited access to care?

The conclusions reached were fundamental to understanding global health system reform. Regardless of the organizational model described (traditional hospital, home care, community centers, nursing homes, other long-term care alternatives), the experience of each nation was based on two factors: funding and culture. First, the finance system does not matter. What matters is that money is available as an incentive to develop an organizational model. Second, differences between nations with the same healthcare finance system can best be understood in the context of cultural differences between nations, even more so at the regional/local level. At the local level, innovative healthcare solutions are accomplished and encouraged by, or despite, national healthcare policy.

The Home Care Matrix: The Scope of Home Care Practice

Home care stands as one appealing organizational model competing with others for limited financial resources in global healthcare reform. Growth in home care is being driven by the increasing percentage of older persons in the total population, although children with chronic disease/disability are the fastest-growing segment.[3]

Home care can be defined as the provision by one or more organizations of physician-prescribed nursing care, social work, therapies (physical, occupational, nutritional, speech), vocational and social services, homemaker services, home health aide assistance, and/or personal assistance services to disabled, sick, or convalescent persons in the home. Home care has three dimensions: (1) duration of care, (2) support by others, and (3) application of technology.[4]

The following is a clarification of these dimensions:

1. The duration of care is as follows:
   - Acute (0 to 7 days)
   - Subacute (1 to 6 weeks)
   - Long term (more than 6 weeks)

2. The level of professional/personal support ranges from none (self, family member) to intermittent skilled professional visits to continuous (private duty nursing/personal attendant).

3. The involvement of technology ranges from none to low technology (aids for daily living, communication, mobility) to high technology (life-sustaining devices). People who require prolonged use of HTHC must anticipate dramatic changes in public policy and new dynamics of marketplace forces early in the twenty-first century. The population at greatest risk for service denial is MF/TD children.

The Home Care Culture: How It Differs from the "Medical Model"

Home care should not be considered an extension of the medical model into the home. In the medical model, the physician commands the situation, with the patient/family dependent on professional authority for decisions and actions. Thus, when receiving care in a hospital or ambulatory care setting, the patient and family are at a power disadvantage and are not in control. Technical and scientific information predominates in the making of decisions, and these decisions might not take into account the patient's and family's wishes. In these settings, physicians and other health professionals control decisions and plan implementation subject to patient compliance. The goal is the reversal of illness and, when possible, a cure.

All service providers involved with home care must accept a different mindset from this institutional way of thinking and relating to patients. Home care culture has different attitudes, beliefs, values, and norms of behavior than the traditional medical model. It demonstrates a person-centered social concept typified by the independent living of persons with disabilities. In this model, physicians serve as collaborators of care and are invited partners with a patient/family active in decision making, plan implementation, and outcome evaluation.

In family-centered care, the patient/family is central and in charge; properly prepared patients/families consider multiple options because they have been empowered and have the resources necessary to make good decisions. Much of their information comes from self-help and mutual aid groups. The

Table 18–1 Healthcare Models

	Medical Model	Home Care Model
Process	Command/control	Collaboration
Focus	Professional focus; patient focus	Person-centered; family-centered
Emphasis	Illness (episodic)	Health-wellness (continuous); health promotion/prevention
Goal	Cure	Caring
Fosters	Dependency	Independency
Decisions	Receptive	Participatory
Communication	One-way	Two-way
Response	Reactive	Proactive
Respect	Professional wisdom	Personal/family insights
Environment	Clinical, invasive	Dignified, private
Ethical foundation	Beneficence	Autonomy

patient/family focuses more on wellness and a desire to improve their health status and life situation rather than expecting a total cure. Patients and their families are active participants, taking responsibility for their own health. Patients/families have important management insights and can make decisions to enhance safety, reduce risk, improve quality, and reduce costs. This makes them essential participants in catastrophic care management (see Table 18–1).

UNDERSTANDING THE PAST

In order to understand the present, one must understand the past. This section presents a history of the events that helped to create populations of MF/TD children. It also provides information on how the medical system tried to respond to the changes in this population.

The Polio Era: Creation of the First Population of MF/TD Children

The pandemic of polio affected infants, children, and even young adults. In response, technology was advanced to reduce the mortality of this disease. Organizations were founded to address the needs of those afflicted with the disease. In addition, communities began to address the special needs of the MF/TD children who survived.

Technological Advances

Technological breakthroughs in health care often result from catastrophic events. Many advances in modern medicine, surgery, and anesthesia were in response to the carnage of World War II. However, another global crisis provided the stimulus to the life-supportive technology that is the concern of this chapter.

During the pandemic of poliomyelitis in the 1950s, countless infants, children, and young adults were stricken with paralytic respiratory polio. Universal panic ensued, and the medical community faced a plague-like crisis of catastrophic proportions.[5] The polio crisis prompted medical advances in upper-airway management (tracheostomy) and mechanical ventilation.[6] Technology reduced mortality of bulbar polio from 90 to 20 percent.[7]

Organizational Advances

Significant organizational response to the polio pandemic of the 1950s included the creation of designated respiratory polio centers.[8] In the United States, the National Foundation for Infantile Paralysis, a voluntary organization, established these centers. Americans gave millions of dollars of support through the March of Dimes. Polio centers were unique because they featured interdisciplinary teams of healthcare professionals, including physicians, nurses, social workers, and therapists—all working together. Among the new professions were rehabilitation (physical) medicine and respiratory (inhalation) therapy, which were formed during World War I. These centers focused not only on acute survival, but also on long-term rehabilitation and education. Hence, the team included physical, occupational, speech, and vocational professionals as well as social support and educators.

Community-Based Solutions

The leadership begun by Franklin D. Roosevelt and the research efforts of Dr. Jonas Salk at the National Foundation for Infantile Paralysis resulted in nationwide immunization and eradication of the threat of polio in 1956. Leaders also established HTHC, which was made possible with the invention of portable home respirators. Engineers designed these life-sustaining devices in response to thousands of polio victims with respiratory insufficiency who preferred life in the community with their families rather than long-term institutional care. Consumers working with their doctors and manufacturers helped design the technology and the home care programs from which they benefited.[9] Gini Laurie, noted historian of the poliomyelitis era, stated, "the centers and home care resulted in tremendous financial savings and a greater degree of independence and self-sufficiency than was ever dreamed possible for people so severely disabled. The average hospital time was cut from more than a year to seven months; the home care costs were one-tenth to one-fourth of hospital costs."[10]

Home care was not a new concept in America. From colonial times, the home was the traditional site of health care.[11] Furthermore, the United States had long experience with home visiting to support the health, social, educational, and other needs of children.[12] However, with HTHC life could be sustained/supported on a prolonged basis at home by augmenting or replacing a person's ability to breathe with a machine. Partnerships involving patients/families, physicians and other healthcare professionals, and organizational leaders all working together on a local basis, developed these home care programs. Creative people designed cost-saving solutions that made

HTHC less expensive and more desirable than institutional care (e.g., the use of personal care attendants/alternative care providers).[13]

The Critical Care Era: Creation of the Next Generation of MF/TD Children

The polio era laid the foundation for the creation of neonatology, critical care units, and rehabilitation. Emphasis also moved from polio to birth defects which created different solutions and experiences for both the system and families. Home care was added as a better option for children and their families.

Advances in Neonatology, Critical Care, and Rehabilitation Medicine

The technological and organizational advances of the polio era laid the foundation for the development of neonatology, critical care, and rehabilitation medicine. After the eradication of polio, many physician leaders began to apply their new knowledge and skills to other challenges. Founders of intensive care units for neonates and children often had experience with polio. Other leaders developed neonatology or critical care because of advances in their specialties and the need for units to concentrate on technology and interdisciplinary teams. In the 1960s at the Children's Hospital of Philadelphia, C. Everett Koop, M.D., established the first neonatal intensive care unit (NICU) in the United States. Jack Downes, M.D., created one of the nation's earliest pediatric intensive care units (PICUs).[14] Advances in pediatric medicine, surgery, and anesthesia led to remarkable results, such that critically ill neonates, infants, and children could recover from life-threatening acute illnesses with dramatically improved survival rates and recovery.

In the late 1950s, the National Foundation ended support for the respiratory polio centers and redefined its focus to birth defects.[15] Some centers remained with support of public monies, including Goldwater Memorial Hospital (New York), Texas Institute for Research and Rehabilitation (Houston), and Rancho Los Amigos (Downey, California).[16] Although acute care physicians no longer had experience with long-term mechanical ventilation, physicians at these former polio centers applied long-term mechanical ventilation for chronic ventilatory insufficiency to patients with spinal cord injuries and other neuromuscular-skeletal disorders in the hospital and even at home.

Initial Hospital-Based Solutions

The "price to pay" for the miracles in the intensive care unit (ICU) was the simultaneous survival of a small number of infants and children who could not be removed from medical technology. Almost all concerned considered such ventilator-dependent patients "failures of treatment," and the setting of their care received much criticism. The children also failed to thrive. When taken off technology, they became medically unstable, decompensated, or died in the hospital or at home.

Attempts to wean these children from mechanical ventilation failed. Occasionally, some pediatric residents just "let a month go by without weaning." This resulted in medical stability, enhanced energy and vigor, and improved eating and participation in therapy and play due to augmented functional reserve.

Furthermore, autopsies of some of these children sent home without mechanical ventilation revealed potentially reversible narrowing of small pulmonary blood vessels, usually observed at high altitude, suggesting that such children needed ventilation. Evidence from young laboratory animals (anatomical studies) and humans (functional studies) suggested that the pediatric lung had potential for growth and development during the first decade of life. Children with chronic respiratory insufficiency, if provided optimal ventilation, might not only do better (become more active, alert, and aware), but also might even grow and develop to the point that they would no longer require life support at all.

The initial hospital-based efforts to address these children with special needs focused on the creation of "step-down" units. Solutions required an integrated team approach involving patients and families in self-care. Optimal support (optimal ventilation, pharmacology, nutrition, and developmental stimulation) changed the outcome and proved that special needs children could thrive. The first specialty-designated units featured patient-centered team approaches led by primary care nurses. They emphasized child development and a team organization. Families took an active role in learning skills, adapting procedures, providing care, making management decisions, and, eventually, if they chose, planning transitional care. In these units, parents and other family members could be thoroughly prepared for roles and responsibilities as caregivers, which one day would help them feel ready for care at home.

Over time, evidence suggested that additional solutions were necessary for other transitional care settings. Several pediatric centers with expertise in chronic illness/disability considered MF/TD children a challenge worthy of the extension of their mission and devoted part of their resources to their needs. These centers included Seashore House in Philadelphia; AI DuPont in Wilmington, Delaware; LaRabida in Chicago; Mt. Washington in Baltimore; and the Hospital for Sick Children in Washington, D.C. In these centers, physicians focused on chronic care and the family as a social unit and addressed long-term developmental, social, and educational needs.

Initial Home Care Experiences

Parents encouraged the first home care initiatives for MF/TD children as a better option for families with children who required prolonged mechanical ventilation; physicians saw this as a way to reopen limited ICU capacity for more acute-care needs. By the mid-1980s, the pediatric literature reported several home care discharge experiences.[17] The first reports came from the earliest developed units responsible for major advances in neonatology and critical care pediatrics. Each report described organizational and funding concerns. Hospital care for MF/TD children was reimbursed (retrospective cost-plus); home care was not. However, early demonstrations determined that resources could be found and "creative financing" arranged by establishing working relationships among healthcare providers, administrators, and funding sources.

The Recent Past

More recently, there has been a change in the view about care of MF/TD children. Healthcare planners and legislators began to see home health as a viable care option for these children. Public funding was made more readily available for the care of these children and some insurance companies explored solutions for providing care. In addition, the HTHC industry flourished as a response to changing attitudes about home care and the increased availability of funds.

Bringing Public Attention to the Population of MF/TD Children

U.S. Surgeon General C. Everett Koop (1981–1989) advocated for the care of life-supported children in the home. Moreover, he shared the vision that responding to the needs of technology-dependent children and their families stimulated solutions that were global in nature and could be applied to all special-needs children with disabilities and/or chronic illness. As a result, the U.S. Public Health Service, Division of Maternal Child Health, sponsored the "Surgeon General's Workshop on Children with Handicaps and Their Families: Case-Example—The Ventilator-Dependent Child."[18] Conference planners invited a broad spectrum of actors who had been impacted by the issues at hand. The planners thought that if all of the system's stakeholders could be present, they would become participants in planning and implementing that system and ensuring its success. A small task-group format encouraged interaction among national leaders of relevant programs/policies, healthcare professionals, and organizational leaders, and, most important, informed consumers (parents and ventilator users).

Public Policy Responses to Meet the Needs of MF/TD Children

By the early 1980s, ventilator-dependent children were not rare. One example was Katie Beckett, a young child from Cedar Rapids, Iowa, who was evaluated in Illinois for medical technology special needs. Julie Beckett, mother of Katie, learned that home care for children like hers was possible in Illinois. Katie's mother and pediatrician sought funding support for home care, but they came across bureaucratic red tape with Iowa Medicaid. With resourcefulness, determination, and conviction, Katie's mother contacted the appropriate politicians, who brought the plight of these children and the barriers created by government policy and practice to the attention of then–Vice President Bush. President Reagan highlighted the case of Katie Beckett at a 1981 press conference; Katie was sent home as "an exception to policy."[19]

When the president makes an exception to policy, it can stimulate an urgency to deal with anticipated future cases. Thus, U.S. Health and Human Services Secretary Schweiker established an ad hoc task force, and Congressman Henry Waxman charged his healthcare committee staff members to design a public policy response: community-based "waivers" to existing policy determined by strict criteria with financial risk limited to a defined number of children. Since 1982, public funding for MF/TD children has been obtained as a waiver from Medicaid policy. States can apply to the Health Care Finance Administration for approval of a community-based waiver for a limited number of beneficiaries. The waiver provides a mechanism to utilize Medicaid funds without requiring a copayment by families that essentially reduces their financial assets to poverty level. However, not all states applied for waivers, and those that did were as relevant as the insights and understanding of the authors who submitted them. Furthermore, waivers limited the number of beneficiaries and took an excessive amount of time for approval. Once waivers were approved, restrictive policies and procedures replaced what had been more innovative creative financing negotiated for individual cases.

Private Reimbursement Practices

Not all technology-dependent children required Medicaid funding. Some had limited private indemnity benefits, often with major medical insurance. Although these policies did not cover this new category of patient, insurance company administrators (medical directors) and employers who determined benefit selection were open to direct dialogue for creative solutions to utilize the remaining funds that they were obligated to spend. They were less restricted by rules and regulations, which permitted more flexibility to meet the individual needs of employees' families. However, physicians still thought it wise to involve all public payers (especially Title V agencies) who were knowledgeable about both community-based resources and access to public funds to supplement private benefits.

Service Delivery

When the first attempts were made to discharge MF/TD children to their homes, home care equipment providers and home health agencies were hesitant to provide high-technology devices and supportive personnel in the home due to potential medical liability risk and lack of funding. However, as insurance companies and waiver cases began to provide a potentially limitless funding stream, home care agencies and vendors began to develop pediatric programs. Families could obtain equipment, supplies, and support, but they faced fragmented service programs in the community. Payers soon realized that HTHC, previously delivered at significant cost savings compared to hospitalization, started to approach or exceed costs of institutional care. This resulted, in part, from inadequate coordination or integration of service delivery and from funding approaches that did not incorporate cost-management mechanisms. The availability of funding without adequate cost controls encouraged development of an HTHC industry, resulting in an explosion in costs and utilization.[20] This excessive growth in costs and utilization has become a major public policy concern.[21] Families are at risk for denial of home care, because public policy requires that home care must by law be less expensive than institutional care.

ANALYZING THE PRESENT

Today, parents and professionals concerned about MF/TD children face a disorganized array of fragmented sources of funding/services to meet these children's healthcare, social, educational, and developmental needs. The cost of this lack of integrated management of services required by these children is high; the needs of these children might not be met or, if met, the actual expenditures can be excessive. Children and families are victims of cost/operational inefficiencies that might put the option of home care as a viable option at risk, because cost might exceed institutional alternatives. The situation will become more critical with managed care/capitation.

Current Reimbursement Policies and Practices for HTHC

The ability to fund care for MF/TD children comes from a variety of sources. States have different guidelines for the use of Title V funds, but this can be a resource for community-based services. Although private insurance regards these children as "catastrophic costs" cases, some companies using innovative case management practices to assist in financial their care. In addition, alternative funding sources such as managed care organizations (MCOs), family contributions, and voluntary/community agency assistance are being explored.

Public Sector

Not all MF/TD children at home require Medicaid (Title XIX). However, with time, those with finite private indemnity insurance will require a public funding alternative. Over a lifetime, insurance policy limits are commonly exceeded, and home care benefits will be restricted by Medicaid policy with or without waiver exceptions. Community-based waivers are highly variable from state to state.

Each state also has a designated program for "children with special needs" (Title V). These funds have defined categorical criteria with or without additional Social Security benefits. Compared to funds available from Medicaid, Title V funding is far more restricted. Title V programs provide involvement by concerned professionals who want to meet the comprehensive needs of these special children. In Illinois, for example, Title V has been a valuable resource for information about community-based services and as a case manager of Medicaid waiver funds.

Other public funds have been identified and applied toward MF/TD children. For example, underutilized budgeted state funds identified by resourceful parents have funded a statewide case-management program for ventilator-dependent children in Pennsylvania. This was accomplished by a family who had chosen home care on a ventilator for their developmentally delayed MF/TD child as a preferable situation to prolonged institutionalization.

Private Sector

Private sector funding from traditional indemnity insurance commonly pays for healthcare costs retrospectively "at cost." "Cost shifting" by healthcare providers has placed an added burden on private insurers to compensate for underfunded public payment. For private insurers, a MF/TD child represents a "catastrophic cost" case. As early as 1983, private insurers (Aetna and later Blue Cross/Blue Shield) responded with case-management strategies that required a healthcare professional (nurse/physician) to review and approve costs for these exceptional cases. Despite policy restrictions, these case managers have been approachable as colleagues to develop flexible, individualized programs. Employers who have developed self-insurance Employee Retirement Income Security Act (ERISA) programs both with and without third-party administrators also utilize case management for exceptional cases.

Health maintenance organizations (HMOs) assume full financial risk for enrolled members by accepting premiums for total comprehensive care. They attempt to locate and contract with hospitals and healthcare providers who will agree to financial arrangements that assume part or all of the financial risk for providing services. The line between funder and provider can become fuzzy, depending on the contract. Arrangements vary among contracts, which often incorporate exceptions to deal with catastrophic cost situations. Funding systems are not designed for many of the health needs or the social support and educational/developmental needs for MF/TD children. Costs, not care, drive these financial considerations.

HMOs also have designed programs incorporating case management as a strategy to limit financial exposure that might exceed anticipated expenditures. In some cases, "benefit management" is interpreted very narrowly, limiting or rejecting payment for needed services for MF/TD children. However, some HMOs have demonstrated remarkable innovations in case management/program design that have led to significant cost saving and enhanced quality for MF/TD children.[22]

Alternative Funding Sources

Because the need is great and the care expensive, alternate sources of funding for MF/TD children's care are being considered. MCOs are attempting to control costs and provide medically-necessary care. Families are responsible for several areas of direct and indirect costs for the care of their MF/TD children. In addition, nonprofit and voluntary/community agencies may be called upon to raise funds for care and research.

Managed Care Practices.   MCOs apply funding practices that have become more prominent for MF/TD children and their families. In fact, managed care has become the dominant delivery system for Medicaid. Medicaid managed care programs operate on primarily two options in their attempt to manage care by managing costs. They try to contain costs by using volume discount contracts with providers and by favoring provider networks that can provide comprehensive services. In some cases, MCOs can transfer all financial risk to providers by capitation—paying providers a payment "per patient, per month" for all healthcare needs. Although the intent is to provide incentives for health promotion/prevention, it also provides incentives to limit expenditures, because cost overruns are liabilities to the provider. Providers then might consider health promotion costs for MF/TD children to not be medically necessary.

In addition, MCOs attempt to control costs by determining "medical necessity" and requiring approval of all benefits by a gatekeeper, who is often a primary care physician (family physician/generalist). Because MF/TD children potentially represent catastrophic costs, MCOs also use case managers. Gatekeepers and case managers may or may not be sensitive to the medical necessity of many services that would improve the well-being and promote the health of their beneficiaries. This program is gaining in popularity with states as budgets become tighter and tighter.

Family Contributions.   Families are exposed to both direct and indirect costs for their MF/TD children. Many reimbursement programs require annual deductibles and copayments for covered benefits that might also have finite limits requiring major medical coverage, which also might be limited.

(MF/TD children and families sometimes find even million-dollar coverage insufficient.) Furthermore, the family must face many uncovered health-related expenses that are often not considered: the need to expand/modify the house, increased energy costs/taxes, the loss of earnings due to providing direct care, the need to buy new means of transportation and mobility, and payments for technical aids for education/developmental purposes. Although they might not seem medically necessary, they promote health and indirectly affect healthcare expenditures. They permit continuity of home health care that, when properly designed and managed, can limit healthcare costs and/or extend benefits.

Voluntary/Community Agencies.   Some nonprofit and voluntary/community agencies provide funding for "categorical" needs. For example, organizations that address a particular medical condition raise funds for research/services directly or via the United Way (e.g., Muscular Dystrophy Association, United Cerebral Palsy, Easter Seals). Such agencies will not fund catastrophic health costs; rather, they may choose to provide supplementary funding for designated purposes (purchase of devices). Community agencies have been more helpful in responding to developmental and educational (health-affecting) needs. Some charitable organizations (e.g., Rotary International) have raised funds designated for individual children and special populations. In addition, creative financing (combining funding from private, public, community sources) designed by concerned professionals, organizations, and parents working together has funded extraordinary costs of MD/TD children on an individual case basis.

Current Service Provision

Services for complex chronic conditions are provided without a coordinated, integrated management approach. This fragmentation frustrates all of the participants and actors involved in the MF/TD child's care.

Health Care Needs

MF/TD children being cared for at home require a variety of services for their medical, psychosocial, developmental, and educational needs. These services all promote the child's general health. Few resources target the pediatric population only or provide "one-stop shopping," including case management. Thus, families and professionals must work within a fragmented and uncoordinated service system that features gaps, duplications, and inefficiencies.

Psychosocial/Developmental Needs

The psychosocial/developmental needs of MF/TD children affect their health. Sometimes services that meet these needs are available from home health agencies, but they also can be found in other community agencies designated for other purposes. Many community agencies have "home visiting" as part of their programs.[23] However, they are not integrated with the services provided by home health agencies.

Families often find that they can get more support for health and related needs by turning to other families and concerned persons who join together as self-help or mutual aid groups.[24] Self-help groups such as SKIP (Sick Kids

[Need] Involved Persons) are a major source of support for families; these groups supplement professional care and provide assistance not available in the professional sphere. Other self-help groups (e.g., Family Voices) provide advocacy and serve as catalysts for social change.

Educational Needs

As MF/TD children have become more prevalent in the community, educational systems have found these children to be a major challenge beyond current special-educational programming. In some school districts, developmental therapies (physical, occupational, and speech therapy) prepare children for school; these services do not depend on health insurance. Recently, MF/TD children have benefited from federally-mandated early intervention programs for birth to age 3 and 3- to 5-year-old children. In Illinois, families, health, and funding agencies have joined in local area councils to facilitate case finding, system design, and coordination of services to prepare children for entry into the school system.

APPROACHING THE FUTURE

The future of MF/TD children is closely tied to the future of HTHC. Due to the unconstrained growth of the home care industry and the increasing costs of HTHC, the future of HTHC has now been questioned on ethical grounds.[25]

The Ethical Framework

Ethical conflicts result when multiple ethical principles reflecting different perspectives must be considered. In terms of HTHC, conflict may arise regarding what the professional wants to do, what the patient/person/family wants to have done, and what society can afford to do. Because one option demands trade-off with another, HTHC can give rise to an ethical debate.

Before engaging in that debate, it will be worthwhile to lay out groundwork for considering the ethical issues involved here, to avoid the trap of giving ready answers to objections whose implications brook no such answers. Judgments about right and wrong must always be arrived at by (1) considering the various human values involved in a complex life situation, (2) assigning these values proper weight with the help of agreed-upon criteria, and (3) resolving value conflicts in light of that assessment. Each of these steps needs clarification.

Considering Human Values in a Complex Life Situation

Precisely because life situations are complex, they must be analyzed carefully for what is really at issue. Sorting out the underlying problems, within the global problem, requires rigorous analysis of the various physical, spiritual, psychological, and social realities presented. It is important to know the medical facts in a case and the conclusions that can be validly drawn from them. Hunches or guesses, much less wishes, cannot validly ground ethical decisions. The spiritual and psychological state of a person must be questioned carefully, which can make a profound difference in the weight assigned to various values. Relationships, family attitudes, finances, and the larger social situation all require careful investigation before any decision can be prudently made.

Assessment of Values with Agreed-Upon Criteria

Values are of varying importance in common human estimation. For example, survival is more crucial than comfort; good health is more valued than material possessions. However, "common human estimation" can also be controverted. Therefore, an agreed-upon criteria is needed to assess the relative importance of human values.

In the Western tradition, the so-called natural law was for many people the norm for human values. It was thought to be inscribed in the heart of every human being, and it based conscience as the individual's practical judgment of right and wrong. For some, it is still the surest criterion of true value.

Resolving Value Conflicts

Values sometimes appear to be in conflict. Safeguarding one value might entail risk for another value or values. When this is the case, criteria are needed to determine which value should be given priority. In recent discussions of values in the medical field, there has been widespread use of some value-based principles that, many would agree, provide guidance for deciding the correct resolution of ethical dilemmas. These principles have to do with the overall welfare of the patient (beneficence), the appropriate freedom of the patient for self-determination (autonomy), and the rights of everyone connected with the patient's care (justice). HTHC poses some ethical questions that differ in detail, but not in substance, from questions posed by health care in general. Therefore, it might be helpful to use these principles in making ethical value judgments about various aspects of HTHC.

Principle #1: Beneficence.   This principle asserts that the healthcare provider should always act in the patient's best interest. Not only should the caregiver not do the patient harm (something often formulated in a separate principle of nonmaleficence, but in fact included in this principle implicitly), but should always strive to achieve overall good for the patient.

Home health care is intended to further the patient's overall good. It is, when properly administered, care for the whole person: psychological, spiritual, and social, as well as physical, well-being. The very notion of the word *home* implies this. Home is commonly thought of as the place where we feel most comfortable: in the midst of family, surrounded by familiar things that call up memories of past happiness, with easy access to friends and the normal business of everyday life, and with none of the institutional trappings and timetables that are necessary in hospitals.

Applying Ethical Principles Using Adult Case Examples.   Technological breakthroughs have made it possible to care at home for patients who, until recently, would have had to be hospitalized in order for their medical needs to be addressed. In itself, this is obviously a good thing for patients. Of course, in concrete instances, such high-tech home care entails aspects that call into question its being the ethically correct thing to do.

A clarifying case is in order. Fred Marks is a 49-year-old victim of non-Hodgkin's lymphoma and is diagnosed as terminal. He has been released from the hospital so that he can live out his remaining days at home, in accord with his and his family's wishes. Now bedridden, he requires periodic injections, dressing changes, and enteral feeding, in addition to personal care.

His wife, Mary, has learned to manage all this, with the help of a married daughter who comes in from some distance away every other day for a few hours. But Mary is very worried about what might be in the offing as Fred's condition worsens: Catheter tubes that will need unclogging, the suctioning of secretions, perhaps even monitoring a portable ventilator if her husband needs help in breathing, and so forth. Doctors assure her that the technology is available to enable Fred to stay at home, as they both wanted, and as he desperately hopes to—but Mary secretly dreads the responsibilities this will impose on her. She is not sure she can cope. Just the other day the feeding tube was almost jarred loose, and she panicked until she managed to get it stabilized.

Meanwhile, her two younger sons, 12 and 16, are spending more and more time out with their friends. They tell Mary they cannot bear to be around their father for more than a short time, they do not want to bring their buddies over, and they feel ashamed of themselves for this. What used to be a lively, happy home for them is now a real downer.

So far, HTHC has been a helpful means to ensure the best interests of the patient (beneficence). If Mary manages to master the intricacies of further technology as it becomes necessary, then this will continue to be the case. If not, then Fred's best medical interests might be in jeopardy. However, there is a further complication with ethical ramifications: the possibility that Mary and Fred may end up disagreeing about what is in fact possible with regard to his care. This brings in the second basic principle.

Principle #2: Autonomy. According to this principle, the patient's freedom should be respected in all healthcare decisions. Not only should doctors not impose treatment or measures that are not absolutely indicated medically, or otherwise preempt the patient's own choices (behavior often spoken of in terms of paternalism), but all caregivers should acknowledge the patient's right to decide the direction and extent of her or his care within the parameters of medical correctness and real possibility.

Up to this point, everyone concerned has been able to respect Fred's wishes without any difficulty: They were precisely what doctors judged reasonable, and exactly what Mary wanted for the husband she dreaded losing and wanted to stay close to as long as she could. Now the situation may be changing.

Fred insists that he is not bothered by the possibility that Mary will not be able to manage further technology with perfect assurance. He would rather be "less well-cared for" at home, he says, than "perfectly cared for" in a hospital. Mary cannot make him understand the absolute panic she feels at the thought of being responsible for something that harms her husband. She does not even want to mention the strain she knows the situation is putting on their younger children.

It is clear that Fred's freedom is beginning to be a problem in the larger picture of things because Fred is not the only person involved in his illness; though, of course, he is the central figure. There are other persons to consider, starting with his family, who have certain rights as well. These rights, among others, are the concern of the third principle.

Principle #3: Justice.   Human situations always involve relationships, and relationships entail mutual rights and responsibilities. The balancing of rights and responsibilities is, at its most basic level, the sphere of justice: giving to each person that person's due. There are microrelationships, such as those in a family, and macrorelationships, involving a person and society.

In this case, Mary is owed some consideration that Fred might not be giving her. She has a right to her own health, physical and psychological, and the latter may be endangered by Fred's demands. Then there are the younger children. On the one hand, learning to care for their father can be a maturing factor for them and stand them in good stead when they assume adult responsibilities. On the other hand, it can be unjust to ask of them more than adolescents can bear. Clearly, the situation needs discussion.

The case of Mary and Fred is one possible scenario for HTHC. It shows the tensions that can be involved and highlights the sensitivity needed to be aware of danger spots. However, other scenarios emphasize other dimensions.

Take the situation of Priscilla Smith. At the age of 13, Priscilla, who was a good swimmer, dove headfirst into what she thought was deep water. It turned out to have large rocks in it, and she hit one solidly, breaking her neck. Saved from drowning by the quick thinking of her companions, she regained consciousness in a hospital bed only to find herself a quadriplegic for the rest of her life. She is able to move only her head, nothing else. From the hospital, she was transferred to a nursing facility, where she lived for the next 15 years. She needed total care; she could do nothing for herself. Even her breathing was difficult, but she refused any thought of a ventilator. She wanted no part of a machine that would, she felt, create the ultimate dependency.

Fighting a continual battle with despair, at age 28, Priscilla had the good fortune to meet a physician who was convinced that she could live outside an institution, given new technological possibilities for home care. With the help of friends, she found a suitable apartment and soon discovered that she was able to do much more than the limitations of the nursing facility had ever let her imagine. A motorized wheelchair that she learned to control by puffing and sipping on a plastic straw gave her new mobility. The clinic she visited for occupational therapy put her in touch with people looking to develop new technologies for home care. She was able to help them understand what the needs of a consumer like her really were, as well as what forms of technology were actually practical for her situation. Out of that came a job as a consultant that, in turn, expanded into speaking engagements: She was actually a wage earner!

Moreover, though still in need of 24-hour care, she found no lack of volunteers willing to take a turn helping her. Even if her apartment was equipped with sophisticated devices that enabled her to turn the TV on and off, unlock the door, even activate and use a computer—it looked like a cozy apartment, not a clinic! When one visits her today, there is no machinery evident apart from the motorized wheelchair in which she spends most of her day. A portable ventilator (recognized, in the end, as a means of independence, rather than its opposite) is neatly tucked under its seat, and her tracheostomy tube is artfully concealed by a lovely silk scarf. Priscilla is living a life amazingly close to normal, thanks to the miracles of HTHC.

This case gives another view of HTHC. HTHC can enable a person to be productive and happy despite fearful physical limitations, because technology has found a way to compensate for such limitations. If the same ethical principles are applied to Priscilla's situation, the following conclusions can be made:

1. The ethical principle of beneficence is at work here. The volunteers Priscilla has attracted and the doctors and therapists who have helped her achieve so much demonstrate this. It also is found in the public sector through the various programs that contribute to the costs of maintaining her health. Beneficence also is demonstrated by the private sector, which has found ways of using and paying for her services, thus enabling her to provide in good part for herself.

2. In terms of autonomy, Priscilla has been able to make choices about how to live her life that no one could have imagined at the beginning of her quadriplegia. Despite her dependence on caregivers—or perhaps because of her willingness to accept such dependence consciously and without resentment—she lives a dignified, useful, and fulfilling life. Without the technology to support her decisions, this would remain forever a pipe dream.

3. How is the justice principle addressed? In terms of family, there is no issue; she is not asking for care from them. The volunteers who help her do so because they want to, not out of any sense of obligation. What is the role of society in this case? Are the costs involved in giving Priscilla the care she needs an imposition on other taxpayers? Given her ability to work and contribute to society, it is not difficult to answer "no" to this question. However, the question is a valid one, and in other situations, the answer may be more difficult to formulate.

Pinpointing Ongoing Ethical Issues

These two cases begin to illustrate the variety of ethical choices in HTHC situations. Each individual case requires its own special analysis; generalizations are, as always, dangerous. In a 1994 book, *Bringing the Hospital Home: Ethical and Social Implications of High-Technology Home Care*, edited by John D. Arras, one can see the broad spectrum of HTHC in the results of a project that involved a working group of clinicians, scholars, and policy analysts who reviewed specially commissioned papers. They also listened to the narratives of patients, healthcare professionals, family caregivers, and involved friends, as they related their own experiences of HTHC.[26] Five of the major papers have been published in abridged versions in a special Supplement to the Hastings Center Report (September–October 1994), furnishing a convenient collection of reflections on various aspects of HTHC, both positive and negative.[27] Most are thoughtful and many would seem correct, but some raise questions from the viewpoint of this chapter.

For instance, the novel element of HTHC is "the hypermedicalization of the home, the extension of medical dominion to the heretofore private sphere of family and friends."[28] This is based on a questionable assumption about the nature of HTHC. If the mindset of service providers is institutional and the model for home care is medical, then perhaps the statement stands. However, it could be contended that proper home care represents a social concept that is person-centered and that is best understood from the independent living model of persons with disabilities (see Table 18-1 for the ramifications of these two models); thus, home hypermedicalization is not appropriate.

In the independent-living model, it is rather the radically changed roles, relationships, and responsibilities of physicians, patient/family members, and care partners that are the truly novel elements. The home is not hypermedicalized; there is no question of medical dominion invading the private sphere of the home. Or, if in a given case there is, then precisely for that reason ethical questions must be raised about the true good of the patient and his or her autonomy, as well as about justice to everyone concerned.

Arras described HTHC as "a complex social phenomenon that improves life for many while threatening to erode for others the conditions that tend to foster important social goods and opportunities. . . ." [29] Some of the antinomies involved include home versus miniature ICU and the gift of easy breathing versus being tethered to a machine. The real importance to caregivers of being given the opportunity to care versus the sometimes-crushing burden for laypeople of having to perform functions that were once the exclusive province of trained medical personnel also is involved.

In addition, important cost-containment factors for hospitals versus escalating (and sometimes highly inflated) costs at home and efficient high-tech versus human high-touch for patients needs to be considered. Arras raised the immensely complex issue of public costs and national priorities, noting that although the distinction between high-tech and low-tech is not necessarily important for public policy, there is an anomaly apparent in pouring huge sums of money into HTHC when "the basic needs of many patients for nonmedical community support often go unmet." [30]

There may well be an anomaly in the cost of HTHC, and the question needs continual investigation and monitoring. However, as mentioned earlier in this chapter, the reasons for the escalation of costs from initial experiences with pediatric HTHC to the current situation raise a whole other category of ethical questions regarding public policies of control, regulation, and integration of production and delivery. The principle of justice can be useful in assessing when profits ought to be subject to governmental control to ensure that the consumers of HTHC not become victims of a kind of "blackmail" made possible by the dire need in which they find themselves, together with the monopolistic character of the industry that is serving that need. Are excessive costs due to lack of system design, operational inefficiencies, fragmentation of service delivery, and lack of coordination of the continuum of care just?

All of these points need to be considered when assessing the ethical aspects of decisions about a given case involving HTHC. They can be examined under the categories of beneficence, autonomy, and justice, but such categories can only structure the analysis of what is at stake, They cannot promise easy, preset solutions to complicated human situations. Beyond that, the considerations raised by examining HTHC suggest an increasing necessity of public policy decisions about health care in general.

These decisions include such thorny questions as whether there is a need to create a whole category of intermediate-care institutions. There is also an issue of whether there is a need to institute more effective monitoring and control of the health-technology industry, as well as technology assessment. In addition, society must decide whether there is a need to impose global limits on health-care spending, even rationing quotas about who gets what kind of care.

These are not new issues, but they grow in importance and assume ever-new complexity as HTHC becomes a more prominent aspect of our healthcare landscape. People, both lay and professional, with a stake in HTHC are increasing exponentially. They must continue to wrestle with the issues, attempting to hold in proper tension their many and varied needs that clamor for recognition and respect. This will be necessary if they are to be able to shape a future society in which HTHC's obvious benefits can be reaped in a way that enables all to be truly human and responsible in caring for one another.

What Will the Future of Reimbursement Look Like?

Healthcare cost expansion exceeding the general rate of inflation cannot continue unabated. For over a decade, various strategies have been attempted in the United States to control costs. These include cost-plus retrospective reimbursement, case-mix average prospective payment for diagnosis-related groups (DRGs), volume-discount contracting with preferred providers, cata-strophic complex-care case management, regulation of physician fees determined by resource-based relative value scales (RBRVS), and others. They limit expenditures, and potentially, quantity and quality of care. All of these tactics are part of the universal rubric of managed care that up to now has focused more on managing costs than on maintaining or improving quality.

The attempts at federal healthcare reform will not end. Instead of being comprehensive, political healthcare reform will likely be incremental, focusing more on financial reform than system delivery. Instead of federal reform, states are likely to be the sites of experimental programs. One can see the beginnings of these changes in the health insurance mandates in Tennessee and Massachusetts.

Market-driven healthcare reform has really been taking place for some time and will only intensify. Many of the players are publicly traded (investor-financed) private sector organizations that are developing the means to deliver basic healthcare services and financing. To realize potential return on investments, rigorous cost management will be put in place. Ultimately, all payers—and the public—will realize that capitation is inevitable. All health care will be delivered within a total finite amount of expenditures (global budget). Those receiving HTHC represent complex expensive care that are "outliers" to any managed care approach, and payment for their healthcare costs will be at risk without special "carve out" considerations.

The needs of MF/TD children include family social support as well as developmental and educational services. However, constraints on public healthcare expenditures extend to social and educational budgets as well. All politicians are conscious of the need to reduce government expenditures. Budgets for all federal programs are at risk. State and local budgets will also be strained as never before. State/local governments have responded to public referenda to limit debt and tax financing and have already put in cost controls (balanced budget requirements) that demand fiscal responsibility. Public sector funding for all services will be constricted and growth will be limited.

What Organizational Strategies Make Sense in This Future Funding Environment?

Market/political healthcare reform, proposed or real, has already resulted in market-driven responses that can help predict future realities. In the future, health care will be delivered by comprehensive community-based integrated delivery systems (IDSs). These systems will provide acute, subacute, and long-term care in institutional settings and nonfacility-based alternatives, including the home. All system components will have to operate within financial constraints that will encourage cost saving (e.g., replacement of professionals with paraprofessionals, nonprofessionals, and volunteers; substitution of human resources with advanced medical information and communication technologies).

Health care is not the only need of MF/TD children. Other community-based services (social support, developmental, and educational) also under funding/budgetary constraints must also consider integration and cost-limiting strategies. Volunteer and self-help organizations should realize the value of resource sharing and the synergy that is possible through organizational interdependency. Case management and home visiting, currently used by many agencies, will be an essential component of future organizational growth. Many community-based service organizations that already use cost-management approaches (e.g., case management) will coordinate services, meeting multiple needs simultaneously. In the future, they will find that integration of services from multiple sources enhances client benefit and maximizes resource utilization. Public funders providing oversight will contract with social agency preferred providers that implement these strategies (public sector integration of social agency funding).

What Organizational Planning Approaches Will Make Them Happen?

Organizations wanting to serve MF/TD children and their families in the future will require systems thinking. The complexity of changes in the political, market, and public policy environments will require our responding as learning organizations that are utilizing systems approaches. Meeting the multiple needs of MF/TD children with fragmented, isolated, and competing services will no longer be a possibility. Today HTHC is a nonsystem. Tomorrow, a systems approach will be mandatory. Organizations will entertain considerations of strategic alliances in a variety of forms, including joint ventures on a program/organizational basis, staged mergers, or provider-payer-consumer system development. In this way, complementary services can be better coordinated and managed (e.g., home visiting can serve multiple purposes, including medical/social service delivery, technical support, and case management).

Future action planning should consider a process whereby all stakeholders in systems development, including consumers, will be identified and invited into the process of system planning, implementation, and evaluation; outcome analysis will be used as feedback for further system development. These systems will be in the form of stakeholder partnerships, each representing unique perspectives essential for the successful operation of the system. The ultimate partnership will link healthcare consumers (patients), providers, and payers who design, use, and develop the systems together.

UPDATE FROM A PRACTITIONER'S VIEW

An increasing number of elderly and disabled children are living longer, but with greater disabilities because of advances in technology that increase longevity regardless of the patient's medical status. The societal costs of futile and end-of-life care have created conversation about this problem while offering few solutions. The conversation is not limited to those who receive home health care, but includes those whose care is provided through institutions. It is important to look at the implications of living longer with disabilities for the current and future generations of consumers of healthcare services.

Today, nearly 27 percent of Medicare's budget is spent on end-of-life care for America's seniors.[31] There are wide geographical variances in per-patient costs and views of what end-of-life care encompasses. Standard of care practices vary based on the number of hospital beds and physicians available in different parts of the country. There are considerable differences in healthcare practitioners' philosophical approaches to death and dying. These views generally mirror the local societal values of these issues. Oregon openly encourages discussion of end-of-life issues between physician and patient in a pragmatic approach to utilization of comfort/palliative treatments with less emphasis on curative protocols. In contrast, Florida has an aging, transplanted multicultural population that demands high-tech solutions for their end-of-life care.[32]

Beginning in 2011, the baby boomers will be entering the Medicare system at a rate greater than 10,000 persons per day for the next 18 years. This huge number of new beneficiaries will create an even greater strain on Medicare/Medicaid budgets and on the home health industry. Younger wage earners will be forced to take on this societal financial burden not of their making. Simultaneously, this generation will be concerned about paying for a social security and healthcare system that they believe will be nonexistent when they reach retirement age. As these costs to society increase, the inevitable response will be to bring costs under control through managed care and rationing. Hopefully, health status and the patient's ability to benefit from treatment will be the measure of availability and not the patient's chronological age or disability.

The cost of high-technology care outside of acute care facilities continues to be a major issue. Third-party payers have the same quality-of-life expectations for home care patients as hospitalized patients in futile-care situations. However, there is a need to balance benefit with burden. Society is also entitled to a return on its investment. So who pays for high-technology home health care and for how long? Let the deliberations begin.

CONCLUSION

What will the future for MF/TD Children and HTHC be like? Will they survive in a rationed care or managed care world? What can be established? How will it be established?

1. An integrated family-centered service delivery system will operate within finite predetermined financial constraints. The financial risk to manage available resources and respond to the multiple needs of all beneficiaries will be the burden of the system. Community-based alternatives (e.g., HTHC) cannot survive if they cost more than institutional-based alternatives.

2. The system must be operated by an integrated management approach that involves and links all stakeholders in system development. Stakeholders include healthcare, social service, developmental and educational professionals, patients/families, payers, community-based providers/agencies, and lenders. A process of planning, implementing, evaluating, and modifying the system that respects and incorporates multiple perspectives can resolve ethical/management conflicts. In this way, the evolution of the system will be flexible, meeting needs of each individual participant and group while maximizing the utilization of resources. The system will not survive if it is fragmented or unable to innovate.

3. The system must be designed "smartly," using available management-information systems and advanced communications that can extend the impact of each player. The central role must be given to the people/families at home, who have valuable insight and skills in self-management and management of their own program needs.

4. The system must integrate a variety of services targeted to meet multiple needs. The system must present a total service package that will offer options, depending on the needs of each individual situation. Such an integrated system must be designed and operated locally, because its success will be based on dedicated collaborative efforts of professionals, parents, providers, and payers who will all benefit if given the opportunity to work together within the constraints of managed care/capitation.

5. The system must responsibly accomplish multiple goals: universal access, medical necessity as determined by system criteria, quality improvement, and cost containment. It must prove itself by presetting desirable outcomes and acceptable indicators of variance. Only by achieving desired results as determined by rigorous outcomes research will the system justify the resources required for survival.

SUMMARY

This chapter deals with high-technology home care, an issue that challenges the healthcare system on many levels. The author reviews past issues that resulted from the creation of populations of MF/TD children. The complexity of concerns for parents, healthcare systems, and communities who care for these children is explored. Ethical issues for the future are also explored in this chapter. Finally, in the practitioner's update, the costs of technology and its relationship to MF/TD children and adults at the end of life are discussed. The ethical issues created will affect current and future members of society.

QUESTIONS FOR DISCUSSION

1. How has technology increased the benefits and burdens for the parents of MF/TD patients?
2. What is society's role in providing care for patients with disabilities who require expensive technology-based care? Should such care be rationed?
3. What do you think will be the impact of healthcare cost reforms on the HTHC industry?
4. What principles of ethics can be used to make a case for HTHC?
5. What aspects of social justice could be used to defend using resources for MT/TD patients?

NOTES

1. Institute of Medicine, *Assessing Medical Technology* (Washington, D.C.: National Academy Press, 1985); U.S. Congress, Office of Technology Assessment, *Life-Sustaining Technologies and the Elderly* (OTA-BA-306) (Washington, D.C.: U.S. Government Printing Office, 1987); B. A. Weisbrod, "The Health Care Quadrilemma: An Essay on Technology Change, Insurance, Quality of Care, and Cost Containment," *Journal of Economic Literature* 29 (1991): 523–552.

2. J. R. Hollingsworth and E. J. Hollingsworth, *Care of the Chronically and Severely Ill: Comparative Social Policies* (New York: Aldine de Gruyter, 1994).

3. B. C. Vladeck, "Home-Based Care for a New Century" (keynote address given at the Arden House Milbank Memorial Fund and Visiting Nurse Service of New York, Harriman, New York, 1993).

4. A. L. Goldberg, "Can High-Technology Home Care Survive in a World in Search of Health Care Reform?" in *Home Mechanical Ventilation*, D. Robert, et al., eds. (Paris: Arnette-Blackwell, 1995).

5. G. Laurie, "Introductory Remarks," in *Whatever Happened to the Polio Patient? Proceedings of an International Symposium*, A. L. Goldgery and E. A. M. Faure, eds. (Chicago: Yearbook, 1981).

6. C. G. Engstrom, "Treatment of Severe Cases of Respiratory Paralysis by the Engström Universal Respiratory," *British Journal of Medicine* 2 (1954): 666.

7. H. S. Kristensen and F. Neukirch, "Very Long-Term Artificial Ventilation (Twenty-eight Years)," in *Clinical Use of Mechanical Ventilation*, C. C. Rattenborg and E. Via-Reque, eds. (Chicago: Yearbook, 1981).

8. Laurie, op. cit.

9. "Roundtable Conference on Poliomyelitis Equipment" (paper presented at the National Foundation for Infantile Paralysis, New York, May 28–29, 1953).

10. Laurie, op. cit.

11. E. Ginsberg, et al., *Home Care: Its Role in a Changing Health Services Market* (Totawa, NJ: Roman and Allanhead, 1984), 6.

12. D. S. Gomby and C. S. Larson, eds., *The Future of Children: Home Visiting*, vol. 3, no. 3 (Los Altos, CA: The David and Lucile Packard Foundation, Center for the Future of Children, 1993).

13. Laurie, op. cit.

14. A. L. Goldberg, "Pediatric High-Technology Home Care," in *Intensive Homecare*, M. N. Rothkopf and J. Askanazi, eds. (Baltimore: Williams & Wilkens, 1992), 199–214.

15. Laurie, op. cit.

16. A. L. Goldberg, "Home Care for a Better Life for Ventilator-Dependent People," *Chest* 84 (1983): 365–366.

17. B. H. Burr, et al., "Home Care for Children on Respirators," *New England Journal of Medicine* 309 (1983): 1319–1323; A. L. Goldberg, et al., "Home Care for Life-Supported Persons: An Approach to Program Development," *Journal of Pediatrics* 104 (1984): 785–795; R. G. Kettrick and M. Donar, "The Ventilator Dependent Child: Medical and Social Care," in *Critical Care, State of the Art*, vol. 4 (Fullerton, CA: Society of Critical Care Medicine, 1985), 1–38; R. C. Frates et al., "Outcomes of Home Mechanical Ventilation for Children," *Journal of Pediatrics* 106 (1985): 850–856.

18. Report on the *Surgeon General's Workshop, Children with Handicaps and Their Families: Case Example—The Ventilator-Dependent Child* (PHS-83-50194) (Washington, D.C.: U.S. Department of Health and Human Services, 1993).

19. "Girl Cited by Reagan Received Medicaid under a Special Rule," *New York Times*, (November 11, 1981).

20. J. D. Arras, *Bringing the Hospital Home: Ethical and Social Implications of High-Technology Home Care* (Baltimore: The Johns Hopkins University Press, 1995).

21. "Caring for an Aging World—Allocating Scarce Resources. The Technology Tether: An Introduction to Ethical and Social Issues in High Technology Home Care," *Hastings Center Report* (September–October 1994): S1–S28.

22. A. L. Goldberg and M. J. Trubitt, "An Integrated Approach to Home Health Care," *Physician Executive* 20, no. 1 (1944): 45–46.

23. Gomby and Larson, eds., op. cit.

24. A. H. Katz, H. L. Hedrick, D. H. Isenberg, L. M. Thompson, T. Goodrich, and A. H. Kutscher, *Self-Help: Concepts and Applications* (Philadelphia: The Charles Press, 1992).

25. Goldberg and Trubitt, op. cit.; Katz et al., op. cit.

26. Arras, op. cit.

27. "Caring for an Aging World," op. cit.

28. J. D. Arras and N. N. Dubler, "Bringing the Hospital Home: Ethical and Social Implications of High-Technology Home Care," in *Hastings Center Report, Special Supplement* (September–October 1994): S20.

29. Arras, *Bringing the Hospital Home*, S20.

30. Ibid., S27.

31. J. Apply, "Debate Surrounds End-of-Life Health Care Costs," *USA Today* (October 19, 2006). Available at http//:usatoday.com/money/industries/health/2006-10-18-end-of-life-costs_x.htm.

32. Ibid.

CHAPTER 19

Spirituality and Ethics in Healthcare Organizations

Dexter Freeman and Eileen E. Morrison

OVERVIEW

A generational shift is occurring in healthcare organizations. Baby boomers are aging and beginning to confront the daily struggles of living with chronic diseases. At the same time, members of the Millennium Generation (those born between 1979 and 2001) are entering the healthcare fields. This skeptical generation is more concerned about the quality of their lives than the amount of their paychecks.[1] These two generations are asking similar questions: Why am I here? Why am I doing this job? What does it mean to have a quality life? How can I make a difference?

Of course, these heartfelt questions are at the core of motivation for patients and healthcare providers. However, because of our system's ignorance and patients' lack of opportunity to discuss their thoughts, these questions are rarely verbalized. As a result, patients, providers, administrators, employees, and entire organizations search for something they cannot describe. Nevertheless, they believe that if they find it they will be more complete, fulfilled, and healed. Some writers have described this state of being as a sense of authenticity,[2] a journey to spiritual healing,[3] spirituality at work,[4] and the practice of the soul at work.[5]

In this chapter, Freeman and Morrison provide information about the role of spirituality in healthcare work settings. The concept is important to consider in a text on healthcare ethics, because it affects all aspects of delivery. Patients are no longer satisfied with reductionist views of curing. Professionals are desperately seeking a sense of fulfillment that is greater than their paycheck. Even the Joint Commission on the Accreditation of Healthcare Organizations has responded by mandating that healthcare institutions incorporate spiritual assessments into their medical practice.[6] With such a change in emphasis, one must question whether it is unethical not to incorporate spirituality into the healthcare work environment.

The authors' primary objective in this chapter is to help the reader understand the ethical prudence of spirituality in the healthcare work environment, whether as spirituality relates to the process of practitioners interacting with patients or organizational leaders interacting with employees. This chapter presents working definitions of spirituality and spirituality at work. It then provides an overview of how spirituality affects the healthcare environment, with an emphasis on leadership, employees, and patients/clients. Finally, in keeping with the theme of this text, the critical ethical issues presented by spirituality in the healthcare workplace are addressed.

INTRODUCTION

Graber[7] notes that a spiritual ethos continues to be antithetical to most healthcare organizations, even though Americans typically value selfless and compassionate healthcare service. Moreover, a spiritual ethos often serves as the impetus for many people entering the healthcare professions. Dr. Rachel Remen, a Clinical Professor of Family and Community Medicine at the University of California in the San Francisco School of Medicine, identified that countless numbers of scientifically competent students pursue careers in medicine because they are filled with gratitude and have an overwhelming desire to help others.[8] Although these future physicians might be scientifically gifted, they also are spiritually inspired.

Thus, both America and the U.S. healthcare system are in the midst of a transformation. Historically, people have sought the aid of physicians so they could experience healing, not just the absence of physical symptoms. However, the advent of biomedical research, with its emphasis on symptom management and a reductionist approach that treats diseases, rather than whole people, changed the system. The current perspective in health care has caused healthcare organizations to place more emphasis on accountability and empiricism in healthcare practice. This nonpersonal approach to healthcare practice has not only brought about dehumanization, depersonalization, and organizational isolation, it also justifies the necessity of healthcare practitioners' codes of ethics.

Over the years, physicians and healthcare administrators have stopped seeing themselves as facilitators of healing. Many entered the profession with idealistic hopes and dreams of being able to make a difference. Yet, the indoctrination they get in higher education and their work environment teaches them that "real professionals" do not have time for matters as abstract and obtuse as exploring their patients' sense of existentialism or spirituality. Healthcare administrators also disregard the spirit that compelled them to serve others who were seeking to be whole. As a result, we have spiritless organizations and professionals who are seeking to help those who desire not only physical, but also spiritual transformation.

However, over the past two decades a transition has been occurring in the healthcare industry; people are starting to express an interest in healing again. Of course, when we discuss *healing* we are referring to it with its old English derivative, "to make whole," acknowledging that healing cannot occur without recognizing it as a spiritual process.[9]

Because of this new interest, attitudes toward spirituality in the workplace appear to be changing. Although today's information age, with its emphasis on facts, brevity, and the security of depersonalization continue to be prevalent, a transition to a deeper calling is becoming apparent. This also shows in patients' desires. Research suggests that patients desire and feel more comfortable with physicians who are not only open to their own humanity, but who also are willing to allow patients to discuss their spiritual proclivities.[10]

The past two decades have revealed a resurgence in the need to embrace the whole patient in the healthcare system, but organizations also have started to recognize the importance of addressing their workers' spiritual needs. Books such as Briskin's *Stirring of Soul in the Workplace*, Bolman and Deal's *Leading with Soul*, and, more recently, Benefiel's *Soul at Work* affirm that the business world has recognized people's need to pursue a profession for more than a salary or prestige.

Ashmos and Duchon[11] associate this amplified interest in spirituality in the workplace to several factors. First, the spread of worker demoralization, brought about by massive layoffs, downsizing, and workplace reengineering, has left employers empty and apathetic. Second, baby boomers are aging and beginning to recognize their impending mortality, generating greater interest in the meaning of life. Third, social isolation and the decline in neighborhood organizations have increased the need for workers to feel connected in their work environment. Thus, spirituality is not just something that is nice to recognize; research and anecdotal evidence reveals that it is essential to acknowledge its presence in order to promote the well-being of everyone involved.

SPIRITUALITY: A REVIEW OF DEFINITIONS

A universal force compels humans to express compassion for the helpless and to search for a more complete state of existence. This force is so multifaceted, dynamic, and unique that it is nearly impossible to completely describe, measure, or define. Our best efforts to define it, which some refer to as *spirit* or *soul*, often are feeble and inadequate; nevertheless, no one can ever doubt the reality of its existence.

Carl Jung said, "I do not hold myself responsible for the fact that man has, everywhere and always, spontaneously developed religious (spiritual) forms of expression, and the human psyche from time immemorial has been shot through with religious (spiritual) feelings and ideas."[12] No one can truly explain where this universal force originates or how to control it; however, research is beginning to show that its presence has a positive effect on recovery from illness, organizational performance, and the relationship between healthcare practitioners and their patients. Yet, how do we define this nebulous force that we call *spirit* or *spirituality*?

McBride et al. define *spirituality* as an intrinsic experience that goes beyond a belief in God or a higher power; it is an internal perspective that inspires one to believe in a force greater than themselves, and it serves as a guide for providing meaning to one's life.[13] Ashmos and Duchon[14] describe the spiritual dimension as a universal state of human existence that involves a search for a desire to experience a sense of meaning and purpose. Neck and Milliman[15] define *spirituality* as an expression of one's desire to find meaning and purpose in life. It is a process of living out one's deeply held personal values. Handzo and Koenig state that it is a personal quest for understanding answers to ultimate questions about life, its meaning, and the one's relationship to the transcendent.[16] In summary, although spirituality can incorporate the practice of one's religious faith, it includes much more than religion. In fact, one can be religious and not spiritual, as well as be spiritual and not religious. Spirit or spirituality is the force or source that inspires an individual, community, or organization to seek its meaning, purpose, and a connection with all things. When an individual or an organization is open to spiritual potential, that individual or organization is multidimensional and capable of embracing a sense of duality. Conger defined *spirituality* as the source of one's values and meaning, a way of understanding the world, an awareness of one's inner self, and a means of integrating the various aspects of oneself into a whole.[17] If an individual or organization is estranged from the spirit, that organization or individual becomes estranged from values, meaning, and a sense of humanity. The person or entity begins to function in an unethical manner. The following case scenario depicts the spiritual transformation that often occurs as one is confronted with a medical crisis and connects with the concept of spirituality.

SHARON'S STORY: FINDING PEACE LIVING IN THE IN-BETWEEN

Sharon is a 53-year-old African American female who has relied on hard work and determination to combat fear, helplessness, skepticism, and social injustice. Despite the resounding complaints of those around her, she has never used her birth in poverty, the illiteracy of her parents, or existence of racial injustice as an excuse for not achieving her goals in life. In fact, Sharon frequently used these ostensible barriers as motivations to work harder. She was the first member of her family to receive a college education, a Masters degree, and now people call her "Dr. Sharon," because she now has her PhD. However, it was shortly after Sharon reached the ultimate goal in her life that her world came crashing down.

Sharon suffered with headaches, high blood pressure, and fluid retention in her legs while she was finishing her PhD. Visits to her doctor resulted in the use of medication to lower her blood pressure, and she was encouraged to modify her diet. Sharon attributed her symptoms to the stress of working a full-time job while trying to complete her dissertation; a feat that many of her family, friends, and so-called well-wishers said could not be done. She assumed that once she completed her studies, she would be back to normal again. This did not prove to be the case; within a couple of months after she received her doctoral degree, she was diagnosed with chronic kidney disease.

She now receives dialysis three days a week, is confined to a strict diet, is waiting for a suitable kidney donor, and is filled with countless questions, including: Why did this happen to me? How did this happen to me? How can I have a quality life when I am always hooked up to this machine? Will I ever be free from this pain? Each time Sharon goes into the dialysis center she confronts the harsh cold reality of her current condition. Her endless questions follow her everywhere she goes. However, no one in the bastion of compassion and hope, better known as the dialysis clinic, asks her about her day. No one questions her about her apprehensions or what she relies on to make it through the day. She even wonders if they would notice if she did not show up. As she observes the robotic manner in which many of the technicians, nurses, and social workers perform their duties, she wonders if these people even believe in what they are doing. One part of Sharon would like to believe the doctors and providers are working hard and really care about what is happening to her. Another part of her says that she is only a body count, an insurance claim, and a name waiting on a list. Yet, Sharon has always been the eternal optimist, and she hates to see things this way. She has never had much patience for whiners, and her greatest fear is to be viewed as a whiner herself.

Sharon has worked most of her life to be free to pursue the life the desires. In most cases, every goal that she sought she has accomplished; that is until now. The pain she feels is more than physical—it is the pain that comes from acknowledging the presence of two worlds; neither of which she can totally embrace. For years, she chose to believe in the value of hard work, commitment, and dedication. She felt that if a person is willing to dedicate him or herself to succeed, there is nothing that he or she cannot overcome. She refused to believe that oppressors and social injustice could hold her down. She refused to be part of a world of oppression and victimization that is filled with pain, hopelessness, and feelings of personal and social inadequacy.

However, Sharon now is feeling oppressed and victimized by this disease that she cannot conquer. She desperately needs the assistance of someone, or to go someplace where she can recapture her hope, joy, and passion for life again. She is living between hope and despair; fear and certainty; anger and faithfulness.

SPIRITUALITY AND LIVING IN THE IN-BETWEEN

Many people and organizations are like Sharon, in the process of transformation; however, most are not even aware of it. People, organizations, and societies invariably grapple with who they really are, what is most important, and what is the best way to satisfy the mutual needs of everyone involved. Does one rely on policies and programs that were devised according to empirical wisdom? Does one allow the conscious to be his or her guide? Is it best to do that which is most expedient? Does one do that which is the most cost-efficient? In the case of Sharon, does she continue to work hard and do what she has always done? Should a healthcare organization, physician, or administrator be concerned with helping Sharon answer her questions? Carol Pearson and Sharon Seivert[18] described the transition from one paradigm, or personal perspective, to another perspective as a time of living in the "in-between."

During times of living in-between, individuals, organizations, and communities begin to uncover their deepest truths. For individuals who have always been in control, their moment of living in-between occurs when they become aware of their helplessness. Other individuals may have lived their entire life nurturing and serving others; their time of living in-between occurs when they must seek the assistance of others and allow others to see their pain. Living in the in-between demands that individuals embrace the shadowy aspects of their souls. In the case of Sharon, she must learn to acknowledge her sense of helplessness as part of herself as much as she views her belief that she can control her fate through hard work. When she learns to acknowledge that she is weak as well as strong, initially she may feel more vulnerable. However, eventually she will develop a greater sense of completeness.

SPIRITUALITY: NURTURING THE WHOLE PERSON

William Miller and Carl Thoresen[19] discuss the perpetual pendulum that swings from scientific-based secularism to spiritually-based holistic treatment in health care. They described how, long before the proliferation of subspecialties and the emergence of the medical-technological model, healthcare delivery systems utilized culturally-defined healers who blended spiritualism to promote health. During this time in history, a lack of scientific knowledge about the disease process resulted in more reliance on spiritual and religious resources. It would not have been uncommon to rely on a shaman, *curandero*, priest, or pastor to assist or in some cases serve as the primary healthcare provider. However, as the healthcare system has become more specialized, knowledgeable, and focused on understanding the organic origins of diseases and illnesses, it has become more dichotomous. In an effort to become more scientifically grounded and medically proficient, many healthcare delivery systems have thrown out the spiritual baby with the bathwater. As a result, we have people who work, manage, and seek services in healthcare delivery systems who only recognize part of the person.

Whether one is addressing the needs of people with cancer, AIDS, chronic kidney disease, diabetes, the death of a loved one, or a multitude of medical problems, the literature consistently confirms that illness is fraught with spiritual concerns and issues.[20] In her book, *My Grandfather's Blessings*, Rachel Ramen makes the following remark:

> Through illness, people may come to know themselves for the first time and recognize not only who they genuinely are but also what really matters to them. As a physician, I have accompanied many people as they have discovered in themselves an unexpected strength, courage beyond what they would have thought possible, an unsuspected sense of compassion or a capacity for love deeper than they had ever dreamed. I have watched people abandon values that they have never questioned before and find the courage to live in new ways.[21]

The research, anecdotal accounts, and literature all agree that it is impossible to treat the whole person without acknowledging the spiritual aspects of the healthcare consumer. Larimore, Parker, and Crowther examined the literature pertinent to incorporating spirituality into medical practice, and they discovered the following: (1) a positive relationship frequently exists between spirituality and physical and mental well-being; (2) most patients desire to discuss and be offered basic spiritual care by their healthcare provider; (3) most healthcare providers believe that spiritual interventions would help healthcare consumers, but they feel inadequately trained to deliver such care; and (4) most healthcare consumers (patients) censure healthcare delivery systems for ignoring their spiritual needs.[22] Moreover, a plethora of data supports that individuals who are spiritually connected have fewer physical health problems, recover from illness quicker, and experience less stress during serious illness than those who are not.[23] Thus, it is clear that providing appropriate, competent, effective, and ethical care to consumers of healthcare delivery systems demands that the spiritual aspects of the healing process be incorporated. Moore and Casper conclude that caring for the whole person begins with the organization, or in this case the healthcare delivery system, recognizing that those who deliver care have an inner life that needs to be incorporated into the work they do.[24] The next section of this chapter will address the importance having a spiritually-oriented organization that enables consumers, workers, leaders, and communities to reach their ultimate goal in life. However, before discussing incorporating spirituality into the work environment, let's discuss the history of work in America.

A HISTORY OF ATTITUDES TOWARD WORK

Attitudes toward work in America can be traced to the Industrial Revolution and the development of Taylor's Scientific Management.[25] During the Industrial Revolution, the United States transitioned from a primarily agrarian and cottage-industry culture to an industrial model. In response to this change, Frederick Taylor sought to make the workplace more efficient and profitable. In his view of efficiency, people worked the same way machines did, producing the same quality work through standardization of the work process.

Harmony in the work setting was achieved by adhering to the rules and being organized. If workers thought about the task and deviated from the prescribed best way to approach it, then efficiency and productivity were decreased. In short, workers were paid to work, not think. Thinking was the role of the manager.

Taylor believed that the ideal employee was one who did as he was told (gender selection deliberate) and submitted to regulations. He was an employee who could control himself and his emotions. This self-control was acquired by maintaining diligence when completing tedious work. In addition, Taylor expressed paternalistic attitudes toward the worker. He believed that the poor must be managed by those who had knowledge (management) for their own good. Individuals should be willing to sacrifice for the corporation and accept a day's pay for a day's work, as determined by managerial formulas.

The legacy of Taylor's work is alive and well in today's workplaces. Management often speaks of reengineering to increase the clockwork order of the work process and to remove human interference. There is an increasing need to standardize and to pay for performance, even in healthcare delivery systems. Management laments that it cannot get employees to "think right" or that employees are "not paid to think, just to get the work done."

The idea of employees as machines also is alive and well. Employees still work to the limits of their resiliency, through 12- to 15-hour daily work schedules. Although the workplace has become increasingly stressful by its requirements for high-level performance, increased pace, and intensity of work, management often discourages time off and time outs. Taylor's idea of a day's pay for a day's work has evolved into the idea that bonuses and higher pay will keep employees' efficiency high for tedious or even dangerous jobs. The human element is ignored in order to get the work accomplished, and money is used to "rent souls."[26] Employees are finding that their jobs are increasingly regimented, less in tune with who they are as human beings, and requires that they sacrifice who they are or what they believe to become proficient at delivering the product that management has deemed to be most important.

Taylor is not the only influence on the American attitude toward work. As early as 1933, Eton Mayo[27] offered a different idea of how work should be viewed. Based on his work at Harvard and the now famous Hawthorne Studies, he postulated that work and productivity were influenced by humane variables such as job satisfaction and teamwork. The nature of work came to include psychological factors, and the field of industrial psychology took on new meaning. Attempts were made to better understand the balance between these humane factors and the work itself.

The legacy of Mayo's work also is seen in the twenty-first-century work-place. Influential writers such as Peter Drucker and Peters and Waterman explored the humane side of work, including how feelings affect morale. Humane areas became linked with productivity and the need to find meaning in life. The tension between working for money and finding the passion in work was explored, as well as strategies for blending the soft, or humane, side of management with the hard side of productivity and efficiency.

Organizational research conducted over the past two decades shows that blending of the two paradigms is not only good idea, but it also has a positive impact on organizational performance. Jurkiewicz and Giancalone[28] found that organizations that embrace spirituality grow faster, have larger increases in efficiency, and have higher rates of return than those that do not embrace spirituality. Rick Chamiec-Case and Michael Sherr[29] identified that, even though there remains a strong bias against organizational leaders incorporating their spiritual beliefs and values into the workplace, the literature has clearly identified benefits in three areas of organizational growth when spirituality is incorporated. These benefits include: (1) increased productivity, worker motivation, and creativity; (2) increased overall performance of the organization and the likelihood of developing a more ethical organization; and (3) increased the job satisfaction and level of worker commitment. These findings and other factors have increased the receptivity toward incorporating spirituality into the workplace.

WHY A CHANGE IN ATTITUDE?

Over the past 10 to 12 years, awareness of the need for attending to the spirit in the work setting has increased. At one time, effective organizational leadership was based on how efficient a manager was at accomplishing a particular task. Now, effective leadership entails responding to an individual's four basic needs: (1) the need to be unique, (2) the need to be in union with something greater than oneself, (3) the need to be viewed as useful, and (4) the need to be understood by others, as well as to understand how one fits into a greater context.[30]

Another reason for the heightened interest in recognizing the humane needs of workers is related to the needs of employees now entering the workforce. Research on attitudes of those from the Millennium Generation (those born between 1979 and 2001) discovered that most of them believe that the quality of their job, not their salary, is most important.[31] This idealistic generation questions authority and seeks to make a difference with their lives. Given their attitudes, many from this generation choose to work in various healthcare delivery systems. They are not going to be motivated by adhering to the status quo. They are looking for more than a job that pays; they are seeking a vocation or a calling.

Employers also are beginning to be interested in the spiritual nature of work, but not just for altruistic motives. Spirituality in the workplace is believed to benefit the organization at a societal, organizational, and individual or employee level.[32] Organizations that incorporate spirituality into their values and practices often are perceived as operating according to deontological principles—that is, emphasizing the "power of goodness"—and the teleological principles that help workers and consumers understand the purpose and meaning related to their current plight. When a healthcare organization appears to be working toward meeting a universal need, society believes that the organization is more competent.[33] From an individual perspective, employees who work in spiritually-focused organizations have better physical and mental health, a greater sense of self-worth,[34] are more tolerant of their personal failures at work,[35] and are better able to realize their full potential.[36]

In summary, a number of factors have influenced the change in attitude toward embracing spirituality in the workplace. Both individuals and employers have discovered that spirituality in the workplace can boost employee loyalty and increase worker morale. This is a significant influence given the needs of the employment force that comes out of the Millennium Generation. The next section will further examine how spirituality in the workplace is defined.

SPIRITUALITY AT WORK DEFINED

The extent that spirituality exists in the workplace is contingent on the degree to which one immerses the whole self in one's work. It also is contingent on the degree of interconnectedness that a worker experiences in the work setting. *Interconnectedness* is the extent to which people view themselves as being part of something that is larger than they are. In addition, *spirituality at work* is the extent to which work relates to accomplishing one's full potential.[37] Marques, Dhiman, and King[38] suggested, based on their extensive analysis of the literature, that a comprehensive definition of *spirituality in the work setting* is possible. They conceptualize it as an experience that includes being connected to others through common factors. These factors include beneficence, fidelity, compassion, leadership, integrity, and creativeness. Spirituality in the workplace begins by understanding that all employees have a spirit as well as a body. It is fostered by leadership that can sustain the connectedness between people through effective communication, role-modeling, the creation of teams that actually work, and a willingness to honor employees as more than just full-time equivalents (FTEs).

Groen found that common factors for the expression of spirituality in organizations included a sense of calling, creativity, balance between home and work, an investment in employee welfare through appropriate benefits, a sense of community, and evidence that articulated values were practiced on a daily basis.[39] Justice, stewardship, altruism, and tolerance also seem to be factors that define spirituality at work. Some authors go as far as providing a prescription for managers who want to define their leadership as fostering such practices. These concepts include defining their personal model of spirituality and work, acting true to themselves, respecting others beliefs, fostering trust, and maintaining their own spiritual practices.[40] The next section will further examine the essence of creating a spiritual environment at work and spiritual leadership.

Spirituality and Leadership

Considering the work environment and the services provided in health care, the concept of spirituality in the work setting should be a significant area of concern and study. When the nature of the work involves caring for patients/clients and their needs and working with families in distress, it is difficult to "check one's spirit at the door." In fact, most people who are served by healthcare organizations do not want their care to be provided in a robotic, spirit-bereft manner. They seek providers who are compassionate, understanding, and empathically centered on their needs. In addition, employees want to contribute to patients' healing and seek an environment that recognizes their value.

In *The Thief of the Spirit*, Carl Hammerschlag tells of his encounter with a famous 93-year-old Mayan healer in Belize by the name of Don Eligio Panti. The Belizean government regards this man as a national treasure, and he was the only healer in this Mayan community that still used traditional methods of healing. As Hammerschlag sat on a bench waiting to see Don Eligio, he reflected on the austere environment in which this elder statesman was treating others, in comparison to the sterile environment that most Western medicine is delivered. When Hammerschlag finally was able to see Don Eligio, he noticed his simple physical appearance. After exchanging pleasantries, he asked Eligio what was the most important thing he had learned about being able to heal. Eligio responded, "You can't heal if you have Bad Belly."[41]

"Bad belly" occurs when an administrator, leader, doctor, or any healthcare provider loses contact with the spirit that has compelled him or her to serve and that enables him or her to join the patient or consumer in the healing journey. In order for a healthcare leader (this also includes the other categories of providers previously mentioned) to create an environment that invites the spirit, he or she must do as Don Eligio. In order for one to be an effective spiritual leader, one must be visionary and willing to challenge the status quo, which in some cases may be devoid of spirit and lacking in authenticity. In addition, an effective spiritual leader must also inspire others and share their vision, enable and encourage others to follow their passion, enable others to live in the moment, and model the principles and values in a congruent manner.[42]

In an attempt to be more efficient, to see more clients, to make more money, to protect itself from future litigation, and to be more scientific, a number of healthcare delivery systems have developed "bad bellies." Administrators develop and enforce policies that inhibit the consumer from experiencing the healing they desire as they live in-between fear and faith, life and death, and trust and distrust. No one in this system with "bad belly" has time to ask or allow the client to explore what his or her illness means, what he or she relies upon to make sense of the illness or provide support during moments of uncertainty, or how the current situation has strengthened or challenged his or her faith. As a result of not giving patients the opportunity to explore these issues, an individual's physical symptoms might be resolved, but he or she may never experience healing or wholeness.

Dan Wilford, the one-time CEO of Memorial Hermann Healthcare Systems said, "Organizations with spiritual leadership behave different from leaders in other organizations. They employ leadership strategies and practices that create cultures based on moral and ethical values."[43] However, this is not to imply that spiritually-oriented healthcare organizations are perfect and do not confront ethical dilemmas and issues. The final section of this chapter will discuss some of the potential ethical issues that might occur in spiritually-oriented healthcare delivery systems.

ETHICAL ISSUES AND SPIRITUALITY

Ethical Theories and Spirituality

What is the relationship between respecting, and even encouraging, spirituality in the healthcare workplace and theories of ethics? Certainly, elements of each support this practice. For example, if you are a proponent of natural law, you could argue that ignoring spirituality could limit a person's ability to achieve his or her highest potential. This is especially true when you consider that part of your potential is to seek wisdom and to know God. Therefore, to diminish the spiritual component of a person or an organization could be an unethical practice.

Sheep[44] proposes two spiritually-laden questions that every healthcare administrator should consider when attempting to create a work environment that is conducive to nurturing the whole worker: (1) Would this organization be more productive, innovative, and the people feel more satisfied if the workers felt a greater sense of connection to their work?; (2) Does this organization have an ethical responsibility to seek to improve the quality of life of its workers as members of society? If you are a fan of Kantian deontology, you could use the categorical imperative to state that respecting and allowing one to pursue spiritual growth is a moral and ethical duty. Or, one might consider that allowing people to find meaning in their work and life is a universal law. As such, healthcare leaders and administrators have an ethical duty to provide environments where both patients and workers can examine their spiritual needs and desires.

The practical utilitarian view might also consider the ethics of incorporating spirituality into the healthcare workplace. Unlike the deontological approach, which determines the appropriateness of an action based on it being inherently right, morally justified, or a matter of principle, utilitarian theories of ethical decision making often are based on the ethical writings of people such as Jeremy Bentham and John Stuart Mills.[45] These writers suggest that an action or behavior might be justified if it yields the greatest good for the greatest number. Therefore, a utilitarian might support spirituality in the workplace if incorporating spirituality into the workplace resulted in increased worker productivity, decreased worker turnover, increased patient confidence in the provider, and a greater sense of connectedness between administrators and staff. Studies by Lloyd,[46] Jurkiewicz and Giacalone,[47] and Mitroff and Denton[48] have confirmed that it does more than meet the existential desires of workers and patients, it also positively impacts worker performance, organizational growth, and workers' creativity.

Spirituality in the workplace has been discovered to be in the best interests of organizations that promote *egoistic-individual* (the individual's desire to reach their highest potential) desires, as well as organizations that promote *egoistic-local* (organizational success is primary and profit is a primary motivation) desires.[49] Mitroff and Denton[50] conducted a study of spirituality in the workplace by interviewing managers and executives. They discovered that the more spiritual an organization was, the more profitable it was. In addition, the more a worker was able to include themselves in their work, the more creative, emotionally stable, and productive the worker was in the workplace.

Finally, recall the discussion of virtue ethics presented in Chapter 1. Aristotle believed that ethical people will work toward their highest level of excellence and attempt to live virtuous lives. Certainly, some level of spirituality is a part of finding the answers to Aristotle's questions about personal character and living together in community. Healthcare professionals are expected to have high moral character and practical wisdom and to use this philosophy in their daily practice. Including spirituality in the healthcare workplace can facilitate and even honor this practice. If professionals actually demonstrate Aristotle's practical wisdom and high moral character in their practice, they should be better able to assist patients when they are experiencing moments of in-between.

Ethical Principles and Spirituality

Health care calls for the application of ethical principles in day-to-day practice at the patient and organizational level. For example, first you must avoid nonmaleficence or doing harm to patients and/or employees. The story of Sharon comes to mind as an example. The lack of spiritual connection between her and the professionals who were supposed to be serving her needs causes her harm. Simple and cost-free acts, such as asking the appropriate questions and really listening to her responses, could have avoided this harm. In addition, small acts of kindness (beneficence) could have made her life-changing illness easier for her to bear.

Nonmaleficence and beneficence are not limited to patient spirituality. Think of how much more positive and less stressful a healthcare environment can be when professionals truly care about each other. Again, small actions and well-chosen words can provide a refurbishing of the spirit that can only lead to greater quality health care and an increase in organizational loyalty.

Respect for autonomy also relates to spirituality at work. Can you imagine engaging in respect for persons without acknowledging that the spirit is part of who they are? It would seem incredibility disrespectful to do so (Kant would not be happy at all). The same is true for the autonomy of an organization. If you do not feel that you are part of something larger or that work that you do is not valued, then it would be easy to be disloyal to the organization. Imagine the financial and quality implications from the potential lack of commitment, low morale, and high turnover rates.

You also cannot ignore the relationship between ethics and spirituality in the healthcare workplace. In order to assure just treatment, healthcare delivery systems must be willing nurture the whole person, whether the patient or the worker. This includes more than just responding the physical needs of the patient or the monetary needs of the worker; healthcare systems must acknowledge their spirit as well. Just treatment might require a few more minutes of listening, even when you are tired, or asking questions to determine hidden issues or concerns. It is helpful to think about the Kantian question, "How would I like to be treated if I were in this situation?"

Practicing justice that acknowledges an employee's spirituality can take many forms. Perhaps justice means making sure that breaks are a part of the workday or respecting time for renewal. It can also be honoring employees' quests for understanding their purpose and meaning in life by providing them a quiet place to think. Again, acting with justice does not have to add to the cost of health care, but it can positively affect the bottom line.

Embracing the spirit in the workplace begins with spiritual leadership that results in the transformation of the organization and community. Wolf[51] identified several principles that spirit-focused healthcare leaders should use to promote transformation in their organizations. First, the spirit-focused leader is primarily concerned with creating an environment that recognizes and respects the importance of strong moral and ethical values that are exemplified throughout the organization. Second, spirit-focused leaders recognize that healthcare providers enter the field in response to a calling; therefore, they give employees the opportunity to discover and examine their sense of purpose and meaning for the work they have chosen to pursue. Third, spirit-focused leaders recognize the importance of connectedness at both the vertical (with a divine being) and horizontal (between workers and those outside the organization) levels. As a result, spiritual leaders typically plan and encourage community involvement via joint programs and community-oriented activities.

SUMMARY

This chapter examines whether it is unethical to include or exclude spirituality from the delivery of health care. The literature suggests that not only is excluding spirituality unethical, impractical, and counterproductive, but also that it is impossible to exclude spirituality from work that is inherently spiritual. Spirituality will always be paramount to the services that are provided via healthcare delivery systems, as long as the people who pursue careers in the healthcare arena due so in response to a spiritual calling. It will also be significant as long as people seek care because they desire healing (wholeness or a sense of completeness), and not just relief from physical symptoms.

The ultimate role of the worker in the healthcare delivery system is to help communities reconcile the dichotomous thoughts, feelings, emotions, and experiences they encounter during the time of in-between. These times of in-between often occur during physical crises; however, in order to help communities experience healing, the organization must have a "good belly." As described earlier, an organization with a "good belly" is one that recognizes its spiritual calling, employs spirit-focused leadership, and values spirituality at every level of operation.

Although spirituality is multifaceted, and some say nebulous and impossible to define, this chapter provides a brief overview of just how important and relevant it is to the delivery of health care. The chapter presents a number of definitions of spirituality and offers information on how to recognize its influence in the workplace. Even though some might insist that spirituality is antithetical to professional medical care or the healthcare delivery system, this position is contrary to the expressed needs of those who work in health care and those who seek care in healthcare systems. It is clear that healthcare organizations that embrace spirituality tend to be ethically sound and maintain a healthy balance between the needs of the individual and the organization. They also are efficient, productive, and create an environment that connects with patients.

QUESTIONS FOR DISCUSSION

1. How does Conger define *spirituality*?
2. How do Pearson and Sievert define "living in the in-between," and how does this concept relate to spirituality in healthcare organizations?
3. What are some common factors in the ability to express spirituality in the workplace?
4. What factors influence the extent that spirituality can be expressed in the workplace?
5. How might the deontological perspective support spirituality in healthcare organizations? How might the utilitarian perspective support spirituality in healthcare organizations?

NOTES

1. L. Berger, "'Millenials' are Eager but Anxious," *Young Money* (2005). Available at www.young-money.com/careers/career_trends/050315. Accessed December 27, 2006.

2. C. Pearson and S. Sievert, *Magic at Work: A Guide to Releasing Your Highest Creative Powers* (New York: Doubleday, 1995).

3. C. Hammerschlag, *The Theft of the Spirit: A Journey to Spiritual Healing with Native Americans* (New York: Simon & Schuster, 1993).

4. D. Ashmos and D. Duchon, "Spirituality at Work: A Conceptualization and Measure," *Journal of Management Inquiry* 9 (June 2000): 134–145.

5. M. Benefiel, *Soul at Work: Spiritual Leadership in Organizations* (New York: Seabury, 1993).

6. Joint Commission on the Accreditation of Healthcare Organizations, *Comprehensive Accreditation Manual for Healthcare Organizations: The Official Handbook* (Chicago: Joint Commission on the Accreditation of Healthcare Organizations, 2003).

7. D. Garber, "Spirituality and Healthcare Organizations," *Journal of Healthcare Management* 46 (January–February 2001): 39–52.

8. R. Remen, "Clueing Doctors in on the Art of Healing," *Science and Theology News* (July–August 2004): 32.

9. M. Burkhardt, "After All: Reintegrating Spirituality into Healthcare," *Alternative Therapies in Health and Medicines* 4 (March 1998): 2.

10. M. Donnelly, "Faith Boosts Cognitive Management of Cancer and HIV," *Science & Theology News* (June 15, 2006).

11. D. Ashmos and D. Duchon, op. cit.

12. C. G. Jung, *Modern Man in Search of a Soul* (Orlando, FL: Harcourt Brace Jovanovich, 1933), 122.

13. J. L. McBride, G. Arthur, R. Brooks, and L. Pilkington, "The Relationship Between a Patient's Spirituality and Health Experience," *Family Medicine* 30 (February 1998): 122.

14. D. Ashmos and D. Duchon, op. cit.

15. C. Neck and J. Milliman, "Thought Self-leadership: Finding Spiritual Fulfillment in Organizational Life," *Journal of Managerial Psychology* 9 (November 1994): 9.

16. G. Handzo and H. Koenig, "Spiritual Care: Whose Job Is It Anyway?" *Southern Medical Journal* 97 (December 2004): 1242.

17. J. A. Conger, *Spirit at Work: Discovering the Spirituality of Leadership* (San Francisco: Jossey-Bass, 1994).

18. C. Pearson and S. Sievert, op. cit.

19. W. Miller and C. Thoresen, "Spirituality and Health," in *Integrating Spirituality into Treatment*, William Miller, ed. (Washington, D.C.: American Psychological Association, 1999), 3–18.

20. R. Dunphy, "Helping Persons with AIDS find Meaning and Hope," *Health Progress* 68 (1987): 58–63; E. J. Taylor, "Why and Wherefores: Adult Patient Perspectives of the Meaning of Cancer," *Seminars in Oncology Nursing* 11(1995): 32–40; Garber, op. cit., 42.

21. R. Remen, *My Grandfather's Blessings* (New York: Riverhead Books, 2000), 29.

22. W. Larimore, M. Parker, and M. Crowther, "Should Clinicians Incorporate Positive Spirituality into Their Practice? What Does the Evidence Say?" *Southern Medical Journal* 97 (December 2004): 1242.

23. H. Koenig and H. Cohen (eds.), *The Link Between Religion and Health: Psychoneuroimmunology and the Faith Factor* (London: Oxford University Press, 2002).

24. T. Moore and W. Casper, "An Examination of Proxy Measures of Workplace Spirituality: A Profile Model of Multidimensional Constructs," *Journal of Leadership and Organizational Studies* 12 (2006): 111.

25. A. Briskin, *The Stirring of the Soul in the Workplace* (San Francisco: Berrett-Koehler. 1998).

26. Ibid., 155.

27. Ibid.

28. C. L. Jurkiewicz and R. A. Giancalone, "A Values Framework for Measuring the Impact of Workplace Spirituality on Organizational Performance," *Journal of Business Ethics* 49 (2004): 129–142.

29. R. Chamiec-Case and M. Sherr, "Exploring How Social Work Administrators Integrate Spirituality in the Workplace," *Social Work & Christianity* 33 (2006): 270.

30. G. Strack and M. Fottler, "Spirituality and Effective Leadership in Healthcare: Is There a Connection?" *Frontiers of Health Services Management* 18 (2003): 3–18.

31. L. Berger, op. cit.

32. T. Moore and W. Casper, op. cit., 109.

33. Ibid.

34. K. Krahnke, R. Giacalone, and C. Jurkiewicz, "Point-Counterpoint: Measuring Workplace Spirituality," *Journal of Change Management* 16 (2003): 397.

35. A. Mohamed, J. Wisnieski, M. Askar, and I. Syed, "Towards a Theory of Spirituality in the Workplace," *Competitiveness Review* 14 (2004): 102–107.

36. I. Mitroff and E. Denton, "A Study of Spirituality in the Workplace," *Sloan Management Review* 40 (1999): 86.

37. T. Moore and W. Casper, op. cit., 109–118.

38. J. Marques, S. Dhiman, and R. King, "Spirituality in the Workplace: Developing an Integrated Model and Comprehensive Definition," *Journal of the American Academy of Business* 7 (2005): 81–91.

39. J. Groen, "How Leaders Cultivate Spirituality in the Workplace: What the Research Shows," *Adult Learning* (2003): 20–21.

40. J. S. Lewis and G. D. Geroy, "Employee Spirituality in the Workplace: A Cross-cultural View for the Management of Spiritual Employees," *Journal of Management Education* 24 (2000): 682–694.

41. C. Hammerschlag, op. cit., 142.

42. G. Strack and M. Fottler, op. cit., 9.

43. E. Wolf, "Spiritual Leadership: A New Model," *Healthcare Executive* (March–April 2004): 23.

44. M. Sheep, "Nurturing the Whole Person: The Ethics of Workplace Spirituality in Society of Organizations," *Journal of Business Ethics* 66 (2006): 357.

45. F. Reamer (ed.), *Ethical Dilemmas in Social Service* (New York: Columbia University Press, 1990), 15.

46. T. Lloyd, *The Nice Company* (London: Bloomsbury, 1990).

47. C. Jurkiewicz and R. Giacalone, "A Values Framework for Measuring the Impact of Workplace Spirituality on Organizational Performance."

48. I. Mitroff and E. Denton, op. cit., 86.

49. M. Sheep, op. cit., 355.

50. I. Mitroff and E. Denton, op. cit., 83.

51. E. Wolf, op. cit.

PART IV

Critical Issues for Society's Health

Although it is not possible to address all of the ethical and healthcare issues that might affect American society in the twenty-first century, this last section of the text presents a sampling of those issues. Chapter 20 presents a discussion of the equality and inequality of the healthcare system. It explains how these concepts are defined and measured. It also establishes the ethical positions on which Americans base their assessment of health inequalities and inequities. Finally, the author poses some ideas about dealing with inequalities and inequities when they occur.

In Chapter 21, Hackler presents information about rationing health care and discusses its ethical ramifications. After defining *healthcare rationing*, he gives arguments for situations where this action is ethically defensible. He also presents a mechanism for making morally sound healthcare rationing decisions. This chapter certainly has ramifications for health care for the rest of the twenty-first century.

The remaining chapters present issues that affect individuals and the society in general. In Chapter 22, Warshaw writes about the how clinical practitioners address the issue of domestic violence and the limitations in their ability to do so effectively. She also presents some of the ethical dilemmas faced by these clinicians and the need for society to make greater efforts to address this social problem. Chapter 23 is especially germane in light of recent events. It provides an overview of the government, healthcare system, and individual's response to both human-caused and natural disasters. Problems that arise in the planning and response for these efforts are discussed in relationship to ethics theory and principles.

The final chapter (Chapter 24) provides a summary of all four sections. It also presents what the author refers to as "emergent ethical issues." These issues include the continuing effects of technology on society and individuals and the the myriad of potential ethical issues posed by technology diffusion. Another second issue presented in this chapter is that of disease experience, specifically childhood obesity. This condition presents major concerns for the future of both health care and the ethics of treatment for society.

Chapter 24 also discusses patient-focused care with emphasis on the influx of baby boomers and their desires for quality health care. It includes information about the ethics of providing care that emphasizes the patients, their needs, and the maintenance of fiscal responsibility. Finally, the author presents a brief discussion of the environment as an emerging issue for health care and relates this issue to ethical theories and principles.

CHAPTER 20

Health Inequalities and Health Inequities

Nicholas King

OVERVIEW

In this important chapter, King addresses one of the most difficult ethical issues for U.S. society—the nature and extent of health of inequalities or disparities in America. He also discusses health inequities with respect to the population in general and specific groups. King then explains the ethical issues associated with health inequalities and inequities from a theoretical and practical view. Using tables as illustration, he presents some ideas about how to reduce healthcare inequities. This chapter increases understanding about this complex ethical and logistical issue.

INTRODUCTION

People have long recognized that some individuals are healthier than others and that some live longer than others do, and that often these differences are closely associated with social characteristics such as race, ethnicity, gender, location, and socioeconomic status. The introduction of the regular collection of vital statistics by European states in the nineteenth century enabled Edwin Chadwick and other social reformers to quantify and compare the health and living conditions of different social classes. More recently, epidemiologists, sociologists, geographers, and other researchers have used advanced qualitative and quantitative methods not only to identify and track a wide variety of health inequalities, but also to produce increasingly sophisticated models to explain their causes and consequences.

As knowledge and understanding of health inequalities has increased, so too, has the political will to reduce or eliminate them. One of the two goals of the United States' Healthy People 2010 initiative is "to eliminate health disparities among segments of the population, including differences that occur by gender, race or ethnicity, education or income, disability, geographic location, or sexual orientation."[1] In the United Kingdom, the release of successive government reports on socioeconomic inequalities in health in 1980 (the "Black Report") and 1987 (the "Health Divide" report) stimulated increased scrutiny of the National Health Service. Other countries and nongovernmental organizations have undertaken major initiatives to address health inequalities both within and between nations.

This chapter reviews the central ethical issues raised by the existence of health inequalities, their study, and attempts to reduce or eliminate them. These issues can be summarized in a series of basic questions: What are health inequalities? Why are some health inequalities also health inequities? How are they measured? What is the best way to reduce or eliminate health inequities?

WHAT ARE HEALTH INEQUALITIES?

To understand the issues associated with health inequities, it is important to first define how a society defines and assesses health. It is also important to have a concept of what constitutes an inequality as it applies to health care. Finally, since all inequalities are not inequities, one must also take the normative view of ethics to determine what are true health inequities for a society.

Health

In order to define the term *health inequalities*, one must first answer the question of what is *health*? The answers vary considerably, from narrow definitions focusing on the absence of disease to broader ones encompassing a wide range of measures of subjective and objective characteristics. At one end of the spectrum, Norman Daniels advocates the use of a relatively narrow definition of health as "normal functioning, that is, the absence of pathology, mental or physical."[2] By contrast, the World Health Organization Constitution defines it as "a state of complete physical, mental, and social well-being and not merely the absence of disease or infirmity."[3] More expansive definitions of health might include happiness, freedom from disability, quality of life, and the capacity to lead a socially meaningful and economically productive life. Narrow definitions have the benefit of being objectively measurable by biological and physiological characteristics, but fail to capture aspects of human experience that might be more relevant to assuring social justice, such as happiness and capabilities. Broader definitions rectify this limitation, but often involve highly subjective judgments by researchers or patients, and thus are more difficult to adequately measure and compare.

Researchers assess health status in many ways. Under a narrow definition of health, the most common health indicators are mortality, survival, life expectancy, disease incidence, and disease prevalence. Definitions that are more expansive might also include physiological indicators of overall health (e.g., height, weight, body mass index, and blood pressure), symptoms, self-rated health status, sense of well-being, social connectedness, and productivity. Different kinds of health problems have different classification schemes. The *International Classification of Diseases* (ICD) *Manual* provides standard definitions of physical illness based around etiopathies that alter organ function and produce symptoms. ICD classifications are widely accepted and are used in clinical diagnosis and health research. By contrast, the *Diagnostic and Statistical Manual of Mental Disorders* (DSM) defines mental health problems in terms of symptoms rather than etiology, which has been subject to considerable criticism.[4]

Because different populations can have radically different health belief systems, definitions of health, or subjective experience of symptoms, comparing populations to determine the levels of inequality between them can be difficult. This is particularly true when trying to compare rates of mental illness, symptoms, or self-reported health status between nations with widely disparate cultures. For this reason, international health inequalities often are expressed in terms of mortality or infant mortality rates, which—although collected haphazardly in some locations—are thought to be the most objective indicators of health status available.

Discussions of health inequalities might also utilize measures of health care, including rates of diagnosis, treatment, cost, insurance coverage, quality, survival, symptom reduction, or some other health outcome measure. Strictly speaking, *health inequalities* should be distinguished from *inequalities in health care*. Although the two are often linked, this is not always the case. Some inequalities in health care do not necessarily lead to health inequalities, whereas many health inequalities occur in the context of healthcare equality.

Inequality

A *health inequality* is a descriptive term that can refer either to the total variation in health status across individuals within a population or to a difference in average or total health between two or more populations. In Table 20–1, the average body mass index (BMI) of populations A and B are identical, but the variation within population A is clearly larger than that *within* population B. Thus, we may say that there is greater total inequality within population A than population B, but that there is relative equality *between* the two populations. Although there is some debate over which is a more scientifically rigorous measurement,[5] most scholarly work on the topic defines health inequalities as differences in health between populations.

Because health inequalities generally involve the comparison of *population averages* (although other measures can be used), great care must be taken in making inferences regarding individuals. In Table 20–2, the average BMI of population A is lower than that of population B. However, the two individuals with the highest BMI are in population A, and the individual with the lowest BMI is in population B. Thus, benefiting (or suffering) from an inequality is a property of the respective populations, A and B, but *not* a property of individuals selected from those populations.[6]

Why Are Some Health Inequalities also Health Inequities?

In contrast to the descriptive term *health inequality*, *health inequity* is a normative term that refers to a difference that is judged to be morally unacceptable.[7] Although all health inequities are, by definition, health inequalities, not all health inequalities are health inequities. For example, because

Table 20–1   Average BMI—Example 1

	Population A	Population B
	40	30
	38	29
	18	27
	16	26
Average	*28*	*28*

Table 20–2   Average BMI—Example 2

	Population A	Population B
	35	33
	34	32
	22	31
	21	20
Average	28	29

elective cosmetic surgery is generally not considered a necessity for good health and functioning, unequal access to it might not be considered an inequity. Similarly, because skydiving is generally considered to be a freely chosen behavior, the fact that the mortality rate for falls from great heights is much higher among skydivers is generally not considered a health inequity.

Determining whether a particular inequality (or class of inequalities) constitutes an inequity requires a moral judgment based on *a priori* beliefs about justice, fairness, and the distribution of social resources, and thus it is one of the primary areas in which ethical analysis plays a role. Commentators generally define *health inequities* by referring to either the populations affected by inequalities or the causes and consequences of inequalities.

One way of determining whether a health inequality qualifies as an inequity is through reference to the relative social position of different populations. If a health inequality benefits a population that is in some way already socially or economically advantaged, then we may deem that inequality unjust through its association with a prior distributive injustice. This "egalitarian liberal" perspective[8] judges health inequalities to be morally wrong primarily because they suggest that some individual's or groups' rights are being violated, thus negatively impacting their health. Paul Farmer argues that ill health, and health inequalities in particular, are evidence of injustice or structural inequity in the world "even though it may be manifest in the patient."[9] More specifically, Paula Braveman contends that

> [a] health disparity between more and less advantaged population groups constitutes an inequity *not* because we know the proximate causes of that disparity and judge them to be unjust, but rather because the disparity is strongly associated with unjust social structures; those structures systematically put disadvantaged groups at generally increased risk of ill health and also generally compound the social and economic consequences of ill health.[10]

The existence of health inequalities might indicate that a given population has disproportionately suffered international military and economic exploitation,[11] inequitable distribution of economic resources,[12] or historical patterns of race-based economic and social injustice.[13]

This definition of health inequity accords with John Rawls' "difference principle" of distributive justice: that social inequalities should be of benefit to the least-advantaged members of a society.[14] It also has the benefit of using *a pri-*

ori judgments about social or economic inequity as the foundation for adjudicating claims of health inequity. Thus, for example, an economically disadvantaged population does not need to repeatedly prove that every health inequality adversely affecting them constitutes an inequity.

However, this definition also suffers from significant drawbacks. First, the *a priori* identification of disadvantaged populations can be contentious or arbitrary in some situations. Would a health inequality favoring those with annual incomes of $5 million over those with annual incomes of $2 million constitute an inequity? In most countries, despite their lesser social status, women enjoy a longer lifespan than men do. This is possibly because of genetic factors, but also possibly because of lower rates of risk behaviors, such as smoking and alcohol use. Few observers identify this as a health inequity.

At the same time, many observers argue that the dramatically higher rates of morbidity and mortality from HIV/AIDS among women in a number of countries[15] are evidence of serious health and social inequities.[16] By contrast, higher rates of HIV/AIDS among men in richer nations, such as the United States, have seldom been identified as a gendered health inequity (though the delay in devoting health resources to the disease during the 1980s was frequently cited as evidence of a sexual-orientation health inequity). In addition, how might this definition account for novel forms of sociological categorization that may be accurate but do not lend themselves easily to judgments of relative disadvantage? For example, if one makes judgments about race-county combinations that indicate that low-income rural blacks who live in the South have a lower life expectancy than low-income whites in Appalachia and the Mississippi Valley.[17]

This definition also neglects situations in which a genuinely unjust distribution of health might happen to benefit those in socially superior positions—as, for example, when a major pollutant happens to affect disproportionately a nearby wealthy community. Finally, if other social inequities exist and have (rightly or wrongly) been deemed socially acceptable, does this mean that the resultant health inequalities cannot qualify as unjust? Many American cities tolerate a certain level of homelessness as socially acceptable. Are higher rates of tuberculosis and mental illness among the homeless therefore socially acceptable as well?

A more common definition of health inequity focuses on the *causes and consequences* of a given health inequality, rather than the specific populations that it affects.[18] Under this viewpoint, a health inequality qualifies as an inequity if it is *systematic*, *avoidable*, and *unjust*. The most widely-cited example of this point of view is Margaret Whitehead's definition of health inequities as "differences [in health] which are unnecessary and avoidable but, in addition, are considered unfair and unjust."[19]

A *systematic* health inequality is one that consistently affects two or more populations and is not the result of random variation. For example, some so-called "cancer clusters" (elevated incidence of cancer in a community) are in fact the transient result of random variation. This has led to conflicts between community members who feel victimized by an apparent health inequity and health officials who argue that no such inequity exists.[20]

The criterion of *avoidability* has several components.[21] Health inequities must be *technically avoidable*—that is, a successful means of reducing the inequality must exist. They must be *financially avoidable*—that is, sufficient resources exist to rectify the inequality. Finally, they must be *morally avoidable*—that is, rectifying the inequality must not violate some other social value, such as liberty or distributive justice.

The third criterion is an *unjust cause*. Whitehead[22] lists the following determinants of inequality:

1. Natural, biological variation

2. Freely chosen health-damaging behavior, such as participation in certain sports and pastimes

3. The transient health advantage of one group over another when that group is first to adopt a health-promoting behavior (as long as other groups have the means to catch up fairly soon)

4. Health-damaging behavior where the degree of choice of lifestyles is severely restricted

5. Exposure to unhealthy, stressful living and working conditions

6. Inadequate access to essential health and other public services

7. Natural selection or health-related social mobility involving the tendency for sick people to move down the social scale

Whitehead argues that health inequalities resulting from the first three determinants are neither unjust nor unfair, and thus should not be considered health inequities. By contrast, health inequalities arising from the latter four are unjust and unfair, and thus qualify as health inequities. Examples of inequalities that would not qualify as inequitable under this definition would include: Ashkenazi Jews' elevated risk of developing breast cancer, because of their slightly higher rates of carrying the BRCA1 and BRCA2 mutations;[23] the previously mentioned example of skydivers, whose freely chosen behavior elevates their risk of death; the higher rates of some communicable diseases among people living in temperate climates, because the insect vectors for those diseases are more prevalent than in colder climates; and early recipients of a vaccination campaign.

This definition of health inequity avoids the criticisms leveled at the first definition, and it accords with Iris Young's observation that, in general, it is not patterns of inequality *per se* that are morally wrong, but rather those whose causes and consequences we deem to be unjust.[24] However, like the previous definition, it suffers from some significant drawbacks. First, the degree to which many high-risk health behaviors are "freely chosen" is a topic of considerable debate. Three of the top nine "actual causes of death" in the United States—consumption of tobacco, alcohol, and illegal drugs—involve the use of substances that are highly addictive,[25] which might significantly diminish the element of free choice. Both lung cancer rates and cigarette consumption (a primary risk factor for lung cancer) increase as socioeconomic status diminishes.[26] Are the resultant socioeconomic inequalities also inequitable?

A second problem with this definition is that, by favoring cause over population as the deciding factor, health inequalities that benefit otherwise socially-advantaged populations would be deemed inequitable and thus ostensibly in need of social remedy. This result contradicts most peoples' intuition that social justice by definition involves redistributing social resources to the disadvantaged, rather than the other way around.

Perhaps the most significant problem with this definition is that many health problems have multicausal etiologies, and it is difficult or impossible to isolate a single, overriding causal factor. Diseases of the heart and cardiovascular system result from a complex combination of "just" causes, such as genetic predisposition and health behaviors (diet, exercise, smoking, etc.), as well as "unjust" causes, such as stressful living and working conditions and inadequate access to preventive health care. In some cases, it might be possible to quantify the relative contribution of each determinant to a population's health through sophisticated regression analyses. Yet this leaves open the question of whether moral judgments of inequity should be entirely dependent upon the outcome of statistical analyses.

Finally, a health inequality might be judged to be morally wrong not because there is something inherently bad about health inequality, but rather because it is evidence of, or a contributing factor to, some other morally unacceptable situation. A health inequality thus "acts as a signpost—indicating that something is wrong."[27] For example, from an "objective utilitarian" perspective,[28] a health inequality between two subpopulations might be judged bad because it indicates that the sum total of health in the entire population is not being maximized. In this case, inequality *per se* is not seen as morally wrong, and the rectification of the health inequality would simply be a means toward the end of maximizing overall population health.

Similarly, some researchers argue that pervasive health inequalities across the entire socioeconomic spectrum are indications not of injustices directed at particular subpopulations, but fundamental social problems that adversely affect the health of all but those at the absolute top of the social hierarchy. Michael Marmot argues that socioeconomic gradients in chronic disease and life expectancy result from comparatively low levels of autonomy, social engagement, and social gradient.[29] Similarly, Richard Wilkinson argues that low social cohesion and pervasive psychosocial stress in societies with greater income inequality leads to shorter life expectancy.[30] If these authors are correct that almost every member of a society is in some way subject to health inequality, then attempts to encourage health equity could appeal to self-interest rather than social injustice.

HOW ARE HEALTH INEQUALITIES MEASURED?

Regardless of which definition of health inequity one uses, determining whether a specific situation is inequitable requires that the health status of at least two populations be measured and compared. In order to do this, one must determine which *populations* it is most appropriate to compare and the most appropriate *measures* that should be used in comparing these populations. Although these determinations are based primarily on technical judgments to ensure the most statistically valid measurement and data analysis, they also require ethical judgment regarding the appropriate focus of description and intervention.[31]

Populations

By definition, inequalities are differences between groups of people. Specifying the composition of these groups is vital and involves important ethical decisions.

First, the populations chosen should differ from one another in some way that is socially or morally important. We would thus expect that health inequalities among socially important groups. Race/ethnicity, gender, education level, or socioeconomic status (SES) would deserve scrutiny, whereas health inequalities among groups with different hair or eye color—distinctions that carry little social or moral weight—would be of less interest. In general, there is significant overlap between commonly-accepted social and political distinctions and populations of interest to health inequalities researchers. However, the moral relevance of some distinctions—geographic differences between U.S. states, political differences between conservative or liberal governments—are more ambiguous.

Second, health inequalities generally involve establishing a *comparison group* that serves explicitly as a reference against which one or more populations are compared, and implicitly as an ideal target to be achieved by all groups. A number of choices of comparison groups exist, any one of which is technically sound, but each of which carries different ethical implications. Consider the hypothetical example shown in Table 20–3. Clearly, significant health inequalities exist among the different racial/ethnic groups. However, the *amount* of inequality depends on the choice of comparison group. Which is the most appropriate in this case? Several answers are possible:

- We might choose the *total population average* as the reference group. Intuitively, it seems most just to consider the average of the general population as the standard of fairness against which to judge any particular subpopulation, much as we might consider a fair distribution of income to be one in which everyone clustered closely around the average.[32] In this example, the relative risk of the worst-off group (Hispanics) when compared to the total average is 1.75.

- We might choose the *best-off population* as the reference group. Although it is unfeasible to expect that every group in a society might earn as much as the best-off group, often it is possible to expect all groups to enjoy the

Table 20–3   Disease Prevalence, per 100,000

Subgroup	Disease Prevalence
Non-Hispanic White	7.6
Black	12.4
Hispanic	16.8
American Indian/Alaskan Native	6.9
Asian/Pacific Islander	10.2
Total	*9.6*

best possible level of health. Indeed, in some cases—for example, life expectancy, immunization coverage, or access to life-saving HIV medications—it is difficult to justify expecting anything less than the best possible health status as a fair and just outcome. In this example, the relative risk of the worst-off group (Hispanics) when compared to the best-off group (American Indians/Alaskan Natives) is 2.44.

- We might choose the *most socially advantaged population* as the reference group. Under the first criterion, a health inequity is *by definition* a difference that favors a more (or most) socially advantaged population over a less socially disadvantaged one, and we would be less concerned with comparisons between relatively disadvantaged populations. In this example, the relative risk of the worst-off group (Hispanics) when compared to the most socially advantaged group (Non-Hispanic whites, the majority population) is 2.21.

- Finally, we might choose some *independently defined target rate* as a reference category. Many common health indicators, including blood pressure, body mass index, and total cholesterol level, have widely-accepted thresholds separating high and low risk. It might be most just to expect all groups to pass that threshold, regardless of the relative rates of other groups. (The above example is not pertinent to this choice.) Moreover, using this reference category would ensure that all groups use a medically justifiable amount of some healthcare resource, which is useful in cases where some subpopulations "overutilize" that resource.

Measurement

A wide variety of statistical measures of inequality are available, from simple averages to sophisticated measures of total inequality. A comprehensive review of these measures is beyond the scope of this chapter. Instead, it will use the example of absolute and relative measures to illustrate the ethical issues often involved in choosing between different measurement strategies.

Two of the simplest measures of health inequality are the absolute and relative difference between populations. The *absolute difference* (AD) is a *number* resulting from *subtraction* of the numerical measure of one group's health status from another. The *relative difference* (RD) is a *ratio* resulting from *division* of the numerical measure of one group's health status from another. Consider the example shown in Table 20–4.

Clearly, inequalities exist and favor population B for both conditions. Suppose one could fund efforts to reduce only one of these inequalities. Absent

Table 20–4 Mortality rate, per 100,000

	Population A	*Population B*	*AD*	*RD*
Heart disease	80	60	20	1.333333
Cancer	270	230	40	1.173913

Table 20–5   U.S. Infant Mortality Rate, per 100,000 live births

	Black	White	AD	RD
1950	43.9	26.8	17.1	1.6
1998	13.8	6	7.8	2.3
Change	30.1	20.8	−9.3	1.5

Source: Data from D. Mechanic, "Disadvantage, Inequality, and Social Policy," Health Affairs 21, no. 2 (2002): 48–59.

other considerations, one might reasonably decide to fund the larger inequality, but which one is larger? In absolute terms, the inequality in cancer rates is twice as large (40 vs. 20) as that in heart disease; but in relative terms, the inequality in heart disease rates is almost twice as large (33% vs. 17% higher for population A). There is no consistent standard for judging which measure is more appropriate in this case. A reasonable case could be made that the AD is more important, because eliminating it would save more lives in absolute terms, and thus cancer should receive funding. Conversely, one might reasonably argue that the RD better represents the "true" inequity, because it is not affected by the number of cases involved, and thus heart disease should be funded.

The choice of the appropriate measure is particularly important when assessing health inequalities over time, as well as the relationship between *distributive* considerations (in this case, health inequalities) and *aggregative* ones (in this case, overall health). In some cases, measures that improve aggregate health in an entire population and all of its subpopulations might simultaneously increase inequalities between the more and less advantaged members of the population. Consider Table 20–5.[33]

Between 1950 and 1998, overall infant mortality in the United States declined precipitously for all racial groups. The absolute reduction in infant deaths during this period was almost 50 percent higher among blacks than whites (30.1 vs. 20.8), and the absolute difference in rates decreased (from 17.1 to 7.8), which indicates that blacks benefited *more* than whites did from reductions in infant mortality during this time period. However, during the same period the relative difference between the two groups increased (from 1.6 to 2.3), indicating that blacks benefited *less*. So, were racial inequalities in infant mortality better or worse in 1998 than in 1950? Did improvements in infant mortality disproportionately benefit whites or not? Was there a trade-off between overall population health and health inequalities or not?

WHAT IS THE BEST WAY TO REDUCE OR ELIMINATE HEALTH INEQUALITIES?

Even if we can reach agreement that a measurable health inequality exists, that it constitutes an inequity, and that it deserves to be addressed, there is no single rationale for determining the most ethically-sound way to reduce or eliminate that inequity. Several ethical considerations play a role in deciding between possible interventions.

The first consideration concerns the relationship between equality of *treatment* and equality of *outcomes*, embodied in the principles of horizontal and vertical equity. *Horizontal equity* refers to the equal allocation of resources (in this case, health care) across a population. Universal healthcare accords with this principle on the grounds that everyone needs health care, and no individual or group should receive disproportionately better or worse care than another.

Vertical equity refers to the allocation of different resources for different levels of need. Health care or public health programs that target a disadvantaged social group accord with this principle, on the grounds that unequal allocation of resources might be necessary in order to achieve equal health outcomes. An extreme emphasis on vertical equity is liberation theology's injunction that the poorest members of a society should always be accorded preferential treatment, because they bear the greatest burden of social inequality.[34] In choosing between these two principles, it is worth asking: If everyone receives the same treatment, are unequal outcomes ethically problematic? If everyone has the same outcome, are unequal treatments ethically problematic?

A second issue is the aforementioned relationship between distributive and aggregative considerations, and the cases of "leveling up" or "leveling down" to achieve the goal of equity. Consider the following four situations shown in Figures 20–1 through 20–4.

Assume that the rate being measured in these charts is something beneficial, such as access to life-saving medications. Figure 20–1 represents the current situation, in which the total population rate is 27.5, and a simple index of total inequality[35] is 5. Suppose that we wish to *both* improve overall access to life-saving medication *and* reduce the total inequality of access in this population. In Figure 20–2, the total population rate is better (higher), and each subpopulation has benefited, but the total inequality is worse (also higher).

In Figure 20–3, the total inequality has been greatly reduced, but overall access has been slightly reduced; the access rate of the two best-off popula-

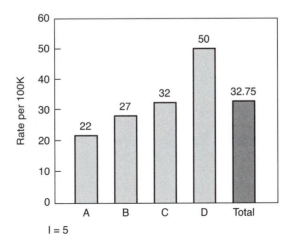

Figure 20–1

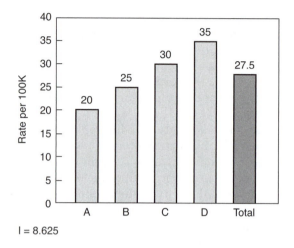

I = 8.625

Figure 20–2

tions has decreased, but that of the worst-off has increased. Finally, in Figure 20–4, total inequality has been reduced to zero, and overall access has dropped slightly, The access of the top two populations has decreased, while that of the bottom two has increased. Which of the other three situations represents the best trade-off between the reducing inequity and improving overall health?

Many other considerations regarding the appropriate distribution of social resources play a role in determining the best approach to reducing health inequities. Given a number of different subpopulations (e.g., multiple racial or ethnic groups or education levels), are some subpopulations more or less "deserving" of direct intervention to reduce health inequalities? Consider another example. Epidemiological evidence indicates that

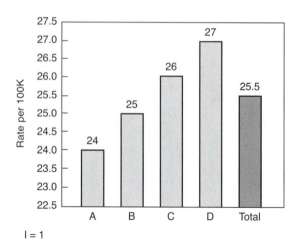

I = 1

Figure 20–3

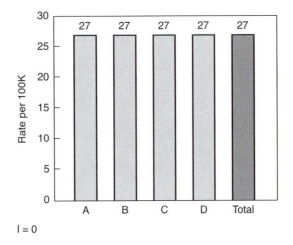

Figure 20–4

differences in socioeconomic status, nutrition, exposure to pathogens and toxic substances, and health care very early in life can have profound impact on health status and inequalities later in life.[36] This raises the possibility that the best way to reduce health inequalities in the long term might be to invest as heavily as possible in pre- and postnatal health care, perhaps at the expense of health care much later in life, when reducing inequalities might be prohibitively expensive. Is this an acceptable triaging of social resources?

CONCLUSION

Despite repeated calls for and considerable resources devoted to their elimination, dramatic health inequities persist and in some cases are increasing. This review might make the task of addressing health inequities seem unnecessarily daunting, or even insurmountable. In some cases, the task is indeed complex. However, the existence and persistence of significant gaps in the health and longevity between the most- and least-advantaged populations worldwide compels us to take action, no matter how challenging the task.

SUMMARY

The author begins by defining the essential concepts for understanding the ethical problem posed in the chapter. He then explores the ethical difference between an inequality and an inequity. King goes further and explains how inequalities are measured and the issues associated with defining populations and measurement standards. Finally, he presents areas to consider in reducing or eliminating health inequalities.

QUESTIONS FOR DISCUSSION

1. What is the difference between health inequalities and inequities in health care?

2. What ethical theories help to define if a health inequality is truly an inequity?

3. How can health inequalities be used as indicators of larger social problems for socioeconomic groups?

4. How do researchers use ethics to specify populations when studying health inequalities?

5. In the author's view, what is the best way to decrease health inequality?

NOTES

1. U.S. Department of Health and Human Services, *Healthy People 2010: Understanding and Improving Health*, 2nd ed. (Washington, D.C.: U.S. Government Printing Office, 2000).

2. N. Daniels, "Equity and Population Health: Toward a Broader Bioethics Agenda," *Hastings Center Report* 36, no. 4 (2006): 22–35.

3. World Health Organization, "Preamble to the Constitution of the World Health Organization," *Official Records of the World Health Organization* 2 (1946).

4. P. R. McHugh, "Striving for Coherence," *Journal of the American Medical Association* 293, no. 20 (2005): 2526–2528.

5. See C. J. L. Murray, E. E. Gakidou, and J. Frenk, "Health Inequalities and Social Group Differences: What Should We Measure?" *Bulletin of the World Health Organization* 77, no. 7 (1999): 537–543; and P. Braveman and S. Gruskin, "Defining Equity in Health," *Journal of Epidemiology and Community Health* 57 (2003): 254–258.

6. Making inferences about properties of individuals form aggregate group statistics is commonly referred to as the *ecological fallacy*.

7. The term *health disparity* often is used interchangeably with *health inequities*, particularly in the United States, but it also is used interchangeably with *health inequality* in other countries. For this reason, I will use the terms *health inequality* and *health inequity* throughout this chapter.

8. M. J. Roberts and M. R. Reich, "Ethical Analysis in Public Health," *Lancet* 359, no. 9311 (2002): 1055–1059.

9. P. Farmer, *Pathologies of Power: Health, Human Rights, and the New War on the Poor* (Berkeley: University of California Press, 2003), 153.

10. P. A. Braveman, "Measuring Health Inequalities: The Politics of the *World Health Report 2000*," in *Health and Social Justice: Politics, Ideology, and Inequity in the Distribution of Disease*, Richard Hofrichter, ed. (San Francisco: Jossey-Bass, 2003).

11. S. Benatar, "Global Disparities in Health and Human Rights: A Critical Commentary," *American Journal of Public Health* 88, no. 2 (1998): 295–300.

12. N. Daniels, B. Kennedy, and I. Kawachi, *Is Inequality Bad for Our Health?* (Boston: Beacon Press, 2000).

13. J. S. House and D. R. Williams, "Understanding and Reducing Socioeconomic and Racial/Ethnic Disparities in Health," in *Health and Social Justice: Politics, Ideology, and Inequity in the Distribution of Disease*, Richard Hofrichter, ed. (San Francisco: Jossey-Bass, 2003).

14. J. Rawls, *A Theory of Justice* (Cambridge: Harvard University Press, 1971).

15. T. C. Quinn and J. Overbaugh, "HIV/AIDS in Women—An Expanding Epidemic," *Science* 308 (2005): 1582–1583.

16. S. Zierler and N. Krieger, "Reframing Women's Risk: Social Inequalities and HIV Infection," *Annual Review Of Public Health* 18 (1997): 401–436.

17. C. J. L. Murray, S. C. Kulkarni, C. Michaud, N. Tomijima, M. T. Bulzacchelli, T. J. Iandiorido, and M. Ezzati, "Eight Americas: Investigating Mortality Disparities Across Races, Counties, and Race-Counties in the United States," *PLoS Medicine* 3, no. 9 (2006): 1513–1524.

18. M. Whitehead, "The Concepts and Principles of Equity and Health," *Health Promotion International* 6, no. 3 (1991): 217–228; O. Carter-Pokras and C. Baquet, "What Is a 'Health Disparity'?" *Public Health Reports* 117, no. 5 (2002): 426–434.

19. M. Whitehead, "The Concepts and Principles of Equity and Health," (Copenhagen: The World Health Organization, 2000), 5.

20. P. Brown, "Popular Epidemiology and Toxic Waste Contamination: Lay and Professional Ways of Knowing," *Journal of Health and Social Behavior* 33, no. 3 (1992): 267–281; A. Gawande, "The Cancer-Cluster Myth," *The New Yorker* (February 8, 1999), 34–37.

21. A. Bambas and J. A. Casas, "Assessing Equity in Health: Conceptual Criteria," in *Health and Social Justice: Politics, Ideology, and Inequity in the Distribution of Disease*, Richard Hofrichter, ed. (San Francisco: Jossey-Bass, 2003).

22. M. Whitehead, "The Concepts and Principles of Equity and Health," *Health Promotion International* 6, no. 3 (1991): 217–228.

23. J. P. Struewing, P. Hartge, S. Wacholder, S. M. Baker, M. Berlin, M. McAdams, M. M. Timmerman, L. C. Brody, and M. A. Tucker, "The Risk of Cancer Associated with Specific Mutations of BRCA1 and BRCA2 among Ashkenazi Jews," *New England Journal of Medicine* 336, no. 20 (1997): 1401–1408.

24. I. M. Young, "Equality of Whom? Social Groups and Judgments of Injustice," *The Journal of Political Philosophy* 9, no. 1 (2001): 1–18.

25. J. M. McGinnis and W. H. Foege, "Actual Causes of Death in the United States," *Journal of the American Medical Association* 270, no. 18 (1993): 2207–2212; A. H. Mokdad, J. S. Marks, D. F. Stroup, and J. L. Gerberding, "Actual Causes of Death in the United States, 2000," *Journal of the American Medical Association* 291, no. 10 (2004): 1238–1245.

26. C. R. Baquet, J. W. Horm, T. Gibbs, et al. "Socioeconomic Factors and Cancer Incidence Among Blacks and Whites," *Journal of the National Cancer Institute* 83 (1991): 551–557.

27. O. Carter-Pokras and C. Baquet, op. cit., 432.

28. M. J. Roberts and M. R. Reich, op. cit.

29. M. Marmot, "Health in an Unequal World," *Lancet* 368 (2006): 2081–2094.

30. R. Wilkinson, *Unhealthy Societies: The Afflictions of Inequality* (London: Routledge, 1996). Also note that the apparent connection between income inequality and life expectancy has been the subject of much debate; see J. P. Mackenbach, "Income Inequality and Population Health," *British Medical Journal* 324 (2002): 1–2; J. W. Lynch, G. D. Smith, G. A. Kaplan, and J. S. House, "Income Inequality and Mortality: Importance to Health of Individual Income, Psychosocial Environment, or Material Conditions," in *Health and Social Justice: Politics, Ideology, and Inequity in the Distribution of Disease*, Richard Hofrichter, ed. (San Francisco: Jossey-Bass, 2003); J. Lynch, G. D. Smith, S. Harper, M. Hillemeier, N, Ross, G. A. Kaplan, and M. Wolfson, "Is Income Inequality a Determinant of Population Health? Part 1: A Systematic Review," *Milbank Quarterly* 82, no. 1 (2004): 5–99.

31. Material in this section draws heavily on Harper and Lynch (2006). See S. Harper and J. Lynch, "Measuring Health Inequalities," in *Methods in Social Epidemiology*, J. M. Oakes and J. S. Kaufman, eds. (San Francisco: Jossey-Bass, 2006).

32. A related problem concerns whether to include the subpopulation of interest in the total population average.

33. The figure was adapted from D. Mechanic, "Disadvantage, Inequality, and Social Policy," *Health Affairs* 21, no. 2 (2002): 48–59.

34. ibid.

35. Average deviation from the total population rate, given by

$$I = [\,|(A - T)| + |(B - T)| + |(C - T)| + |(D - T)|\,] / 4$$

36. E. D. A. Hyppönen, L. M. G. Kenward, and H. Lithell, "Prenatal Growth and Risk of Oclusive and Haemorrhagic Stroke in Swedish Men and Women Born 1915–1929: Historical Cohort Study," *British Medical Journal* 323 (2001): 1033–1034; A. Case, A. Fertig, and C. Paxson, "The Lasting Impact of Childhood Health and Circumstance," *Journal of Health Economics* 24, no. 2 (2005): 365–389.

CHAPTER 21

Is Rationing of Health Care Ethically Defensible?

*Chris Hackler**

OVERVIEW

Hackler, in a logical and well-documented argument, discusses the need for and repercussions of rationing health care in America. Note his clarification of the term rationing and his arguments for a hybrid model of decision making on this issue. Kantian ethics are stressed along with Rousseau's view of democracy in this thought-provoking chapter.

INTRODUCTION

Expenditures for health care constitute a significant portion of the budgets of all industrialized nations. In the absence of cost-control measures, medical spending tends to grow more rapidly than the general rate of economic growth. Increasing demand and the high cost of new medical technologies are only two factors driving healthcare inflation. In several countries, including the United States, substantial portions of the population face difficulty in obtaining medical care. Correcting this situation will mean even greater demand for healthcare services. In these countries, it would seem that the only way to expand coverage while holding costs near current levels would be to reduce per-capita spending.

The problem in the United States becomes even more acute as we plan for the future. Beginning about 2010, the average age of the population will increase dramatically, placing formidable pressure on both healthcare and retirement programs. With continuing inflation and the demand for services increasing yearly, spending on health care will consume a larger and larger portion of the national budget. Unless we find some way to reduce the level of healthcare spending, or at least government healthcare spending through Medicare and Medicaid, little might be left to fund other essential social services. Thus, healthcare spending is a serious and growing problem for which we must find a solution that is both economically sound and ethically just.

The most difficult, painful, and divisive debates about this problem today, at least in the United States, revolve around the issue of rationing. Some say we must never ration health care and that physicians certainly must not do such a thing. Others maintain that soaring health expenditures require us to place significant limits on medical spending, denying some medical services that are

---

*Adapted with permission from C. Hackler, "Is Rationing of Health Care Ethically Defensible?" *Gesundsheitsoeconomica* 1995, Austrian Society for Health Economics.

both beneficial and desired. Still others claim that we are already rationing health care, either by market forces or by denying inclusion or coverage in public programs for the poor. This debate certainly involves serious substantive issues, but some of it also results from lack of clarity about the term *rationing*.

WHAT IS RATIONING?

In the strict sense of the term, we are not rationing health care, and we never have. To ration generally means to give equal portions of a scarce good to everybody. A clear example of rationing is the allotment of goods such as rubber, sugar, gasoline, or gunpowder needed in wartime. The amount needed by the military is set aside, and the remainder is allocated to citizens in equal shares. The term also is used for the fixed (and equal) amounts of food that soldiers are given in battle. Rationing in this sense, which is the common or dictionary definition, does not apply to health care. We have never considered giving our citizens fixed allotments of health care—so many days of hospitalization, so many visits to the doctor, a fixed amount of money to spend on health care, or any such thing. An essential point is that rationing in the ordinary sense is not practiced as a way to save money or decrease expenditures.

Rather, it is a response to a real physical scarcity of goods for consumption. The shortage might be the result of a diversion to war efforts or to export for foreign capital, or it may result from natural events such as crop failures or earthquakes. We have no comparable shortage of medical goods or services in the United States or Western Europe, so it is not obvious why *rationing* would be the term chosen to refer to some of our attempts to limit healthcare spending.

Rationing is essentially a method of distributing resources outside the market system. We in the United States are ambivalent about the status of health care. We think of it both as a commodity to be marketed and as a social good that we ought to supply to those unable to procure it. The result is a complex patchwork of a "system" that leaves many without adequate access to care. That millions of our citizens are not getting the health care they need because they cannot afford it is a deplorable fact and a serious ethical and political problem, but it might be confusing to describe the situation, as many do, as "rationing by price."[1]

One of the first uses of the term in the context of health care was by Aaron and Schwartz.[2] In their view, rationing occurs when "not all care expected to be beneficial is provided to all patients." This is surely too broad a definition of rationing. If this is the meaning of the term, then almost everything is rationed. Most of us would benefit from a new automobile, a new suit of clothes, and perhaps even from extensive cosmetic surgery! Treatment for infertility by in vitro fertilization is rarely provided to patients who cannot pay for it, but it seems odd to say it is being rationed. Aaron and Schwartz claim that denying any potentially beneficial care means, "the value of care is being weighed against its costs, explicitly or implicitly."[3] This seems to equate rationing with cost-benefit analysis, that is, basing the decision whether to provide a certain treatment not just on whether it would be of any benefit, but whether the benefits would be proportional to the cost of the treatment.[4] Cost-benefit analysis is certainly a potential strategy to reduce healthcare spending, but it is not rationing in the customary sense.

A number of practices resemble rationing and are frequently so labeled. Three of these are distribution of scarce goods, prioritization of services, and allocation of financial resources. Distribution of organs for transplantation is a clear example of the first. Transplantable organs are an absolutely scarce resource (i.e., there is no way to produce enough to satisfy all needs). Choices must be made concerning who will get a given organ and who will not.

We all agree that it is ethically acceptable that someone be denied the organ; only one can have it, and it is better that someone gets it than that no one gets it. However, it is not possible for all to share equally in the limited resources, which is the ordinary sense of rationing, but it is possible and ethically necessary to distribute organs fairly. Because someone is denied access to the organ, some will call it rationing, but the expression "just distribution of scarce goods" is quite adequate and less misleading.

The practice of triage in the emergency room is an example of prioritizing access to care. A scarce resource, in this case physician and staff time, is distributed according to urgency of need. This is sometimes referred to as rationing, though it bears almost no resemblance to ordinary rationing. Everybody is served; it is only the order that is at issue. *Prioritizing* is a perfectly serviceable term and more accurate in describing the practice than is rationing. Again, nobody questions the ethical propriety of this practice, because the alternative policy of "first come, first served" would lead to much poorer aggregate outcomes.

Allocation of scarce resources also is often referred to as rationing. Allocating resources means dividing or apportioning them among competing interests. When there is a scarcity of a given resource, then a scheme must be devised to allocate among potential recipients in a way that is efficient, fair, and socially desirable. Rationing in the usual sense, that is, handing out equal shares, is one possible scheme, but not necessarily the best, certainly not in health care.

Money is a scarce resource, though not in the same way as transplantable organs. As a society, we can always find more money to meet the needs of a given group, but we do so at the expense of competing interests. There is a growing consensus that we are spending too much on health care and neglecting other important social needs, and that we must find ethically acceptable ways to limit healthcare spending. We can try to reduce waste and inefficiency, reduce the level of compensation for services, and so on. However, the most direct way to limit spending is to limit consumption or utilization. There are roughly two strategies for limiting utilization: eliminating some of the kinds of services offered or limiting access to the services (or both).

If access is to be limited, the next step is to find an acceptable way to determine who will gain access to the available services. One way to do this is by chance, either first come, first served, or by some kind of lottery. Another way is to identify criteria that will be used to determine when access will be granted. It might be the urgency of the medical need, the potential for medical benefit, the potential for quantity or quality of life, or any combination of factors. It is here that we are most inclined to speak of rationing, but notice that the situation is quite similar to the distribution of transplantable organs; we have too little to go around and must distribute what we have on the basis of criteria that are fair to all. The big difference, and one that calls for ethical justification, is that the scarcity is a matter of policy, a deliberate choice we have made in the allocation of social resources. If the services that are no longer available are ineffective or are of little benefit, then the policy will be relatively easy to justify. If the services are of significant benefit, however, the task of justification will be more difficult.

Though it should be understood as a special use of the phrase, let us use *rationing of health care* for the present purpose to refer to policies and procedures that result in individuals being denied services that would be of significant medical benefit to them for reasons other than absolute scarcity or inability to pay. Again, lack of access because of inability to pay also is a serious ethical issue, but a different one both conceptually and ethically. There are two aspects to rationing so understood: (1) policies that restrict the availability of services and (2) the implementation of those policies by individual gatekeepers who deny patients access to particular services. We turn now to the ethical justification of rationing so understood.

IS RATIONING ETHICALLY JUSTIFIABLE?

The case for the general possibility of rationing health care is quite simple. Life and health are basic goods, and we have a very strong social claim on the means necessary to sustain them. However strong the claim, they must compete with other social goods that in the end might be more important to the flourishing of the community. Under certain circumstances, to be discussed below, we may limit the funds devoted to health care in order to invest in such things as education and cultural enrichment, without which life and health would be hollow possessions, as well as such things as prisons and police activities, which are necessary to the very preservation of the community. To deny that rationing could ever be justified, it would seem necessary to hold that health (or life) is an absolute good or that our moral claim on the means to health is always stronger that any competing claim or need. To compromise that claim for essentially economic reasons could be seen as putting a price on human life, thus contradicting the Kantian maxim. This posits that life has not a price but a dignity, that is, an inner value that takes it out of the realm of things to which we can assign a comparative value or price. We will return to this issue later.

The case for rationing of health care in principle is simple, but that does not mean it will be easy to justify particular rationing schemes. What would be the important considerations in deciding whether a given proposal to ration health care is justifiable? Let us attempt to answer that question by trying to construct an ideal set of conditions sufficient to justify rationing. After surveying the following list, we shall consider how these ideal conditions might be realized in the real world.

1. There are other equally important needs competing for scarce resources.
2. There are no alternative ways to produce equivalent savings.

3. Savings from denied services will benefit other patients or be invested in equally important social needs.

4. Policies and procedures for limiting access to treatment are applied equitably to all.

5. Limits are self-imposed through democratic processes.

If all these conditions were met, then rationing of health care would clearly be justifiable. The trouble is that they are only imperfectly met in the real world, and the degree of approximation varies from place to place. We will have to decide in each case how close to the ideal we must be before a given rationing scheme would be justifiable. There are real budget pressures and competing needs that we must somehow resolve. It is not helpful to insist on the perfect realization of ideal conditions before adopting a policy to deal with a pressing problem. With this in mind, let us examine the criteria in detail and discuss briefly the problems in satisfying them under various social arrangements.

JUSTIFYING RATIONING IN THE REAL WORLD

First, there must be equally important needs competing for scarce resources. The appropriate level of funding for such things as education, housing, and national defense will need to be addressed in concrete terms in a given social context. Is the military budget too big? Are we wasting money on inefficient administrative programs? These are important questions, but, in the end, I believe we will still find far more needs than we can fulfill at current budget levels. In addition, the constant development of new and expensive medical technologies and the aging of the population will continue to increase both the demand for health care and the cost of providing it.

Rationing of care is by no means the only way to control healthcare costs. Before rationing is implemented, every reasonable effort should be made to reduce waste and inefficiency within the system. Unnecessary services should be eliminated and duplication of resources minimized. This is surely easier in more centrally organized systems such as those of Great Britain and Canada than in the fragmented system of the United States. For example, in the United States, there is far more expensive equipment than necessary because of competition among hospitals. Each institution has its own magnetic resonance imaging machine, though it sits unused much of the time. Because the hospital must pay for the machine, the charge for the procedure is artificially high. A study published in 1990 indicated there were 10,000 mammogram machines in the United States, four times the number needed to satisfy current demand and double that needed to satisfy all potential demand if everyone for whom it is recommended had the procedure.[5] More current data is not available, but there is no reason to think that the proportions have changed. Inefficient deployment of resources is a serious structural problem that is difficult to attack in a decentralized and fragmented system.

Another structural problem for the justification of rationing within the United States system concerns the proper transfer of savings. The justice of the practice of distributing organs for transplantation is apparent because we can see that someone benefits from the organ that is denied to someone else. It is likewise important in the justification of healthcare rationing that savings stay within the system and benefit other patients, though the trade-offs might be less visible. The trade-offs are much easier to accomplish and to demonstrate in a unified system than in a fragmented one. It is quite possible for savings to be directed to the salaries of healthcare or insurance company executives or to corporate profits. As private hospitals and health maintenance organizations increase their share of the United States healthcare system, the potential for misdirection of savings grows. Where we have insufficient guarantees against such results, we have a strong argument against rationing measures.

The fourth item on the list of ideal conditions for rationing is the equitable application of rationing policies. If one person sacrifices a beneficial and desired treatment, then others in the same situation should make the same sacrifice. Once again, this criterion is much more easily satisfied within a unified system than a fragmented one. If the system is unified, then the same policies should apply to everyone. If there are many separate and independent units, there is no assurance that their policies will be similar. Similarity of policies, however, is not the only issue. Policies need to be applied similarly by individual physicians within the same system. Because the traditional role of the physician is patient advocate, an understandable temptation will be to "game the system" for one's own patients, that is, to bend, manipulate, or bypass rules that deny a needed resource. Because clinical judgment is necessary in any rationing scheme, we probably will have to live with this problem and just try to minimize it.

The fifth ideal condition for rationing is that limits to health care are freely adopted rather than imposed. Clearly, it is better to be denied a service because of a policy one has adopted rather than because of a policy that has been imposed by others. Limits can be self-imposed in two ways: by participating in the formation of policies and by accepting the results of the process. Direct citizen participation in policymaking can be cumbersome, but it was an important element in the development of Oregon's prioritized list of healthcare procedures.[6] Rationing policies developed openly by politically accountable representatives would also carry a presumptive legitimacy that secretly developed plans would lack.

In addition to the process of development, the fairness of the result is of great importance. If limits are to be freely adopted in the sense that they are accepted, those who are affected must perceive them as fair. It will be no small task to create policies that are universally perceived as just, especially in nations with diverse populations and historic inequities.

It would be difficult enough if there were general agreement on the criteria for making rationing decisions, but the American philosopher Norman Daniels has argued persuasively that there is no consensus on this matter and that none is likely. In distributing organs for transplantation, for example, should we favor those who will live longest and thus benefit most, or should we give each individual a fair chance by means of a lottery? We have neither consensus nor a demonstrable theory that would yield a convincing answer to the question. Nor is there consensus on the matter of aggregating benefits.

Prolonging a life for a year has a higher priority than providing routine dental care for one person, but if the funds saved by allowing the person to die can provide dental care for 600 people during that year, is that an appropriate trade-off? We do not now have answers to these questions, and there is no good reason to think a philosophical theory is about to be produced that will enable us to resolve such issues with confidence.[7]

It is unfortunate that such fundamental issues are unresolved, but it need not paralyze public policy. We do not have a theory that guides our trade-offs in other areas of social policy either, but we manage to make difficult decisions nonetheless. We should not expect a system that everyone agrees is perfectly just. What we should expect is a system that is created openly; that tries to be fair, and succeeds in large measure; and that is open to continual improvement. Designing a workable system that is "just enough"[8] is a matter not only of ethics, but also of economics, history, psychology, and politics.

WHO MAKES RATIONING DECISIONS?

The realization that we do not have an adequate and agreed-upon theoretical basis for rationing decisions makes more poignant the issue of who is making the decisions and how they make them. It was suggested in the previous section that open procedures that are broadly inclusive are best. However, an opposite view also deserves consideration. In their book *Tragic Choices*, Guido Calabresi and Philip Bobbit argue that public involvement in rationing decisions would be unwise.[9] Every open society adheres to a set of fundamental values that is not internally consistent; that is, the values may come into conflict with one another. Tragic choices are those that bare the inconsistencies and force us to choose between cherished values, thus eroding our commitment to the dishonored value.

Rationing decisions are among the most dangerous of tragic choices because they expose our willingness to make trade-offs with human life and in some sense to set a price on it. Thus, these decisions compromise our commitment to the Kantian principle that human life does not have a price, but rather a dignity that gives it inestimable value and incomparable worth.[10]

Of course, we regularly make public policy decisions that in effect price human life, but only if they are the lives of unknown future individuals. We may refuse to invest in mine safety, knowing that lives will be lost as a result, but we will pay whatever it takes to rescue a trapped miner. To do otherwise would be to acknowledge our willingness to price life. That is the essence of rationing decisions, so the argument goes. These decisions expose the conditional nature of our commitment to the sanctity and equality of human life.

In addition to being psychologically painful to individuals, there may be two truly serious consequences of rationing decisions. We may become too willing to price and trade in human life, and social cohesion might suffer. Our shared values provide the moral foundation of social collaboration. As tragic choices expose the contradictions among our values and erode our commitments to them, the foundation will begin to crumble. To preserve social cohesion, according to Calabresi and Bobbit, societies must mask their tragic choices. A policy-making elite should make rationing decisions. They will be sophisticated enough to realize that necessary compromises do not truly diminish the value of life, whereas the larger group "may not be able to make such nice distinctions."[11]

Although we should be sobered by the possibility that public participation in rationing decisions might produce moral and political decay, it is by no means clear that this would result. It is an empirical claim for which evidence is scant. In fact, we have no more evidence for this pessimistic and anti-utopian vision than we do for the idealistic strain in Rousseau's view of democracy (Rousseau was, characteristically, capable of deep pessimism at the same time).

The primary value of democracy for Rousseau was not what it does for us (by producing good laws), but what it does to us. By participating as a member of the Sovereign an individual's "faculties so unfold themselves by being exercised, his ideas are so extended, his sentiments so exalted, and his whole mind so enlarged and refined," that he is transformed "from a circumscribed and stupid animal into an intelligent being and a man."[12]

Surely the truth lies somewhere between the deep skepticism of Calabresi and Bobbit and the soaring faith of Rousseau in human reason. It would be wrong to rely solely on any one source for rationing policies. Open and democratic procedures should be employed, though their exact nature and role in the overall process is not clear. Citizen opinions and preferences should be taken into account, though policy experts (a point acknowledged by Rousseau as well, in the figure of the Legislator) must do the actual formulation of policies. The potential role of citizen groups is very much an open question that deserves further study.

An important lesson to learn from Calabresi and Bobbit, however, is that we should frame the debate in such a way that allegiance to the basic conflicting values is preserved as much as possible, consistent with effective and responsible decision making.[13] Although choices might need to be formulated in terms of monetary value, this does not mean that the ultimate trade is lives for money. Money is only the medium of exchange that allows us to purchase one good at the expense of another. The real trade is, for example, the last two remaining months of a person's life, which would cost $200,000 to prolong for the many infant lives to be saved by a citywide inoculation program that would cost $200,000. Thus understood, it is not life for money, but life for life, which is still in a sense a tragic choice, but one that is perhaps not so ethically suspect or socially corrosive.

CONCLUSION

Rapidly increasing spending on health care can threaten a society's economic and cultural vitality by decreasing savings and investment and draining funds from other social services. Governments are seeking to limit the growth of health spending by promoting greater efficiency and limiting reimbursement for physician and hospital services. A further step is to limit utilization of services, first by discouraging marginally beneficial treatments, and then, if necessary, by denying some costly treatments that would be of substantial benefit. Adopting policies that limit access to treatments of significant medical benefit is commonly called *rationing of health care*, although this use is somewhat at odds with the ordinary meaning of the term.

Rationing will be defensible to the extent that funding is truly needed for other essential social goods and services, that alternative ways of limiting medical spending have been attempted, that money saved will be directed to more compelling needs, and that limits are applied equitably to everyone. It is also important that limits be self-imposed in the sense that they are openly developed and generally accepted as fair. Accepting rationing will be painful because it calls into question our conviction that human life is priceless. We must guard against the potentially corrosive effects of overtly making comparative judgments about human lives.

SUMMARY

As the cost of healthcare delivery increases, the issue of rationing of will become more and more important and increasingly difficult. After defining the concept of rationing, Hackler argues that it may be ethically justified under certain conditions. He also discusses the ideal conditions for rationing in the real world and provides cautions about who should make decisions about this practice. Finally, he stresses that while rationing of healthcare spending may be necessary and could be defended, trading lives for money should be avoided.

QUESTIONS FOR DISCUSSION

1. How does Hackler define rationing when it concerns healthcare products and services?
2. What is the impact of a market-driven economy on the rationing arguments presented here?
3. How does a fragmented healthcare system negatively affect the ethical and procedural decisions to be made in a rationing plan?
4. How can having a foundation in Kantian ethics help to limit the potential for making tragic choices in rationing health care?
5. Given the changes that are projected in the twenty-first century for America (including increasing numbers of elderly, changing demographics, etc.), do you think rationing of health care will be inevitable?

NOTES

1. For example, L. Churchill uses this terminology in his excellent book *Rationing Health Care in America* (Notre Dame, IN: University of Notre Dame Press, 1987), 14.
2. H. J. Aaron and W. B. Schwartz, *The Painful Prescription: Rationing Hospital Care* (Washington, D.C.: The Brookings Institution, 1984).
3. Ibid.
4. M. D. Reagan, "Health Care Rationing: What Does It Mean?" *New England Journal of Medicine* 319, no. 17 (October 27, 1988): 1150.

5. M. L. Brown, et al., "Is the Supply of Mammography Machines Outstripping Need and Demand? An Economic Analysis," *Annals of Internal Medicine* 113 (1990): 547–552.

6. M. Brannigan, "Oregon's Experiment," *Health Care Analysis* 1, no. 1 (1993): 15–28.

7. N. Daniels, "Rationing Fairly: Programmatic Considerations," *Bioethics* 7, no. 2–3 (1993): 224–232.

8. I borrow this term from L. M. Fleck, who has used it in a number of works. See, e.g., "Just Caring: Lessons from Oregon and Canada" in *Health Care for an Aging Population*, C. Hackler, ed. (Albany: State University of New York Press, 1994), 193.

9. G. Calabresi and P. Bobbit, *Tragic Choices* (New York: W. W. Norton & Company, 1978).

10. J. J. Rousseau, *The Social Contract* (New York: E.P. Dutton, 1913).

11. G. Calabresi and P. Bobbit, op. cit., 69.

12. Rousseau, op. cit.

13. J. L. Nelson, "Publicity and Pricelessness," *The Journal of Medicine and Philosophy* 19, no. 4 (August 1994): 340.

CHAPTER 22

Domestic Violence: Changing Theory, Changing Practice

Carole Warshaw

OVERVIEW

This chapter deals with an issue that is often viewed as a social problem rather than a healthcare issue. However, as Warshaw points out, the medical community deals with the aftermath of this issue on a daily basis. She provides a thorough discussion of the personal, social, and systemic barriers that affect interactions between victims of domestic violence and the physicians who treat them. Warshaw also makes a cogent argument about the limitations of current clinical practices, including mental health models. She offers implications for training and practice to assist clinicians in their response to this serious problem for the twenty-first century.

INTRODUCTION

Despite widespread recognition of domestic violence as a public health problem, many clinicians still have difficulty integrating routine intervention into their day-to-day work with patients. This is in part because domestic violence raises a distinct set of challenges for both providers and the institutions that shape clinical practice. Domestic violence is a complex social problem rather than a biomedical one; addressing it means asking clinicians to step beyond a traditional medical paradigm to confront the personal feelings and social beliefs that shape their responses to patients and to work in partnership with community groups committed to ending domestic violence. In addition, addressing domestic violence raises important challenges to the healthcare system itself—to its theoretical models, to the nature of medical training, and to the structure of funding and service delivery. If, as physicians/healthcare providers, we truly want to play a role in preventing domestic violence rather than just treating its consequences, we also need to play a role in broader community efforts to transform the social conditions that create and support this kind of violence in the first place.

Over the past 20 years, it has become increasingly clear that domestic violence carries not only serious health consequences for women, but many hidden social costs as well. As clinicians, we see the profound effects of this violence on a daily basis.[1] We often are deeply affected when we allow ourselves to listen, understand, and grapple with issues that require far more than our medical expertise.

However, efforts are being made to address domestic violence. For example, through the combined efforts of the domestic violence advocacy community, individual practitioners, and numerous professional societies, standards of care have been developed. In addition, major initiatives have been launched to increase provider awareness, establish and distribute clinical guidelines, and offer strategies for improving institutional responses to domestic violence.[2] Innovative hospital-based advocacy programs have increased in number, and 60 percent of medical schools, 80 percent of family practice residencies, and approximately 70 percent of obstetrics/gynecology residencies have developed models for incorporating training on family violence into standard curricula.[3] Yet despite widespread recognition of domestic violence as a public health problem, many clinicians still have difficulty integrating routine inquiry about domestic violence into their day-to-day/ongoing clinical work.[4] Understanding the difficulties faced by healthcare providers as they attempt to address this issue can help not only to improve the practice of medicine, but also to develop more realistic strategies for prevention and social change.[5]

Domestic violence raises a distinct set of challenges for both providers and the institutions that shape medical practice. Because domestic violence is, in fact, a complex social problem rather than a biomedical one, addressing it requires more than simply adding new diagnostic categories to differential diagnoses or new technical skills to clinical repertoires. It means asking clinicians to step beyond a traditional medical paradigm to confront the personal feelings and social beliefs that shape their responses to patients and to work in partnership with community groups committed to ending domestic violence. In addition, the healthcare system itself, through its theoretical framework, the nature of its training process, and the changing structure of clinical practice, presents another set of barriers that profoundly affect the ability of individual providers to respond to women (or men) who have been abused.[6]

PERSONAL AND SOCIAL BARRIERS

As Holtz et al. have reported, the majority of healthcare providers have not learned about domestic violence during their training. Although more recent trainees have been exposed to the topic during their graduate and postgraduate years, the amount of time devoted to it is limited.[7] As a result, "clinical" responses often are shaped by an interplay of the physician's own personal experiences and social, cultural, and religious beliefs.[8] Many factors combine to shape the ways we interpret and respond to life events, including both our individual experiences and the social contexts in which they take place.

Koss et al.,[9] Johnson,[10] Brown,[11] Rieker and Carmen,[12] and Miller[13] have described the psychological impact of gender socialization, the traumatic effects of social disenfranchisement, and the ways in which the denial of intolerable feelings can shape our perceptions and lead to protectively rationalized ways of viewing ourselves, other people, and the world. For instance, the psychological need to protect ourselves from certain feelings in order to ensure psychic survival combined with social or cultural explanations of our experiences can solidify into beliefs and values that may then appear to us as "givens."[14] Clinicians absorb a range of societal views regarding gender and power, around which their own identities are constructed. Assumptions about gender, race, and class so permeate our culture that they often provide an unconscious backdrop through which we come to understand our own experiences and interpret those of others.

In addition, listening to women describe the violence in their lives can have a significant psychological impact on providers.[15] When physicians are not specifically trained to deal with psychological trauma, they are forced to rely on their own capacities to address painful and potentially overwhelming issues. In addition, given the prevalence of violence against women in this society, a significant number of physicians will have experienced or witnessed abuse in their own lives.[16] These issues touch too close to home for many healthcare providers, who may be understandably reluctant to have their own painful experiences evoked while trying to function in a professional capacity.[17]

SYSTEMIC BARRIERS

This section addresses the lack of medical training to support physicians in their efforts to deal with those patients who have experienced domestic violence. It describes how physicians interact with these situations and the limitations of their interactions. In addition, the section will discuss the effect of the physician's educational and training environment on their ability to be empathetic towards others who experience abuse.

Impact of Medical Training

Once they enter the healthcare arena, clinicians are faced with a new set of forces that shape their perceptions and responses.[18] A number of authors have described the gaps in medical education that influence psychosocial aspects of care.[19] Not only is medical training often lax in equipping physicians to deal with difficult social and personal issues, but more insidiously, the process of professional socialization can actually diminish the capacities they already have. Pain, anger, frustration, and sadness are common responses to hearing about abuse. Without specific training and support, many clinicians find themselves dealing with these situations through a variety of techniques designed to protect and distance themselves from potentially distressing encounters.

In a field where competence and mastery are highly valued, it is difficult to risk venturing into areas that make clinicians feel less competent. They may find it easier to focus on problems where interventions lead to outcomes that are more predictable or where it is possible to retain a greater sense of control. These difficulties are only magnified by increasingly time-pressured working conditions.[20]

Professional Socialization and the Intergenerational Transmission of Abuse

Extrapolating from the work of Richman et al.,[21] Baldwin et al.,[22] and others,[23] we can see how abusive training environments might also affect clinicians' abilities to deal with abuse among the women they see as patients. Medical training can be physically punishing, emotionally draining, and socially isolating. Trainees often report feeling humiliated and controlled as well as anxious, exhausted, depressed, overwhelmed, and traumatized.[24] Over time, both students and house staff begin to reorient their identities in terms of medicine's values, to internalize its constructs and judge themselves by its terms. Thus, medical training itself can create some of the same dynamics as abuse. In addition, the structure of medicine is hierarchical and, as such, reflects the gendered power arrangements of the larger society.

In their review of the sexual harassment literature, Schiffman and Frank found that sexual harassment and gender discrimination were common experiences among women physicians, adding yet another layer of abuse for women working within that system.[25] Clinicians' inabilities to recognize abuse in their own lives, whether personal, social, or professional, or to tolerate acknowledging their own vulnerability, make it more difficult for them to empathize with a woman who is struggling in an abusive relationship. The need to maintain a sense of power and control in order to be recognized as competent within that system, and the pressure to avoid feelings that might arise when one cannot, reinforce this dynamic on both individual and systemic levels. Although there has been much discussion about how abuse is transmitted intergenerationally in families, the process of professional socialization within the current structure of medicine can also serve as a vehicle for the intergenerational transmission of abuse.[26]

IMPACT OF THEORY ON CLINICAL PRACTICE

The theoretical foundations of medical education also affect the physician's ability to treat patients affected by domestic violence. For example, social problems are often connected to clinical diagnoses even though they are much more complex than any clinical label. In addition, traditional mental health models may be as a limited as clinical models in providing a framework for recognizing and treating domestic violence. In fact, the mental health system may actually retraumatize the patient. The healthcare system is beginning to understand that a new paradigm may be necessary for addressing this critical problem.

Medicalization of Social Problems

One aspect of medicalization involves the reduction of complex social problems into distinct clinical diagnoses.[27] One of the clearest illustrations of the need to shift from a standard problem-oriented framework to a more comprehensive model involves our evolving understanding of the role domestic violence plays in the lives of women with human immunodeficiency virus (HIV). Several studies have reported that many HIV-positive women either are or have been abused by partners.[28] Many "discrete" medical problems are, in fact, intimately connected to domestic violence, but because we think of them as separate issues, their interrelationships are more likely to be missed. For instance, one might easily generate a problem list that includes HIV infection, substance abuse, pregnancy, depression, and domestic violence without necessarily seeing the connections among them.

Initial recognition of domestic violence among HIV-positive women led to appropriate concerns about reducing risk for further violence, particularly around partner notification.[29] It took longer for domestic violence education and intervention to be incorporated into risk reduction counseling for HIV, pregnancy, and substance abuse. There are significant implications for funding, education, and prevention given that coerced sex within the context of an abusive relationship is a risk factor for HIV transmission and the other consequences of unprotected sex. In addition, substance abuse among women, the other major risk factor for HIV, also increases in the context of domestic violence.[30] In fact, recognition of these connections has led a number of comprehensive HIV programs to integrate screening and counseling for domestic violence into the preventive as well as treatment services they provide.[31]

Limitations of Mental Health Models

The process of stripping away context and transforming lived experience into disorders also occurs within the major mental health models and affects the nature of both diagnosis and intervention. For example, clinicians who work within a purely biological or disorder-specific framework run risks similar to medical and surgical colleagues of failing to recognize and respond to the ongoing violence in a patient's life. They may also see the abuse as being caused by a particular woman's increased vulnerability or as only a secondary problem—a social stressor affecting the course of her primary biological or developmental disorder.

Traditional psychoanalytic theory historically has presented a different set of limitations. The context of ongoing violence and danger that creates and perpetuates a woman's symptoms might not be addressed or might be regarded as symptomatic rather than etiologic. In addition, a clinician bound by the constraints of remaining true to the neutrality of a psychodynamic framework might find it difficult to play a more active role in advocating for safety and in helping women gain access to community resources. Of course, other models—both feminist and psychodynamic—do recognize the importance of social and intersubjective contexts.[32]

When domestic violence is framed solely under the rubric of "family violence," it obscures the gendered aspects of this problem and is more likely to be seen in terms of dysfunctional couple or family dynamics. In doing so, clinicians can lose sight of the larger social dynamics that shape gendered behaviors in families, and are thus less able to help women to gain perspective or mobilize necessary resources. A family systems approach can present even greater dangers to battered women. Assuming equal power within and responsibility for relationship dynamics, it inadvertently holds a battered woman responsible for her partner's criminal behavior and keeps her engaged in the countertherapeutic task of trying to change herself in order to get him to change. In addition, counseling sessions often precipitate further threats or violence. Andersen et al.[33] and Walker[34] have described the dynamics of battering in terms of ongoing domestic terrorism, akin to hostage situations.

In that kind of setting, particularly when her partner continues to engage in violence, controlling behavior, or threats, it is not safe for a woman to be honest or to assert herself. Nor is she likely to be free to make her own choices.[35] Again, newer models of family and couples therapy are being developed that specifically address domestic violence.[36] However, limited data is available on the effectiveness or safety of these treatment modalities, and they have been studied in couples where the level of violence is low.[37]

The emergence of trauma theory over the past three decades has created a significant shift in the ways mental health symptoms are conceptualized and in our understanding of the role abuse and violence play in the development of psychological distress and mental health conditions. Arising out of the experiences of survivors of civilian and combat trauma, it views symptoms as survival strategies. They are adaptations to potentially life-shattering situations that are made when real protection is unavailable and normal coping mechanisms are overwhelmed. Trauma models, although immensely helpful in understanding the impact of domestic violence and other types of victimization, also have limitations in the context of ongoing domestic violence. For many women, symptoms are not "post"; rather they reflect survival strategies needed in the face of ongoing danger. In addition, therapies that focus on helping survivors understand why they unconsciously "chose" an abusive partner, that label them as "codependent" or "enabling," or that hold them responsible for their partner's abusive behavior and for stopping it could be undermining and potentially endangering[38] to someone who is currently entrapped or unsafe.

These models are limited precisely because they are clinical models. They do not provide a framework for recognizing that it is the combination of the abuser's use of violence, threats, and intimidation with the social conditions that support gender inequality and limit options for safety that keeps women trapped in abusive situations and restricts their possibilities for change.[39] These same gender biases also contribute to the reduced likelihood that the small percentage of men abused by a female partner will receive services and to the homophobia that impedes recognition of domestic violence in LGBTQI (lesbian, gay, bisexual, transgender, queer, questioning, and intersex) relationships.

Inadvertent Retraumatization

Inadvertent retraumatization of patients through disempowering interactions within the health and mental health system is another crucial issue. The pressure under current practice arrangements, particularly in managed care or under-resourced public sector environments, to make rapid assessments, diagnoses, and treatment recommendations can push clinicians into taking a more controlling stance in their clinical encounters. For someone whose life is already controlled by another person, the subtly disempowering quality of many clinical interactions can serve to reinforce the idea that adapting to another's controlling behavior is both expected and necessary for survival. In fact, over the past 10 years, guidelines for creating trauma-informed services have been developed precisely to address these concerns.[40]

Changing Theory and Incorporating Context

Clearly, a purely clinical framework limits our ability to respond to abuse. In fact, maintaining such a stance would require that we "diagnose" and find ways to "treat" a pervasive, long-standing form of normative social pathology characterized by a gender socialization process. This process (in its most polarized form) has taught women to focus their identities on meeting men's needs and on maintaining relationships at all costs. It also teaches men that it is both necessary and legitimate to sustain their sense of self at the expense of those with less power, often women and children.[41] This belief is produced within the context of a socioeconomic system that frequently leaves women, particularly those with small children, increasingly fewer options for living independent lives[42] and a criminal justice system that often fails to protect or does so in discriminatory ways.

Although the healthcare system is finally beginning to face the consequences of a problem rooted in centuries of social and legal tradition, it also is important for us to address the more difficult task of transforming gender socialization patterns and to recognize that gender equality is an essential component of primary prevention.[43]

We also stretch the boundaries of the healthcare system when we work with the domestic violence advocacy and criminal justice systems. For example, many women are in danger at the time they seek health care, yet the danger itself is not something amenable to "medical" intervention. By becoming informed of options available in their communities for increasing women's safety, clinicians can help women get the services they need and begin to understand the complexity of their situations. Will a woman risk losing her children in a custody battle? Will she risk losing her means of providing for them? Will she risk deportation if she seeks help? Does she qualify for immigration remedies under the Violence Against Women Act? Will she risk losing someone she loves and who might act lovingly toward her much of the time? Will she risk being killed if she leaves? A more comprehensive model provides a framework for understanding responses to not only trauma, but also, more significantly, to ongoing danger, and for mobilizing the social and legal resources that can increase safety, expand options, and ultimately prevent further violence.[44]

STRUCTURAL CONSTRAINTS

Healthcare providers also face a number of structural constraints that affect their ability to provide appropriate care to women dealing with ongoing abuse. In the current healthcare climate, cost containment often is achieved at the expense of care, and clinicians' needs are placed in conflict with patients' for access to diminishing resources.[45] This is a problem for primary care providers, who often are penalized for spending too much time with patients and for making too many referrals. This is even more problematic for patients, however, at a time when reimbursement for social and mental health services continues to shrink.

Micromanagement strategies devised by insurance companies to reduce "unnecessary" mental healthcare utilization (e.g., continuous intrusive demands to justify treatment) can be disruptive and traumatic in themselves. They create an environment in which short-term medication management or potentially retraumatizing directive treatments focused on symptom reduction rather than healing have become the standard of care, making the consistency and safety required for long-term trauma recovery less likely to be reimbursed.

It is unfortunate that, just when an expanding body of research is clearly delineating the impact of trauma on the human psyche and the need for more intensive treatment for many survivors,[46] market forces are decreasing the likelihood that these kinds of services will be available. This becomes increasingly true as managed care further erodes the possibility of choosing one's provider and type of treatment, removing even the consumer-based economic power from individuals seeking care. For low-income women whose only access to services has been through the public mental health system, this lack of choice has been the norm.[47]

Although providing short-term cost reductions, these policies do not address the long-term personal, financial, and, ultimately, social costs of failing to provide appropriate intervention.[48] In this type of set up, cost containment is seen only in terms of direct individual costs to a given healthcare corporation or system, whereas the exponential, but indirect, personal and social costs that could be prevented by early intervention are not considered part of the relevant financial equation.

A diagnosis-driven reimbursement system poses yet another set of problems for battered women. In order for a woman to use mental health services, she has to be given a diagnosis. But for battered women, the very diagnosis itself can create new dangers.[49] Batterers often use their victims' psychiatric diagnoses to "prove" that they are right, that the problems are her fault, that she is crazy, or that she is an unfit mother. In seeking treatment, a battered woman potentially risks losing her children in custody battles and losing her credibility in court. However, appropriate documentation of the mental health impact of domestic violence can help a survivor to build her legal case. For some women, "psychiatric" symptoms disappear once they are out of danger, but many women continue to be threatened and stalked long after they have left the relationship.[50] For others, symptoms of posttraumatic stress disorder may not begin until they are relatively safe.[51]

In the past, women were refused health insurance for having the preexisting condition of being battered and disability or life insurance because they were considered at higher risk for injury and death.[52] In addition, if a woman is insured on her husband's policy and the bills are sent to him, she is likely to be placed in further jeopardy when he discovers she is seeking outside help.

Nonetheless, strides have been made in both of these arenas. Since 1994, 41 states have enacted legislation prohibiting discrimination against victims of domestic violence and HIPAA regulations allow bills to be sent to a safe address at a patient's request.[53]

In some states, laws that require mandatory reporting of domestic violence can again place the clinician's legal obligations in conflict with the wishes and the safety of his or her patients. Not only do these policies potentially destroy the ability of clinicians to provide a safe place for women to discuss their most pressing concerns, they violate women's rights to choose what they feel will be safest and most helpful to themselves and their children. Under these conditions, both clinicians and patients may avoid raising concerns about abuse, thus losing important opportunities to intervene.[54]

Listening to patients, learning about the repercussions of our interventions, and working to prevent revictimization within the systems survivors interface with become important components of our roles as healthcare professionals practicing preventive medicine. Without a clear institutional commitment to address these issues, however, the pressures to continue practice as usual may be greater than the ability to change.

IMPLICATIONS FOR TRAINING AND PRACTICE

Experience has led many clinician-educators to realize that new training strategies must be developed in order to change attitudes and behavior on the scale that is required to address domestic violence.[55] Standard didactic formats, for example, do not provide sufficient opportunity to address the attitudes and feelings that might interfere with a clinician's ability to provide appropriate care, nor do they offer room to acquire the interviewing skills necessary for an optimal response. Training environments that offer the emotional safety to explore personal and cultural responses to abuse and the opportunities to discuss individual, professional, and institutional obstacles can provide a vehicle for generating change within the healthcare community. Although one-time trainings might raise awareness, ongoing feedback and support are necessary to sustain provider response.[56]

Providing quality health care involves integrating routine inquiry about domestic violence into ongoing clinical practice. This means asking all women patients, including women in lesbian relationships, about abuse and violence in their lives. Whether or not a woman chooses to use services or leave her partner, our intervention is very important. Women often return to violent partners many times before they feel safe enough to leave, feel that they can survive on their own, or can accept that the person they love will not change. When we fail to ask about abuse, we inadvertently isolate women who are living in danger.[57] Just by inquiring and expressing concern, we begin to build bridges, decrease isolation, and create hope.

For a person who lives in an atmosphere of ongoing threats, intimidation, and violence, being treated with respect and taken seriously and feeling free to make her own choices lets her know supportive experiences are possible. By asking women to describe the pattern of their abuse and level of danger and to discuss their options for safety, we provide a place for women to reflect on their situations and consider their choices. By providing access to resources and by facilitating a woman's own decision-making process rather than attempting to direct her to change, we help her shift the balance of power in her life. When we work collaboratively with other members of our communities, we not only help individual survivors rebuild their lives, but also help to change the conditions that allow domestic violence to exist.

In order for clinicians to develop and sustain appropriate responses to domestic violence, however, they must also have the support of the institutions in which they practice. Thus, addressing this issue requires some fundamental changes in the nature of most medical training and in the culture of medical institutions. Creating practice environments and policies that model nonabusive ways of interacting, that support clinicians' efforts to address complex issues with skill and compassion, and that reimburse the more labor-intensive tasks of listening and advocating for change are important components of institutionalizing effective responses to domestic violence.[58] Refocusing our priorities is particularly important in a health-care climate where administrators, insurers, and those who influence healthcare policy must begin to recognize that the long-term consequences of nonintervention far exceed the costs of investing in appropriate intervention and prevention.[59]

In addition, providers acting alone, no matter how motivated, cannot meet all the needs of battered women and their children. An optimal response requires the efforts of all members of the community. Developing interdisciplinary teams within the healthcare setting and creating collaborative partnerships between the domestic violence advocacy community, the mental health and healthcare systems, the child protective system, and the legal system serves a number of functions. It not only provides referral networks for patients, it also creates support networks for providers. More important, it is only by working together that we can begin to develop the kinds of intervention strategies that will be appropriate for and respectful to all victims of domestic violence, while laying the groundwork to develop effective prevention strategies as well.

CONCLUSION

When we ask what battered women need from individual providers, we must also ask what providers need from their training institutions and practice environments in order to respond to those needs. When we do not address the denial of intolerable feelings at a personal level, we are in danger of recreating them not only in individual relationships, but also on social and political levels. Further, when socially-sanctioned abuses of power are not acknowledged, they often are internalized and reproduced through individual interactions. If we truly want to play a role in preventing domestic violence, rather than just treating its consequences, it is important to work together to address the social conditions that create and support this kind of violence in the first place.

SUMMARY

Domestic violence is widely recognized as a social problem that affects both the family and the community. Clinicians deal with the effects of this issue on an almost daily basis, but often find it beyond their medical expertise. This chapter presents a discussion of why physicians may not be prepared to address the needs of those affected by domestic violence and the need for changes in physician training and practice. In addition, it suggests strategies for institutions and communities' engagement in better addressing the challenges of this significant social issue.

QUESTIONS FOR DISCUSSION

1. How does the training environment influence future physicians' position on responding to survivors of domestic violence? How does it influence how they address domestic violence?

2. What is the connection between social justice and the treatment of the aftermath/traumatic effects of domestic violence?

3. What is the moral duty of physicians to the victims of domestic violence?

4. Does a utilitarian approach help or hinder treatment for victims of domestic violence?

5. How do the principles of beneficence and nonmaleficence relate to the issue of dealing with domestic violence?

NOTES

1. E. Stark and A. Flitcraft, "Violence Among Intimates: An Epidemiologic Review," in *Handbook of Family Violence*, V. N. Van Hasselt, et al., eds. (New York: Plenum, 1988), 293–317; D. Dossman, et al., "Sexual and Physical Abuse in Women with Functional or Organic Gastrointestinal Disorders," *Annals of Internal Medicine* 113 (1990): 828–833; J. Domino and J. Haber, "Prior Physical and Sexual Abuse in Women with Chronic Headache: Clinical Correlates," *Headache* 27 (1987): 310–314; M. Koss and I. Heise, "Somatic Consequences of Violence against Women," *Archives of Family Medicine* 1 (1992): 53–59; M. Koss, et al., "Deleterious Effects of Criminal Victimization on Women's Health and Medical Utilization," *Archives Internal Medicine* 151 (1991): 342–347; J. Fildes, et al., "Trauma: The Leading Cause of Maternal Death," *Journal of Trauma* 32 (1992): 43–45; L. McKibben, et al., "Victimization of Mothers of Abused Children: A Controlled Study," *Pediatrics* 84 (1989): 531–535; E. Stark and A. Flitcraft, "Women and Children at Risk: A Feminist Perspective on Child Abuse," *International Journal Health Services* 18 (1988): 97–118; E. Stark and A. Flitcraft, "Killing the Beast Within: Woman Battering and Female Suicidality," *International Journal of Health Services* 25 (1995): 43–64; A. Jacobsen and B. Richardson, "Assault Experiences of 100 Psychiatric Inpatients: Evidence of the Need for Routine Inquiry," *American Journal of Psychiatry* 144 (1987): 908–913; L. S. Brown, "The Contribution of Victimization as a Risk Factor for the Development of Depressive Symptomatology in Women," (paper presented at the 97th Annual Convention of the American Psychological Association, New Orleans,

Louisiana, August 1989); J. A. Hamilton and M. Jensvold, "Personality, Psychopathology and Depression in Women," in *Personality and Psychopathology: Feminist Reappraisals*, I. S. Brown and M. Ballou, eds. (New York: Guilford Press, 1992); J. Herman, *The Aftermath of Violence: from Domestic Abuse to Political Theory* (New York: Basic Books, 1992); B. M. Houskamp and D. Foy, "The Assessment of Posttraumatic Stress Disorder in Battered Women," *Journal of Interpersonal Violence* 6 (1991): 367–375; A. Kemp, et al., "Post-traumatic Stress Disorder (PTSD) in Battered Women: A Shelter Sample," *Journal of Traumatic Stress* 4 (1991): 137–148; L. E. Walker, "Post-traumatic Stress Disorder in Women: Diagnosis and Treatment of Battered Woman Syndrome," *Psychotherapy* 28 (1991): 21–29; J. C. Campbell, "Battered Woman Syndrome: A Critical Review," *Violence Update* (December 1990): 1, 4, 10–11; J. C. Campbell, "Post-traumatic Stress in Battered Women: Does the Diagnosis Fit?" *Issues Mental Health Nursing* 14 (1993): 173–186; C. R. Figley, "Posttraumatic Stress Disorder Part 2: Relationships with Various Traumatic Events," *Violence Update* (May 1992); C. Warshaw and S. Poirier, "Case and Commentary: Hidden Stories of Women," *Second Opinion* 17 (1991): 48–61.

2. A. Flitcraft, et al., *Diagnostic and Treatment Guidelines on Domestic Violence* (Chicago: American Medical Association, 1992); C. Warshaw, et al., *Improving the Health Care Response to Domestic Violence: A Resource Manual for Health Care Providers* (San Francisco: Family Violence Prevention Fund and Pennsylvania Coalition Against Domestic Violence, 1995); C. J. Scott and N. Matricciani, "Joint Commission on Accreditation of Health Care Organizations Standards to Improve Care for Victims of Abuse," *Maryland Medical Journal* 43 (1994): 891–898; W. K. Taylor and J. C. Campbell, "Treatment Protocols for Battered Women," *Response* (1992): 1–21; A. Flitcraft, "Commentary: Physicians and Domestic Abuse: Challenges for Prevention," *Health Affairs* 12 (1993): 156–161.

3. L. K. Hamberger, "Preparing the Next Generation of Physicians: Medical School and Residency-Based Intimate Partner Violence Curriculum and Evaluation," *Trauma, Violence, and Abuse* 8 (2007): 214–225; E. J. Alpert, "Family Violence Curricula in U.S. Medical Schools," *America Journal of Preventive Medicine* 14 (1998): 273–282; S. Rovi and C. P. Mouton, "Domestic Violence Education in Family Practice Residencies," *Family Medicine* 31 (1999): 398–403; R. A. Chez and D. L. Horan, "Response of Obstetrics and Gynecology Program Directors to a Domestic Violence Lecture Model," *American Journal of Obstetrics and Gynecology* 180 (1999): 496–498; Curricular Principles for Addressing Family Violence: Conference Report (Oklahoma City, OK: Robert Wood Johnson Foundation, 1995); S. Hadley, "Working with Battered Women in the Emergency Department: A Model Program," *Journal of Emergency Nursing* 18 (1992): 18–23; C. Warshaw, et al., "An Advocacy-Based Medical School Elective on Domestic Violence" (class offered at the National Conference on Cultural Competence and Women's Health, Curricular in Medical Education, Washington, D.C., October 1995).

4. L. R. Chambliss, et al., "Domestic Violence: An Educational Imperative?" *American Journal of Obstetrics and Gynecology* 172 (1995): 1035–1038; I. S. Friedman, et al., "Inquiry about Victimization Experiences: A Survey of Patient Preferences and Physician Practices," *Archives of Internal Medicine* 152 (1992): 1186–1190; E. Gondolf, *Psychiatric Responses to Family Violence: Identifying and Confronting Neglected Danger* (Lexington, MA: Lexington Books, 1990).

5. N. K. Sugg and T. Inui, "Primary Care Physician's Response to Domestic Violence: Opening Pandora's Box," *Journal of the American Medical Association* 267 (1991): 3157–3160; D. H. Gremillion and G. Evins, "Why Don't Doctors Identify and Refer Victims of Domestic Violence?" *North Carolina Medical Journal* 55 (1994): 428–432; C. Warshaw, "Limitations of the Medical Model in the Care of Battered Women," *Gender and Society* 3 (1989): 506–517; id., "Domestic Violence Challenges to Medical Practice," *Journal of Women's Health* 2 (1993): 73–80.

6. Warshaw, "Domestic Violence."

7. H. A. Holtz, et al., "Education about Domestic Violence in U.S. and Canadian Medical Schools: 1987–1988," *Morbidity and Mortality Weekly Report* 38 (1989): 17–19; E. J. Alpert, "Family Violence Curricula in U.S. Medical Schools," *America Journal of Preventive Medicine* 14 (1998): 273–282.

8. S. K. Burge, "Violence Against Women as a Health Care Issue," *Family Medicine* 21 (1989): 368–373; A. Kramer, "Attitudes of Emergency Nurses and Physicians about Women and Wife Beating: Implications for Emergency Care," *Journal of Emergency Nursing* 19 (1993): 549; D. R. Langford, "Consortia: A Strategy for Improving the Provision of Health Care to Domestic Violence Survivors," *Response to the Victimization of Women and Children* 13 (1990): 7–18; N. S. Jecker, "Privacy Beliefs and the Violent Family: Extending the Ethical Argument for Physician Intervention," *Journal of the American Medical Association* 269 (1993): 776–780; D. Kurz and E. Stark, "Not-so-Benign Neglect," in *Feminist Perspectives on Wife Abuse*, K. Yllo and M. Bograd, eds. (Newbury Park, CA: Sage, 1988), 249–266.

9. M. Koss, et al., *No Safe Haven: Male Violence against Women at Home, at Work and in the Community* (Washington, D.C.: American Psychological Association, 1994).

10. K. Johnson, *Treating Ourselves: The Complete Guide to Emotional Well-Being for Women* (New York: Atlantic Monthly Press, 1990).

11. L. S. Brown, "A Feminist Critique of Personality Disorders," in *Personality and Psychopathology: Feminist Reappraisals*, L. S. Brown and M. Ballou, eds. (New York: Guilford Press, 1992).

12. P. Rieker and E. Carmen, "The Victim-to-Patient Process: The Disconfirmation and Transformation of Abuse," *American Journal of Orthopsychiatry* 56 (1986): 360–370.

13. A. Miller, *Prisoners of Childhood: The Drama of the Gifted Child and the Search for the True Self* (New York: Basic Books, 1981); id., *Thou Shalt Not Be Aware: Society's Betrayal of the Child* (New York: Farrar, Straus & Giroux, 1984).

14. Rieker and Carmen, "The Victim-to-Patient Process"; Miller, *Prisoners of Childhood*; Miller, *Thou Shalt Not Be Aware*.

15. E. Arledge and R. Wolfson, "Care of the Clinician," in *Using Trauma Theory to Design Service Systems*, M. Harris and R. Fallot, eds. (San Francisco: Jossey-Bass, 2001), 91–98; K. Baird and A. Kracen, "Vicarious Traumatization and Secondary Traumatic Stress: A Research Synthesis," *Counseling Psychology Quarterly* 19 (2006), 181–188; I. Way, K. M. vanDeusen, et al., "Vicarious Trauma: A Comparison of Clinicians Who Treat Survivors of Sexual Abuse and Sexual Offenders," *Journal of Interpersonal Violence* 19 (2004): 49–71; L. H. Madsen, et al., "Sanctuary in a Domestic Violence Shelter: A Team Approach to Healing," *Psychiatric Quarterly* 72 (2003): 155–171; B. Bride, "Prevalence of Secondary Traumatic Stress Among Social Workers," *Social Work* 52 (2007): 63–70; C. R. Figley, "Compassion Fatigue: Toward a New Understanding of the Costs of Caring," in *Secondary Traumatic Stress: Self-care Issues for Clinicians, Researchers, and Educators*, B. H. Stamm, ed. (Lutherville, MD: Sidran Press), 3–28; S. R. Jenkins and S. Baird, "Secondary Traumatic Stress and Vicarious Trauma: A Validational Study," *Journal of Traumatic Stress* 15 (2002): 423–433; G. Iliffe, "Exploring the Counselor's Experience of Working with Perpetrators and Survivors of Domestic Violence," *Journal of Interpersonal Violence* 15 (2000), 393–413; Herman, *Trauma and Recovery*; M. A. Dutton, *Empowering and Healing the Battered Woman: A Model for Assessment and Intervention* (New York: Springer, 1992); M. Koss, "The Women's Mental Health Research Agenda: Violence against Women," *American Psychologist* 45 (1990); 374–380; L. Goldman, et al., *American Medical Association Diagnostic and Treatment Guidelines on Mental Health Effects of Family Violence* (Chicago: American Medical Association, 1995).

16. Sugg and Inui, "Primary Care Physician's Response to Domestic Violence."

17. Warshaw, "Domestic Violence"; Koss, et al., *No Safe Haven*; Johnson, *Treating Ourselves*; Brown, "A Feminist Critique of Personality Disorders."

18. Warshaw, "Domestic Violence."

19. P. Williamson, et al., "Beliefs That Foster Physician Avoidance of Psychosocial Aspects of Health Care," *Journal of Family Practice* 13 (1981): 999–1003; R. Fox, "Training in Caring Competence: The Perennial Problem in North American Medical Education," in *Education: Competent and Humane Physicians*, H. C. Hendrie and C. Lloyd, eds. (Bloomington, IN: Indiana University Press, 1990), 199–216.

20. Warshaw, "Domestic Violence"; Williamson, et al., "Beliefs That Foster Physician Avoidance of Psychosocial Aspects of Health Care."

21. J. A. Richman, et al., "Mental Health Consequences and Correlates of Reported Medical Student Abuse," *Journal of the American Medical Association* 167 (1992): 692–694.

22. D. Baldwin, et al., "Student Perceptions of Mistreatment and Harassment During Medical School: A Survey of Ten United States Schools," *Western Journal of Medicine* 155 (1991): 140–145.

23. B. J. Tepper, "Consequences of Abusive Supervision," *Academic Management Journal* 43 (2000): 178–190; D. M. Elnicki, et al., "Medical Students' Perspectives on and Responses to Abuse During the Internal Medicine Clerkship," *Teaching and Learning Medicine* 14 (2002): 92–97; T. J. Wilkinson, et al., "The Impact on Students of Adverse Experiences During Medical School," *Medical Teaching* 28 (2006): 129–135; L. N. Dyrbye, M. R. Thomas, and T. D. Shanafelt, "Systematic Review of Depression, Anxiety, and Other Indicators of Psychological Distress Among U.S. and Canadian Medical Students," *Academic Medicine* 81 (2006): 354–373; id., "Medical Student Distress: Causes, Consequences, and Proposed Solutions," *Mayo Clinic Proceedings* 80 (2005): 1613–1622; M. Seabrook, "Intimidation in Medical Education: Students' and Teachers' Perspectives," *Studies in Higher Education* 29 (2004): 59–74; D. G. Kassebaum and E. R. Cutler, "On the Culture of Student Abuse in Medical School," *Academic Medicine* 73 (1998): 1149–1158; T. M. Wolf, et al., "Perceived Mistreatment and Attitude Change by Graduating Medical Students: A Retrospective Study," *Medical Education* 25 (1991): 182–189.

24. Warshaw, "Domestic Violence"; Richman et al., "Mental Health Consequences and Correlates of Reported Medical Student Abuse."

25. D. Wear, J. Aultman, and N. Borges, "Retheorizing Sexual Harassment in Medical Education: Women Students' Perceptions at Five U.S. Medical Schools," *Teaching and Learning Medicine* 19 (2007): 20–29; F. M. Witte, et al., "Stories from the Field: Students' Descriptions of Gender Discrimination and Sexual Harassment During Medical School," *Academic Medicine* 81 (2006): 648–654; T. D. Stratton, et al., "Does Students' Exposure to Gender Discrimination and Sexual Harassment in Medical School Affect Specialty Choice and Residency Program Selection?" *Academic Medicine* 80 (2005): 400–408; S. A. Shinsako, J. A. Richman, and K. M. Rospenda, "Training-Related Harassment and Drinking Outcomes in Medical Residents Versus Graduate Students," *Substance Use and Misuse* 36 (2001): 2043–2063; J. Bickel, "Gender Equity in Undergraduate Medical Education: A Status Report," *Journal of Women's Health* Gen-B 10 (2001): 261–270; Richman, et al., "Mental Health Consequences and Correlates of Reported Medical Student Abuse"; Baldwin, et al., "Student Perceptions of Mistreatment and Harassment During Medical School: A Survey of Ten United States Schools"; Wolf, et al., "Perceived Mistreatment and Attitude Change by Graduating Medical Students: A Retrospective Study"; M. Schiffman and E. Frank, "Harassment of Women Physicians," *Journal of the American Medical Women's Assocation* 50 (1995): 207–211; D. A. Charney and R. C. Russell, "An Overview of Sexual Harassment," *American Journal of Psychiatry* 151 (1994): 10–17; M. Komaromy, et al., "Sexual Harassment in Medical Training," *New England Journal of Medicine* 328 (1993): 322–336.

26. Warshaw, "Domestic Violence"; Kurz and Stark, "Not-so-Benign Neglect"; Koss, et al., *No Safe Haven*; Johnson, *Treating Ourselves*; Brown, "A Feminist Critique of Personality Disorders"; Fox, "Training in Caring Competence"; C. S. Widom, "Does Violence Beget Violence: A Critical Examination of the Literature," *Psychology Bulletin* 106 (1989): 437–447.

27. K. Johnson and E. Hoffman, "Women's Health and Curriculum Transformation: The Role of Medical Specialization," in *Reframing Women's Health: Multidisciplinary Research and Practice*, A. Dan, ed. (Thousand Oaks, CA: Sage, 1994), 27–39.

28. A. C. Gielen, et al., "HIV/AIDS and Intimate Partner Violence," *Trauma Violence Abuse* 8 (2007): 178–198; S. Maman, J. Campbell, M. D Sweat, and A. C. Gielen, "The Intersections of HIV and Violence: Directions for Future Research and Interventions," *Social Science and Medicine* 50 (2000): 459–478; A. Raj, et al., "Perpetration of Intimate Partner Violence Associated with Sexual Risk Behaviors among Young Adult Men," *American Journal of Public Health* 96 (2006): 1873–1878; B. Lichtenstein, "Domestic Violence, Sexual Ownership, and HIV Risk in Women in the American Deep South," *Social Science Medicine* 60 (2005): 701–714; A. J. Heintz and R. Melendez, "Intimate Partner Violence and HIV/STD Risk Among Lesbian, Gay, Bisexual, and Transgender Individuals," *Journal of Interpersonal Vio-

lence 21 (2006): 193–208; G. Wyatt, et al., "Does History of Trauma Contribute to HIV Risk for Women of Color? Implications for Prevention and Policy," *American Journal of Public Health* 92 (2002): 660–665; A. Raj, J. G. Silverman, and H. Amaro, "Abused Women Report Greater Male Partner Risk and Gender-based Risk for HIV: Findings From a Community-Based Study with Hispanic Women," *AIDS Care* 16 (2004): 519–529; N. El-Bassel, et al., "HIV and Intimate Partner Violence Among Methadone-Maintained Women in New York City," *Social Science Medicine* 61 (2005): 171–183; J. M. Simoni and M. T. Ng, "Trauma, Coping, and Depression Among Women with HIV/AIDS in New York City," *AIDS Care* 12 (2000): 567–580; S. C. Kalicharan, et al., "Sexual Coercion, Domestic Violence, and Negotiating Condom Use among Low-Income African American Women," *Journal of Women's Health* 7 (1998): 371–379; M. Cohen, et al., "Prevalence of Domestic Violence in Women with HIV" (paper presented at the Midwest Society of General Internal Medicine, Chicago, October 1995); K. Rothenberg, et al., "Domestic Violence and Partner Notification: Implications for Treatment and Counseling of Women with HIV," *Journal of the American Medical Women's Association* 50 (1995): 87–93.

29. Rothenberg, et al., "Domestic Violence and Partner Notification: Implications for Treatment and Counseling of Women with HIV."

30. Stark and Flitcraft, "Violence among Intimates."

31. S. J. Klein, "Screening for Risk of Domestic Violence within HIV Partner Notification: Evolving Practice and Emerging Issues," *Journal of Public Health Management* 7 (2001): 46–50; R. Wolfe, J. Lobozzo, V. Frye, and V. Sharp, "Screening for Substance Use, Sexual Practices, Mental Illness, and Domestic Violence in HIV Primary Care," *Journal of Acquired Immune Deficiency Syndromes* 33 (2003): 548–550; S. Maman, et al., "The Intersections of HIV and Violence"; J. E. Maher, et al., "Partner Violence, Partner Notification, and Women's Decisions to Have an HIV Test," *Journal of Acquired Immune Deficiency Syndromes* 25 (2000): 276–282; S. J. Klein, M. L. SanAntonio-Gaddy, E. L. Berberian, and G. S. Birkhead, "Implementation of Domestic Violence Screening as a Component of HIV Partner Notification in New York State" (paper presented at the National HIV Prevention Conference, Atlanta, Georgia, 1999); Cohen, et al., "Prevalence of Domestic Violence in Women with HIV"; Rothenberg, et al., "Domestic Violence and Partner Notification: Implications for Treatment and Counseling of Women with HIV"; V. Breitbert, et al., "Model Programs Addressing Perinatal Drug Exposure and HIV Infection: Integrating Women's and Children's Needs," *Bulletin of the New York Academy of Medicine* 71 (1994): 236–251.

32. Miller, *Thou Shalt Not Be Aware*; G. Atwood and R. Stolorow, *Structures of Subjectivity: Explorations in Psychoanalytic Phenomenology* (Hillsdale, NJ: The Analytic Press, 1984); L. Brown, *Subversive Dialogues: Theory in Feminist Therapy* (New York: Basic Books, 1994).

33. S. Andersen, et al., "Psychological Maltreatment of Spouses," in *Case Studies in Family Violence*, R. Ammerman and M. Hersen, eds. (New York: Plenum, 1991): 293–328.

34. L. Walker, "The Battered Woman Syndrome," in *Family Abuse and Its Consequences*, G. T. Hotaling, et al., eds. (Beverly Hills, CA: Sage, 1988), 139–48.

35. Brown, "A Feminist Critique of Personality Disorders"; M. Bograd, "Family Systems Approaches to Wife Battering: A Feminist Critique," *American Journal of Orthopsychiatry* 54 (1984): 558–568.

36. M. Hansen, "Feminism and Family Therapy: A Review of Feminist Critiques of Approaches to Family Violence," in *Battering and Family Therapy: A Feminist Perspective*, M. Hansen and M. Harway, eds. (Thousand Oaks, CA: Sage, 1993); M. Harway and M. Hansen, "Treatment of Spouse Abuse," in *Spouse Abuse: Assessing & Treating Battered Women, Batterers, & Their Children*, M. Harway and M. Hansen, eds. (Sarasota, FL: Professional Resource Press/Professional Resource Exchange, Inc., 1994), 57–88; V. Goldner, "Morality and Multiplicity: Perspectives on the Treatment of Violence in Intimate Life," *Journal of Marital & Family Therapy* 25, no 3 (1999): 325–336.

37. K. O'Leary, R. Heyman, and P. Neidig, "Treatment of Wife Abuse: A Comparison of Gender-specific and Conjoint Approaches," *Behavior Therapy* 30 (1999): 475–505.

38. Focusing on how a client should change herself may reinforce a perpetrator's controlling tactics (i.e., "you are the one with the problem") and further undermine her ability to gain per-

spective on her situation or to take steps that would increase the safety of herself and her children. This may be of particular concern for clinicians who conduct couples or family therapy; C. Warshaw, "Women and Violence," in *Psychological Aspects of Women's Health Care: The Interface Between Psychiatry and Obstetrics and Gynecology*, D. Stewart and N. Stotland, eds. (Washington, D.C.: American Psychiatric Association Press, 2001).

39. A. Jones and S. Schechter, *When Love Goes Wrong: What to Do When You Can't Do Anything Right* (New York: Harper, 1993); A. Ganley, "Understanding Domestic Violence," in *Improving the Health Care Response to Domestic Violence: A Resource Manual for Health Care Providers*, C. Warshaw, et al., eds. (San Francisco: Family Violence Prevention Fund and Pennsylvania Coalition against Domestic Violence, 1995), 15–45.

40. M. Harris and R. Fallot, "Envisioning a Trauma-Informed Service System: A Vital Paradigm Shift," *New Directions for Mental Health Services, Using Trauma Theory to Design Service Systems*, 89 (2001).

41. Miller, *Prisoners of Childhood*.

42. A. Brown, "Violence, Poverty, and Minority Races in the Lives of Women and Children: Implications for Violence Prevention," Bridging Science and Program Centers for Disease Control Violence Prevention Conference, Des Moines, Iowa, October 1995.

43. Other forms of inequality also contribute to abusive power dynamics and eradicating those are important aspects of primary prevention.

44. Jones and Schechter, *When Loves Goes Wrong*; Ganley, "Understanding Domestic Violence"; www.womenslaw.org/immigrantsVAWA.htm.

45. S. Woodhandler and D. Himmelstein, "Extreme Risk—The New Corporate Proposition for Physicians," *New England Journal of Medicine* 33 (1995): 1706–1708; S. Glied and S. Kofman, *Women and Mental Health Reform* (New York: Commission on Women's Health, Commonwealth Fund, 1995).

46. L. Mellman and R. Bell, "Consequences of Violence Against Women," in *Violence Against Women in the United States: A Comprehensive Background Paper* (New York: The Commonwealth Fund Commission on Women's Health, 1995), 33–40; L. Innes and L. Mellman, "Treatment for Victims of Violence," in *Violence Against Women in the United States: A Comprehensive Background Paper* (New York: The Commonwealth Fund Commission on Women's Health, 1995), 41–54.

47. E. Carmen, "Inner-City Community Mental Health: The Interplay of Abuse and Race in Chronically Mentally Ill Women," in *Mental Health, Racism, and Sexism*, C. Willie, B. Kramer, and B. Brown, eds. (Pittsburgh: University of Pittsburgh, 1995).

48. T. Miller, et al., *Crime in the United States: Victim Cases and Consequences* (Washington, D.C.: National Institute of Justice, 1995).

49. C. Warshaw, "Women and Violence," in *Psychosocial Aspects of OB*; D. Markham, "2003 Mental Illness and Domestic Violence: Implications for Family Law Litigations," *Journal of Poverty Law and Policy* (May–June, 2003): 23–35.

50. Walker, "The Battered Woman Syndrome"; Jones and Schechter, *When Love Goes Wrong*; Ganley, "Understanding Domestic Violence."

51. Warshaw, "Domestic Violence"; Burge, "Violence Against Women as a Health Care Issue."

52. Women's Law Project and Pennsylvania Coalition Against Domestic Violence, *Insurance Discrimination against Victims of Domestic Violence* (Harrisburg, PA: Coalition Against Domestic Violence, 1995); L. Kaiser, *Survey of Accident and Health and Life Insurance Relating to Insurance Coverage for Victims of Domestic Violence* (Harrisburg: Commonwealth of Pennsylvania, Pennsylvania Insurance Department, 1995).

53. See www.womenslawproject.org/pages/issue_insurance.htm:

> In 1994, in partnership with the Pennsylvania Coalition Against Domestic Violence, the Law Project began its ongoing effort to stop insurers from discriminating against victims of domestic violence. The impetus for this work was the denial of health, life and mortgage disability insurance to a Pennsylvania woman because of medical records revealing an incident of domestic violence. Our advocacy began with administrative and legislative efforts to stop such dis-

crimination in Pennsylvania and expanded to assuming a leading role in efforts nationwide to stop discrimination against victims of domestic violence. At present 41 states have legislation prohibiting insurance discrimination against victims of abuse and efforts continue to insure comprehensive legislation at the state and federal level.

54. A. Hymes, D. Schillinger, and B. Lo, "Laws Mandating Reporting of Domestic Violence: Do They Promote Patient Well-Being?" *Journal of the American Medical Association* 272 (1995): 1781–1787.

55. Warshaw, et al., *Improving the Health Care Response to Domestic Violence: Curricular Principles for Addressing Family Violence*; Hadley, "Working with Battered Women in the Emergency Department"; S. McLeer, et al., "Education Is Not Enough: A Systems Failure in Protecting Battered Women," *Annals of Emergency Medicine* 18 (1989): 651–653.

56. N. E. Allen, et al., "Promoting Systems Change in the Health Care Response to Domestic Violence," *Journal of Community Psychology* 35 (2007): 103–120; D. Minsky-Kelly, L. K. Hamberger, D. A. Paper, and M. Wolff, "We've Had Training, Now What? Qualitative Analysis of Barriers to Domestic Violence Screening and Referral in a Health Care Setting," *Journal of Interpersonal Violence* 20 (2005): 1288–1309; M. J. Zachary, C. B. Schechter, M. L. Kaplan, and M. N. Mulvihill, "Provider Evaluation of a Multifaceted System of Care to Improve Recognition and Management of Pregnant Women Experiencing Domestic Violence," *Women's Health Issues* 12 (2002): 5–15; J. C. Campbell, et al., "An Evaluation of a System-Change Training Model to Improve Emergency Department Response to Battered Women," *Academic Emergency Medicine* 8 (2001): 131–138; G. L. Larkin, et al., "Effect of an Administrative Intervention on Rates of Screening for Domestic Violence in an Urban Emergency Department," *American Journal of Public Health* 90 (2000): 1444–1448; Warshaw, et al., *Improving the Health Care Response to Domestic Violence*; McLeer, et al., "Education Is Not Enough: A Systems Failure in Protecting Battered Women."

57. Jones and Schechter, *When Loves Goes Wrong*.

58. Warshaw, et al., *Improving the Health Care Response to Domestic Violence: Curricular Principles for Addressing Family Violence*.

59. S. R. Dube, et al., "The Impact of Adverse Childhood Experiencees on Health Problems: Evidence from Four Birth Cohorts Dating Back to 1900," *Prevention Medicine* 37 (2003): 268–277; V. J. Felitti, "The Relationship Between Adverse Childhood Experiences and Adult Health," *The Permanente Journal* 6 (2002): 44–47; C. L. Whitfield, "Adverse Childhood Experiences and Trauma," *American Journal of Preventive Medicine* 14 (1998): 245–258; V. J. Felitti, et al., "The Relationship of Adult Health Status to Childhood Abuse and Household Dysfunction," *American Journal of Preventive Medicine* (1998): 245–258; Warshaw, et al., *Improving the Health Care Response to Domestic Violence: Curricular Principles for Addressing Family Violence*.

CHAPTER 23

Ethics of Disaster Planning and Response

Eileen E. Morrison and Karen Bawel-Brinkley

OVERVIEW

In recent times, Americans have experienced a number of disaster situations caused by natural events, such as fires and floods, and by human-caused events, such as terrorist bombings and school shootings. Each of these events presented challenges, both logistical and ethical. All information indicates that the United States will continue to face disasters from various sources throughout the twenty-first century. This chapter presents examples of how government, healthcare organizations, and individuals plan for and respond to disaster situations. Although not all inclusive, these examples provide a framework for a discussion of ethical issues that relate to disaster preparedness.

INTRODUCTION

This chapter begins by reviewing examples of recent efforts by the federal government to prepare for and respond to disasters. The scope of the chapter will not allow a thorough examination of every effort made by governments, including those of state or local entities. However, it will highlight examples of agencies that are attempting to prepare the nation for disasters and to respond when they occur. Examples are included from the Department of Homeland Security (DHS), the Centers for Disease Control (CDC), the Federal Emergency Management Agency (FEMA), and the American Red Cross (ARC). Following this discussion, ethical issues related to these responses are presented. Both theories and principles are used to analyze ethical dilemmas, including logistical problems, loss of privacy and autonomy, and social justice.

Next, the chapter moves to efforts made by the healthcare system to prepare and respond to disasters. Again, examples will be used to highlight what has been done to prepare for natural or human-caused disasters. These examples include information from the Joint Commission on Accreditation of Health Care Organizations (JCAHO), the Agency for Healthcare Research and Quality (AHRQ), and hospital systems. These examples will lead to a discussion of ethical issues surrounding resource allocation, obligations of first responders, and social justice.

Finally, several sources will be used to review the obligations of individuals to prepare for disasters. This section also is a starting point for a discussion of the ethical issues faced by individuals. The chapter concludes with a summary of the critical ethical issues for disaster planning and response in the twenty-first century.

DISASTER RESPONSE AND DISASTERS IN U.S. HISTORY

The healthcare industry and its providers have a daily operational framework of treating individuals based on time, survival resources, and supplies. In one respect, healthcare providers plan, develop, implement, and evaluate services for caring for individuals based on the theory of supply and demand. Therefore, the daily operational framework of the organization must be able to adapt to an unexpected crisis. For example, in an emergency the goal for healthcare facilities would be to treat the most severely injured patient first while providing the highest level of care. The time frame, resources, and services would also have to be adequate to meet the needs of the situation. Therefore, treating and providing the highest level of care depends on time, resources, and supplies.[1]

In a disaster situation, the goal is to provide care for the greatest number of potential survivors without depleting resources or services. A *disaster* can be defined as an unexpected catastrophic event or situation that depletes survival resources and supplies in a relatively short time frame. A disaster tends to increase the individual survivor's vulnerability and to decrease the chance for survival.[2] Disasters can be divided into two categories: natural and human-caused. Both types of disasters have occurred throughout American history. These disasters have not only influenced the environment and U.S. society, but also the human experience in general.

The United States has experienced severe hurricanes (Betsy, Camille, and Ivan), floods (Johnstown, Pennsylvania, in 1889 and the Mississippi River flood in 1993), and fires (Chicago in 1871 and San Francisco in 1906). It has also faced the devastation from human-caused disasters, such as the destruction of Pearl Harbor during World War II and the bombing of the Murrah Federal Building in Oklahoma. Just within the early years of the twenty-first century, the United States has endured the disasters of September 11th in 2001, and Hurricane Katrina in 2005. As a result, Americans are beginning to learn to be prepared for the unexpected.

In the event of a disaster, healthcare providers must suddenly shift from a daily operational framework to one that includes providing care for the greatest number of potential survivors involved in the disaster in an efficient and effective manner.[3] Without adequate disaster planning, chaos can proliferate, leading to poor decision making and unethical behaviors. Can we expect ethical behavior when chaos is prominent? In order to have both an ethical and efficient response to a disaster, order needs to be reestablished and chaos eliminated as soon as possible.[4]

DISASTER PLANNING AND RESPONSE BY THE
FEDERAL GOVERNMENT

According to Redlener,[5] the events of September 11th, 2001, spurred efforts to upgrade America's ability to plan for disasters. However, we remain vulnerable to the effects of major disasters, and increased funding will be required to plan for and prevent them. Governments will have to invest in long-term programs that might not provide a return on investment for decades. In addition, these programs will require partnerships among the government (federal, regional, state, and local); nonprofit organizations; healthcare systems, including first responders; and individual citizens. Americans value autonomy and individualism; however, in a disaster, teamwork is essential. This will be difficult for many Americans to understand because we tend to be a nation of people who favor individualism and quick solutions.

Homeland Security

One response to the events of September 11th has been the creation of the Department of Homeland Security (DHS). Any American who has traveled since September 11th is aware of the many changes in security that are part of the duties of this organization. The DHS is responsible for aircraft security, including crew, cargo, and passengers. It employs professional screeners at airports, uses over 7000 screening devices, and places Federal Marshals on flights.

However, airport security is only one small part of how the DHS uses its $34 billion budget.[6] For example, it is instituting Project Bioshield to develop countermeasures against weapons of mass destruction. It also is responsible for screening goods, securing borders, and maintaining databases of information concerning high-risk persons. It uses biosensors to monitor the air in top threat cities to identify potential threats. It also funds research on new biosensors devices to improve this capacity.

In addition to its many responsibilities, the DHS also provides grants to state and local governments for first responders. These grants help to pay for needed equipment, provide opportunities for coordinating training exercises, and offer specific training to over 500,000 first responders. It also is working to protect the nation's infrastructure by conducting risk analyses involving critical areas such as banks, transportation systems, telecommunications hubs, dams, and national icons.

Centers for Disease Control

Other federal agencies also are involved in planning and responding to natural and human-caused disasters. One such agency is the Centers for Disease Control (CDC). According to the CDC Web site,[7] the agency has been involved in tracking natural and human-caused disasters and conducts research on ways to respond to the aftermath of these events. The CDC also provides information to both professionals and the public for disaster planning and response. The CDC offers guides specifically designed for healthcare facilities, businesses, and individuals. It also provides fact sheets and research reports on many areas, including mass-casualty event preparation and response. For example, one report provides information on the nature and classification of bomb injuries, in particular lung injuries from explosions. The CDC Web site includes an alphabetical list of agents and diseases that might be involved in disasters as well as sections on bioterrorism, chemical emergencies, mass casualties, natural disasters, and mental health issues related to disasters.

Federal Emergency Management Agency

The Federal Emergency Management Agency (FEMA) is the federal entity most responsible for responding to local and national disaster situations. According to the FEMA Web site,[8] the agency works in partnership with government (regional, state, and local branches); volunteer organizations; healthcare systems, including first responders; and individuals. It funds studies on hazard-related topics and on how to deal with repetitive flooding. It also provides education on a wide variety of disasters, including chemical emissions, dam failures, earthquakes, volcanoes, tornadoes, and wildfires. FEMA offers interactive maps to track areas where disasters have occurred. On its Ready.Gov site, FEMA provides kits and plans for both individuals and businesses to assist in preparing for disasters. It even has a Web site for children called Ready Kid that offers information on how families can prepare for disasters.

The most obvious service that FEMA provides is disaster assistance for individuals, families, and businesses that are not covered by insurance. Once a disaster area is declared, FEMA assists victims by providing temporary housing and funds for repair, replacement, and other needed services.

It is also involved in disaster prevention through its mitigation division. The mitigation division assists local and state entities with risk analysis and risk-reduction activities. FEMA also is responsible for the national response plan, which takes an all-hazard approach to dealing with domestic disasters and provides templates for disaster planning to state and local entities.

The American Red Cross

Although not a government agency, the Red Cross[9] is a major resource for disaster-response information. Inspired by the Swiss International Red Cross movement, the American Red Cross (ARC) is a humanitarian organization that was founded in 1881. Since that time, the ARC has provided relief and served as a mode of communication between members of the American armed forces and their families. It also provides national and international disaster relief.

According to its charter, established by Congress in 1905, the mission of the American Red Cross is to relieve suffering, particularly when disaster strikes, which includes education of the public and training. Initially, the ARC established first aid, water safety, and public health nursing programs. As the ARC has grown throughout the years, its services have expanded to include educational programs, such as safety training, HIV education, and so on. During wartime, it has provided services for the military personnel, civilian war victims, and prisoners of war. It maintains the civilian blood program, and provides disaster relief.

The Red Cross is famous for its use of volunteers from both the medical and nonmedical communities. Volunteers are trained by the Red Cross to provide services in a variety of disaster situations. It also has a matching program that coordinates a volunteer's expertise with a particular Red Cross need. Volunteers are an integral part of the success of the disaster relief efforts provided by the Red Cross organization.

The Red Cross disaster relief programs provide for the *immediate* needs of individuals and families affected by a disaster. When a disaster strikes, the ARC provides shelter and food and assists with healthcare issues and mental health services. It also offers support services for those who are part of the disaster relief efforts, including emergency workers.

The ARC also is a great proponent of education. It provides an ample amount of educational information on disaster and disaster preparedness. Its Web site includes articles on family disaster planning, animal safety, helping children cope with disasters, and the special needs of the elderly. In addition, information on disaster preparation kits is offered and links to specialized information are provided. Businesses can also find resources on how to prepare for disasters on the Red Cross Web site.

Improving Disaster Preparedness and Response

These organizations demonstrate only a small portion of how the U.S. government prepares for catastrophic events. They have certainly helped to increase the public's awareness of the potential for such events. However, Redlener[10] suggests that there is still much more to do in preparing the nation for future disasters. He offers a plan that includes setting benchmarks, correcting methods of overseeing disaster planning, creating accountability standards, and making the reduction of threats a priority. In addition, he would support changing the manner in which responses to disasters are made. He suggests increasing the influence of the U.S. Surgeon General, changing FEMA's reporting system, and clarifying the role of the military in a disaster situation. Certainly, the government must continue improving its plans for responding to natural and human-caused disasters.

Another disaster response plan has been offered by a team of experts with the Agency for Healthcare Research and Quality (AHRQ).[11] The team's plan deals specifically with planning for mass casualty events. It also stresses five guiding principles for preparedness, which include making sure that the healthcare system is operational and geared toward saving as many lives as possible and organizing a well-coordinated and comprehensive public health medical response. The plan also stresses protecting the rights of individuals wherever possible and making sure there is communication with the public in all stages of the response. The plan offers a series of recommendations to assist planners in dealing with the allocation of scarce resources in time of disaster.

ETHICS ISSUES AND GOVERNMENT DISASTER PLANNING AND RESPONSE

Government agencies have contributed a great deal of information, plans, and funding to assist in disaster planning and response. However, reports by news outlets and by the government agencies themselves reveal that major issues still exist with both the planning for and response to disasters. Many of these issues stem from ethical considerations. In fact, Roberts and DeRenzo[12] suggest that ethical responsibility begins with the plan itself. Because serious ethical decisions might need to be made once a disaster happens, it is necessary to be prepared ethically as well as logistically in the event of a disaster. This means that ethics needs to be a part of the plan's guiding principles and foundation. The very nature of a disaster presents conflicts of interest that will require a discussion and the formulation of standards that account for the community's interest, as well as of those who respond to the disaster.

A consistent theme in Roberts and DeRenzo's work is the necessity of balancing utilitarian and deontological views. In a disaster situation, many feel that the "greatest good for the greatest number" is the most logical approach, maximizing the benefits for as many people as possible, which usually is defined as the number of lives saved. An example of a utilitarian approach is found when healthcare providers are presented with the challenge of caring for the acutely sick and injured and managing those with chronic illnesses and special needs. In this case, triage provides a strategy for healthcare providers to offer the greatest good for the greatest number of disaster victims. Mass causality triaging was a wartime innovation, and it has evolved into grouping individuals based on medical need to achieve greater survival rates. Baker[13] contends that triage is driven by real-time events, the healthcare setting, and the management options available at the healthcare facility. Situational awareness, decisiveness, and clinical expertise are required in triaging disaster victims. Each healthcare facility should develop and practice a rigorous decision-making criteria for triaging.[14]

One type of triage system places casualties into the following groups: (1) nonsurvivable injuries; (2) those who would benefit from immediate life-saving interventions; (3) those who do not need immediate care; and (4) negligible injuries. This is just one grouping example; multiple systems of triage have been developed. Even though evidence-based research is limited on which type of triage is the most effective during a disasters,[15] its use demonstrates utilitarian ethics theory in action.

However, triage has a number of limitations when one considers the community's view. For example, after Hurricane Katrina a great deal of effort and money was expended to recover the remains of those who had died. Strict utilitarianism would find this to be unacceptable because the dead do not offer much benefit to the living. However, community values made this an effort important.

Some suggest that utilitarianism also needs to be balanced with concerns for Kantian, or duty-based, ethics. In the Kantian approach to ethics, all humans have worth. Therefore, it would be inappropriate to sacrifice some individuals over others, even if it meant ignoring the rule of the greatest good for the greatest number. For example, greater resources might need to be expanded to assist those who were elderly, ill, or otherwise vulnerable. Humanitarianism would not allow us to simply leave these people behind because they lacked economic resources to respond to the disaster in which they find themselves. Such actions would be regarded as a violation of the American sense of universal rights.

Another ethics issue that might emerge during a disaster is respect for autonomy. Individual freedom, which is part of the principle of autonomy, can often come into question. For example, should an individual have the right to build a home on a flood plain and not have flood insurance? If this decision is made, what is the government's responsibility if the person's home is destroyed by a flood? What if an individual has been exposed to a highly infectious disease? Does the community have the right to quarantine this individual against his or her will in an effort to protect vulnerable populations?

In addition, the concept of social justice is a major ethical consideration with respect to the government's response to disasters. When a disaster occurs, Americans expect that the government will do whatever it can to respond to the situation and to relieve the suffering of its citizens. Historically, Americans have been both compassionate and generous when disasters have occurred. However, when large amounts of capital (in the billions of dollars) are involved, the potential for fraud, abuse, and corruption exists. Such actions are not only are illegal, but also violate many ethical principles, including beneficence, nonmaleficence, and justice. When these actions are identified, the level of trust in the government is undermined, and people believe that those in government increase their own wealth by trading on the suffering of others. An example of a way that agencies attempt to prevent this loss of trust is found in the actions of the Red Cross. It attempts to restrict unethical behaviors such as fraud, abuse, and corruption by performing background checks on all employees and volunteers.

Ethics must be part of every agency's disaster plan—from its development to implementation and evaluation—in an effort to prevent fraud, abuse, and a loss of trust. It is helpful if the agency incorporates basic human values into its plan and that its mission statement is aligned with corporate ethics and values. Once disaster plans are developed, they should be reviewed not just in terms of resources, but also with an eye toward ethics and community acceptability.

Once a disaster plan has been developed that is congruent with corporate values and ethics, the second step is to communicate the ethical foundation on which the disaster plan is formulated and is to be implemented. To make sure that the plan's ethics are actually practiced, it should be practiced periodically. Clinical simulations often are used to provide practice and experiential learning. For example, local areas of the ARC periodically hold disaster drills. Volunteers from the community are actively encouraged to participate. This allows them not only to practice logistics, but also to think about ethical issues that they might face.

HEALTHCARE ORGANIZATIONS AND DISASTER PLANNING

The United States has over 7500 hospitals and these organizations represent the front line when a disaster occurs. Therefore, it is necessary for hospitals and the entire healthcare system to be prepared to respond effectively and efficiently when a crisis occurs. Although it is not possible to discuss all of the efforts being made by hospitals and the healthcare system with regard to disaster planning and response, examples will provide a helpful background. Information from the JCAHO and the AHRQ provides some general information on disaster planning and preparedness training in the nation's hospitals.

The JCAHO

The JCAHO is one of the more prominent forces in establishing minimum standards for acceptable practice for hospitals and many other healthcare facilities.[16] The *2006 Hospital Accreditation Standards for Emergency Management Planning*[17] offers standards for emergency management planning, drills, and other disaster-response activities. Standard EC.4 defines an emergency as anything that disrupts care. This disruption can be caused by damage to the hospital building, grounds, power systems, or telephone systems. The definition also includes events that create demand for hospital services, including plane crashes, floods, and accidents. It uses the term *potential injury-creating events* (PICEs) to describe potential emergencies.

One of the requirements under the JCAHO standards is that a hospital must conduct a hazard-vulnerability analysis to identify potential emergencies and their possible effect on hospital operations. This analysis should assist the hospital in developing an emergency management plan that is in accord with national and community responses. The plan must identify strategies for mitigation, response, and recovery when an emergency occurs. It must include plans for evacuation of the building and identify alternative care sites should that occur. Back-up needs for internal and external communication systems must be identified and detailed, and descriptions of staff responsibilities must be included.

Hospitals also are required to test their emergency management plans by responding to an actual emergency or conducting planned drills. These drills are required at least twice a year and must include community-wide practice. In addition to the standards for practice drills, separate standards address power sources, information systems, and patient flow. JCAHO also expects the hospital to prepare for the increased demand caused by an epidemic.

In light of recent events, JCAHO has become concerned about surge hospitals and the quality of care that they provide.[18] The JCAHO defines *surge hospitals* as places that allow a hospital to expand its services to quickly in the event of a major disaster. Facilities in this category include closed hospitals; nonmedical buildings, such as veterinary hospitals; convention centers; airport hangars; and schools. Surge hospitals also include mobile medical facilities and portable facilities sometimes called "hospitals in a box."

The JCAHO guidelines provide extensive information on how to plan for an established surge hospitals. It provides detailed information on code requirements, staffing, communication, and coordination. In addition, it offers discussion about what is considered to be sufficient care given the situation of a surge facility. Safety of care is of particular importance to JCAHO, and additional standards for surge hospitals are being considered.

The AHRQ

JCAHO is not the only organization that provides guidelines to assist hospitals in disaster planning and response efforts. The AHRQ has extensive information to guide healthcare facilities in planning for and responding to a variety of disaster situations. Its Web site[19] provides extensive information and resources for hospitals in designing their disaster response. For example, Web conferences and meetings have presented information on such topics as disaster planning drills, surge capacity assessments, and bioterrorism responses. Reports are provided on training clinicians and hospital staff for mass casualties. In addition, briefings are provided on such topics as smallpox, surge capacity, and mass prophylaxis (community preparedness). The Web site also offers assessment tools, including a resource inventory.

In its *Mass Medical Care with Scarce Resources Guide*,[20] the AHRQ provides a chapter specific to hospital and acute care facilities that presents the major issues and challenges facing these facilities now and in the future. For example, it identifies that hospitals are already near capacity in their ability to respond to trauma events, and that communication systems often are incompatible. Despite these challenges, hospitals and acute care facilities need to take the lead when mass causality events occur. AHRQ offers examples of how to be prepared to respond to mass causality situations, increase the system's capacity, and develop an integrated management system. It even provides a template to facilitate discussion and planning.

Organizations that provide first responders to disasters also are engaged in many planning and training efforts. These organizations include local and state police departments, fire departments, emergency medical care systems, public health departments, and long-term care facilities. These organizations must prepare first responders to handle rescues, mass casualties, and recovery from and mitigation of disaster events. In addition, they need to be sensitive to the mental health of individuals who are the front line when disasters occur. First responders can experience acute stress responses and suffer from posttraumatic stress disorder. Organizations that employ first responders have an obligation to do whatever they can to protect the physical and mental health of these extraordinary individuals.

Ethics Issues and Health Organization Disaster Planning and Response

Development of a systematic infrastructure and superstructure that links healthcare agencies, government entities, and the community together is a complex and complicated task. However, it seems that the individual is the common link (see Figure 23–1). With respect to the ethical aspects of disaster response, the model shown in Figure 23–1 assumes that individuals have ethical reasoning ability. However, no two people are alike; each person has a different perspective due to the influence of culture, religion, and life experiences. When planning for a disaster, healthcare providers must be aware of the individual, not just the organization, and should consider the ethical reasoning and decision-making capabilities of potential team members.[21]

Keeping the model shown in Figure 23–1 in mind, healthcare organizations must be aware that dealing with disasters and mass causality events often requires more than just a logistical response. Disasters challenge the ethical foundations of both healthcare organizations and individuals. Each situation and setting will bring its own ethical challenges for healthcare facilities and providers.

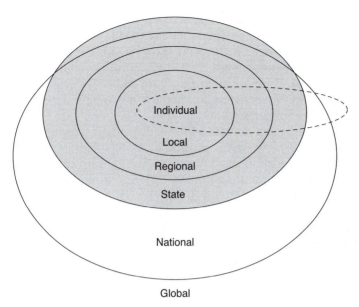

Figure 23–1 Individual as Common Link
Data from S. Sasser, "Field triage in disasters," Prehospital Emergency Care 10 (2006): 322–323, and B. Rogers, and E. Lawhorn, Disaster Preparedness: Occupational and Environmental Health Professionals' Response to Hurricanes Katrina and Rita," American Association of Occupational Health Nurses 5 no. 5 (2007): 197–207.

Obviously, most disaster situations challenge the use of already-scarce healthcare resources. They require an ability to balance the principles of utilitarianism with the ethics of deontology. Hospitals must decide the best use of these scarce resources while remembering to honor the worth of all people. For example, consider a rescue situation. First responders must decide who to save and in what order. This heartrending and difficult decision too often must be made in an instant. Those who are mobile often are rescued first, because they require fewer resources. The elderly, ill, handicapped, or otherwise disabled might be left until later. Although this is an attempt to provide the greatest good for the greatest number when using a scarce resource, it can create situations where professionals are tempted to assist in the death of patients rather than watch them suffer. However, the action of saving the healthy over those who are not would be highly offensive to those who practice Kantian ethics.

Another major ethical dilemma might occur for first responders and hospital staff. A conflict of duty can exist between their duty to the community and to their family. In a disaster situation, these individuals are required by their professional ethics and responsibilities to care for the needs of the community even when their own safety may be endangered. However, they also are human and are concerned about what might be happening to their own families. This causes a conflict and a sense of moral ambiguity. Should they stay and care for the needs of the community, or leave and take care of their own families?

One way a hospital or other agency can assist with this dilemma is to include plans for the families of those who respond to emergencies in the overall disaster response plan. In this way, professionals can be where they are most needed with the knowledge that their families are receiving attention and care, if needed. Such assurance would make it less likely that those charged with disaster response would leave their assignments in order to protect the needs of their families.

Social justice also is a great ethical issue during disaster and mass casualty situations. Emergency systems, including first responders and hospitals, must be aware of the need for fairness. Both in planning for and responding to disasters, they must strive to protect human rights, including the rights of vulnerable populations such as children, the elderly, and the disabled. However, community rights must not be overlooked. They have a right to get assistance in a reasonable amount of time from staff members who are prepared to deal with their needs. They must feel that, when difficult choices must be made, they are made using a plan that considers autonomy, nonmaleficence, beneficence, and justice.

INDIVIDUAL RESPONSE TO DISASTERS

Despite the extensive media coverage of disasters and mass casualty events, the American Red Cross and Wirthlin Worldwide[22] found that the U.S. public is not prepared for disasters. Although the public acknowledges its vulnerability, it has not taken actions to prepare for such events. A study conducted by these two organizations found that only 1 household in 10 followed the Red Cross recommendations for preparedness. Some of the most vulnerable, such as low-income families, are the least prepared to deal with emergencies. Others simply do not feel that it necessary or are too busy to make the effort.

What should individuals do to be better prepared for emergencies? According to the Red Cross[23], people should be "Red Cross Ready" in the event of an emergency. This readiness includes preparing an emergency first aid kit that will enable people to care for their own emergencies. This is especially important because, in the event of a major disaster, government assistance might not be immediate. Preparedness also includes having a least three days worth of supplies for survival. This means have at least one gallon of water and 1600 calories of food that does not require cooking per person per day. These survival materials should be stored in containers that are easily accessible. The Red Cross also asks individuals to include money, a flashlight, a battery-operated radio, and prescription medicines in the emergency kit.

Preparedness also requires that individuals develop a disaster plan. This plan should contain information about what they would do in an emergency. It should identify where they would go and whom they would need to contact. The Red Cross encourages individuals to communicate their plan to family members and friends and even to conduct practice sessions so that they are prepared in an emergency. Finally, individuals should know about the types of disasters that could occur in their area and how to get accurate information pertaining to them. The Red Cross also encourages everyone to learn first aid and CPR because it may take time for emergency medical staff to reach everyone in a major disaster.

The CDC[24] suggests that individuals might have to shelter-in-place when a disaster occurs. This means that people must be able to take steps to prevent contamination if a chemical or radiological disaster occurs. The CDC suggests choosing a room in the home to prepare as a shelter. This room would contain a disaster supply kit and food and sufficient water supply for the family. Businesses should have an emergency plan to get employees to a designated shelter. This shelter should have first aid kits, food, and water. Police or fire departments should have the ability to issue warnings whenever shelter-in-place is necessary.

Redlener[25] suggests that the most important disaster-planning principles are not emphasized in materials that are available to the public. Redlener believes that not only must citizens be physically prepared, they must be mentally ready for disasters and for survival. He stresses that people must be physically fit to survive in a disaster situation. They also need to have considered what they would do in an emergency and how they would survive. This may require devising a plan and practicing it.

Redlener also suggests that citizens receive CPR and first aid training either through the Red Cross or another entity. It also is important to be aware of one's situation at work, home, or in the community. This might include knowing how to exit buildings, being aware of people in your surroundings, and anticipating any dangers in your environment. Redlener believes that Americans need to be more informed about their own communities and the potential for disasters.

In accordance with the Red Cross suggestions, Redlener asks individuals to have a family plan for emergencies. This would include how to care for family members who are elderly, neighbors who might be disabled, or coworkers who might need additional assistance. Plans should address situations that require rapid evacuation and shelter-in-place situations. Communication also is essential during an emergency, so individuals must prepare for situations in which telephones might not be operational. Cell phones and/or two-way communication devices might become lifelines because they can be operated with batteries. Finally, he suggests that families need to realize that this is an age where major disasters can be caused by nature or by human intervention. Citizens and families need to feel that they can control what happens to them by being prepared.

Ethics Implications for Individual Response to Disasters

When a disaster strikes, individuals might face a number of ethical problems. Fear and injury can cause people to act in a survival mode that might not respect the rights and dignity of others. Panic might cause some to harm individuals or property. In fact, disaster survival might cause people to examine their ethics and their behaviors on many levels.

In the United States, individuals tend to expect the government to respond in a timely manner whenever any type of emergency occurs. They put great faith in the ability of the government to handle emergencies. However, individuals are asked to prepare to handle emergencies on their own because government help may not be imminent. Citizens sometimes feel that they are paying tax dollars for these services, and become upset when they are told they are not adequate. Although preparedness is important, individuals can lose trust in their government and begin to question its ability.

Autonomy is another ethical issue for individuals. As government and organizations begin to use high-tech tools to prevent potential disasters, individuals are beginning to question how much of their privacy and autonomy is being lost versus the benefits gained. For example, more and more cities are adding camera surveillance on streets to protect against potential terrorist acts or other crimes. Although this technology benefits the police in terms of crime prevention and prosecution of criminals, some question its value in light of the loss of personal freedom. Others believe that such surveillance is the beginning of a slippery slope where all citizens are watched and autonomy is nonexistent.

Beneficence also is an issue for individuals in both planning and responding to disasters. Without acts of beneficence, many will not survive in a disaster situation. Citizens become truly their brothers' and sisters' keepers in such times. However, in planning for disasters individuals have to consider how far their responsibility goes. Are they going to be responsible for all the elderly in their neighborhood, or just for their immediate family members? Who will be responsible for those in the community who might require extra relief during a disaster? What is the gap between individual beneficence and the government's responsibility? These questions will be troubling for individuals who wish to live an ethical life. They also pose a challenge to an individual's concept of a duty or deontology.

CONCLUSION

This chapter is only a beginning in the study of ethics as it relates to disaster planning and response. The efforts discussed and the ethics issues presented are only a sampling of what occurs when considering this great responsibility. However, the information provided should spark discussion regarding the ethics of government, health care, and individual responsibility for protection from and response to human-caused or natural disasters. It is not possible to predict the types of disasters Americans will face in the twenty-first century. What is true is that others judge this country by how it responds to such events both logistically and ethically.

SUMMARY

The possibility of human-caused or natural disasters is always present. Society expects both government and healthcare institutions to respond to these events in an effective and efficient manner. In fact, as a nation, we are judged on how we respond when these events occur. This chapter provides an overview of some of the government and healthcare disaster preparedness efforts and discusses the ethical issues they raise. In addition, it provides information about individual's responsibility to prepare for the event of a disaster. Certainly, the issue of disaster preparation and the ethical issues it creates is one that will continue into the rest of the twenty-first century.

QUESTIONS FOR DISCUSSION

1. What ethical theories that you have studied apply to the use of scarce resources in a disaster situation?

2. How can individual healthcare professionals prepare themselves to deal with potential disaster situations?

3. Do you think the funds spent on disaster drills are worth the expenditure? How can you defend your answer from an ethics standpoint?

4. Who should be responsible for what happens during a disaster: the individual or the government?

5. Review a disaster plan for a healthcare facility. What is the focus of this disaster plan? On what type of ethical principles is this disaster plan based?

6. When chaos is prominent, can one expect others to demonstrate ethical decision-making abilities? Why or why not?

NOTES

1. M. Baker, "Creating Order from Chaos: Part I: Triage, Initial Care, and Tactical Considerations in Mass Casualty and Disaster Response," *Military Medicine* 172 (2007): 232–236.

2. M. Baker, op. cit.; S. Sasser, "Field Triage in Disasters," *Prehospital Emergency Care* 10 (2006): 322–323; B. Rogers and E. Lawhorn, "Disaster Preparedness: Occupational and Environmental Health Professionals' Response to Hurricanes Katrina and Rita," *American Association of Occupational Health Nurses* 5, no. 5 (2007): 197–207.

3. M. Baker, op. cit.; S. Sasser, op. cit.

4. M. Baker, op. cit.

5. I. Redlener, *Americans at Risk* (New York: Albert A. Knopf, 2006).

6. See www.whitehouse.gov/omb/budget/fy2005/homeland.html.

7. See www.cdc.gov./index.html.

8. See www.fema.gov.

9. See www.redcross.org.

10. I. Redlener, op. cit.

11. See www.ahrq.gov.

12. M. Roberts and E. G. DeRenzo, "Chapter II. Ethical Considerations in Community Disaster Planning," in *Mass Medical Care with Scarce Resources: A Community Planning Guide*, S. J. Phillips and A. Knebel, eds. (Rockville, MD: Agency for Health Research and Quality, 2007), 9–23.

13. M. Baker, op. cit. See also J. T. Ihlenfeld, "A Primer on Triage and Mass Casualty Events," *Dimensions of Critical Care Nursing* 22, no. 5 (2003): 204–207; R. Lanoix, D. E. Wiener, and V. D. Zayas, "Concepts in Disaster Triage in the Wake of the World Trade Center Terrorist Attack," *Topics in Emergency Medicine* 24, no. 2 (2002): 60–70; M. E. Sheeley and N. Mahoney, "A New Reality: Mass Casualty Teams," *Nursing Management* (April 2007): 39B–40H.

14. M. Baker, op. cit.

15. S. Sasser, op. cit.

16. See www.jcaho.org.

17. Joint Commission on Accreditation of Healthcare Organizations, *2006 Hospital Accreditation Standards for Emergency Management Planning, Emergency Management Drills, Infection Control, and Disaster Privileges* (Chicago: Joint Commission on Accreditation of Healthcare Organizations, 2006).

18. Joint Commission on Accreditation of Healthcare Organizations, *Surge Hospitals: Providing Safe Care in Emergencies*, (Chicago: Joint Commission on Accreditation of Healthcare Organizations, 2006).

19. See the AHRQ Web site for information on planning and response information: www.ahrq.gov/prep/.

20. J. L. Hick, G. Kelen, D. O'Laughlin, L. Rubinson, R. Waldhorn, and D. P. Whalen, "Hospital/Acute Care," in *Mass Medical Care with Scarce Resources: A Community Planning Guide*, S. J. Phillips and A. Knebel, eds. (Rockville, MD: Agency for Health Research and Quality, 2007), 53–74. See also A. Katz, A. B. Staiti, and K. McKenzie, "Preparing for the Unknown: Community and Public Health Preparedness," *Health Affairs* 25, no. 4 (2006): 945–957.

21. E. Morrison, *Ethics in Health Administration: A Practical Approach to Decision Making* (Sudbury, MA: Jones and Bartlett Publishers, 2006).

22. American Red Cross and Wirthlin Worldwide, "U.S. Public Unprepared," *The Wirthlin Report* 13, no. 5 (2004).

23. See www.redcross.org.

24. See www.cdc.gov./index.html.

25. I. Redlener, op. cit.

CHAPTER 24

Looking Toward the Future

Eileen E. Morrison

OVERVIEW

This last chapter is reserved for a summary of the themes encountered in the previous four sections of the text. Each chapter in the text presented issues of grave ethical concern and described a world of conflict between the ethical, the clinical, and the financial. However, you should not be alarmed by what you have read. Rather, consider the opportunities each of these themes presents for ethical decision making in your practice.

This chapter also includes some emergent issues not previously addressed. They also have the potential to alter how we think about and practice health care. Although this chapter cannot present every future issue, four have been selected based on their potential impact on clinical practice. They are: the impact of technology; changes in disease experience, including childhood obesity; patient-focused care; and concern about the environment. These areas are discussed in the "Emergent Issues" section of the chapter.

SUMMARY OF SECTION THEMES

Part 1, "Foundations in Theory," provided an overview of the most commonly-held ethics theories and principles used in the American healthcare system. Summers presented a scholarly overview to establish a foundation for further study of the application of ethics to issues for the twenty-first century. The following themes emerged from this part of the text:

1. There is no one theory of ethics that will apply to every situation. Each theory has strengths and limitations.
2. Knowledge of the ethical theories is useful in practice because it allows you to critically think about the issue that you face before you act upon it.
3. Virtue ethics needs to be considered as you build your expertise and practice because it is about your character and your professional presence in the world.
4. The principles of ethics are derived from theory and are useful in making decisions that benefit the individual and the community as a whole.
5. Patients expect you to practice beneficence and nonmaleficence. However, the practice of autonomy and justice often poses difficult choices.
6. The reflective equilibrium model provides a tool for making difficult ethical decisions.

In Part II, "Critical Issues for Individuals," you explored the complexity of ethical issues faced by individuals who use the healthcare system. The chapters were presented in life-cycle order, beginning with the unborn facing the challenge of just how they come to be. You were able to explore the concept of whether those who have not yet been born have rights and the impact of technology on their existence.

Once a person is conceived, the ethics issues continue. In Chapters 6 and 7, you considered the ethical implications of being able to diagnose diseases before birth and its impact on the existence of the individual. You also read about finding a middle ground on the abortion debate. These controversial areas will most certainly continue to be among those you face as you practice in the twenty-first century.

Additional ethical issues arise once a person becomes an adult. Chapter 7 presented an overview of what it means to be competent and to make your own healthcare decisions. Although this might appear simple on the surface, it becomes increasingly difficult when you consider all of the variables that can affect competency. Chapter 8 provided a thorough overview of the Patient Self-Determination Act. Although this law was enacted in the 1990s, it still has the potential to affect how you advise your patients in the future.

Chapters 9 and 10 presented issues related to the elderly and long-term care. The issues presented in these chapters will certainly be of concern in healthcare practice given the potential increase for the need for long-term care services. The aging of the baby boomer generation alone should call your attention to the ethical issues raised in these two chapters.

The last three chapters in Part II dealt with end-of-life issues. These chapters provided both information and ethical challenges. These challenges have been highlighted in recent media-focused cases and are sure to be part of the future of health care. Because of the even greater number of people facing the end of their lives each year, the issues presented must be considered and resolved in an ethical manner.

In Part III, "Critical Issues for Healthcare Organizations," six topics were presented among the many ethical issues faced by healthcare organizations. The topics were selected to represent both critical issues and different types of healthcare organizations. For example, Chapters 14 and 15 were concerned with ethical issues faced by hospitals and hospital systems. These chapters attempted to clarify the differences between institutional ethical positions and clinical ones. In addition, the nature of ethics committees, their decision-making processes, and the current and future issues they face are part of the presentation in Chapter 15. If you plan to practice in a hospital setting, you should find these chapters particularly helpful.

Healthcare organizations other than the hospital also are discussed in Part III. Chapter 16 provided an overview of managed care and discussed its unique ethical issues. It included information on how managed care organizations can decrease conflicts of interest and demonstrate core ethical practices. In light of the potential changes in healthcare financing, including a movement to consumer-driven care, it is important to understand the need for ethical practice among the financial members of health care.

Chapter 18 discussed what happens when technology is introduced to the home care of severely ill children and adults. Although these advances have produced miracles in terms of life extension, they also produce ethical issues for those who must assure access and financing. Finally, Chapter 19 introduced a concept that has been at the core of healthcare organizations, but has come to be less recognized—spirituality in the healthcare workplace. It is important to understand why this issue has become of interest in the twenty-first century and how it relates to the ethics of clinical practice.

Part IV, "Critical Issues in Societal Health," featured selected issues that affect more than the individual or the organization. The selected topics in this section started with an examination of the healthcare system itself, including its inequalities and the ethics of rationing care. Specific issues such as domestic violence and disaster relief also are included as examples of areas that affect all Americans and present serious ethical dilemmas.

EMERGENT ISSUES

A plethora of issues and challenges will be a part of a professional practice as it attempts to provide patient services that are evidence-based, safe, cost-effective, and ethically sound. In addition to having knowledge and skills in their fields, healthcare professionals must plan for these future practice and ethical contingencies. What does the future portend? The only true certainty is change. These changes promise to reach into the core of what it means to practice as a healthcare professional. They will require introspection and action so that the issues they create can be addressed prospectively rather than retroactively. Less "wheel spinning" and more positive actions are needed if healthcare professionals are to maintain their currency and ability to practice care in what could be a vastly different world.

Although it is not within the scope of this chapter to examine every one of the possible changes for health care, it makes sense to examine four areas that seem to be potential change drivers. These four areas include technology, disease experience, patient-focused practice, and the environment. The issues and challenges for healthcare ethics presented by these areas will be discussed.

Technology

Technology is first among the change drivers because it could be seen as the "mother of all issues." It is the overarching issue because its changes are so profound that they can potentially affect all areas of clinical practice, all healthcare organizations, and society. A brief examination of technology's importance to American culture is needed understand the ethics challenges it brings to future healthcare practice.

The more information one learns about technology, the more obvious it becomes that Americans have of love affair with its allure and promises. This fascination with technology is not new. Americans have a long history of developing and embracing technology, beginning with early innovators like Benjamin Franklin and extending to the latest of the creative geniuses. Technology has become so much a part of American culture that many people cannot conceive of an existence without cell phones, iPods, laptops, and HDTV. Many feel that technology has become diffused into the culture to the point that its use is expected by many members of American society.

Of course, this technology love affair is not without its limitations. In fact, it can become a love/hate relationship for some. For example, many Americans do not trust technology and worry about its intrusion into their privacy. In health care, this concern is voiced about the advancement of the electronic medical record (EMR) and what could occur in the event of inappropriate access to patients' most private information. In an age of talented hackers and sometimes-sloppy security, patients' concern might not be completely unmerited. However, many scholars believe that with the Internet and other emerging technologies, privacy is already lost. It is just a matter of how much privacy Americans are willing to give up for the convenience of things such as EMR and what they are willing to do to protect it.

Dependency also is a part of the love/hate aspect of the technology love affair. The expression "technology is great, when it works" is becoming all too common. For the individual technology aficionado, the frustration that occurs when the lover (technology) fails to deliver on its promises causes stress. This makes one wonder if the technology is truly one's friend. However, when there is a technology failure in a healthcare system, the effects can be devastating and have a massive impact on the provision of care. Recent disasters, such as Hurricane Katrina, have exemplified both society's dependency on technology and the profound impact of its failure. Although no one wants to go back to the slide rule and the rotary telephone, the almost complete dependency on technology gives cause for concern and the need for serious back-up planning to reduce its impact when failure occurs.

Whether it is in the love or hate stage, the technology love affair leads to an increase in what has been called the digital divide. Certain members of American society, because of variables such as economics, education, or age, do not have access to technology that can impact their ability to have the same quality of life as other Americans. In addition, even if they have the ability to purchase the latest technology, they might find the required learning curve and new jargon too daunting and simply give up in frustration. In respect to health care, this gap between the "technology-sophisticate" and the "technology-bereft" can seriously impact the individual's ability to access health information, contact health resources, and partner in his or her own health care. It can also affect the overall healthcare system in terms of budget, hiring practices, training costs, and error production.[1]

Because technology is so much a part of the future of health care, and its impact promises to increase exponentially, it seems important to explore a few specific examples of what the future of medical technology could be. These examples illustrate both the impact of technology and serve as a launch pad for a discussion of its ethical challenges. In diagnosis for example, the emphasis will no longer be on the maxim that all disease has the same pattern for the species. Technology such as DNA chips will enable the precise diagnosis for individuals. By using a chip that has known DNA sequences, blood samples can be analyzed to isolate an individual's specific pathogens, cancer cells, and genetic disease potential.

On its surface, this diagnostic innovation appears to be an amazing tool for removing the threat of disease on the quality of life. However, it is not without drawbacks that have ethical ramifications. First, there is the utilitarian issue of cost benefit. Although the cost of DNA chips will eventually decrease, they are projected to cost hundreds, or even thousands, of dollars per chip.[2] Is the cost for this technology worth the benefit it provides for the patient?

Most certainly, the individual benefits. However, this innovation poses a larger ethical issue for society. Which patients will receive the benefit of a DNA chip? Should it be available to everyone, or just to those who have the ability to pay? If one assumes that the market will prevail, than there is certainly an issue with deontology and social justice.

Other computer-related technologies also promise astounding benefits and changes in the healthcare system. For example, Intel is rapidly making progress on radio frequency identification tags (RFID) to assist with the care of elderly patients. These devices could be used in tracking people within their home and determining whether they have taken their medications appropriately. The technology has the potential to actually coach patients on when and how to take their medications, thereby increasing compliance. Research also is being conducted on the use of holograms to detect when patient glucose levels are too high or too low. This technology would provide the practitioner and the patient with the convenience of continuous feedback for monitoring compliance with treatment.

What ethical problems might this new technology create? First is the increasing dependence on technology and the incursion of technology deeper into the personal lives of patients. Despite the benefits of such innovation, the anxiety about loss of personal autonomy could become an issue and limit the use of such technologies. As discussed in the previous example, the utilitarian decision about who would be eligible to receive such technologies and how to pay for this benefit also would become an issue.

Even with these limited examples, it becomes clear that technology is both a boon to patient treatment and a bane to ethics-based practice. The key to successfully implementing technological advances as they are created is to discuss the ethical ramifications and to determine how practitioners and organizations will address them. Without this thought process, technology could overwhelm the ethical foundations on which health care is established.

Disease Experience

Another critical issue that promises profound impact on the delivery of health care in America is the changing disease experience. Although many disease variations have already emerged as issues, including penicillin-resistant staph infections, new viral strains, and the reemergence of tuberculosis, perhaps the most far-reaching problem is the obesity epidemic. In fact, the United States leads all developed nations in the prevalence of obesity. When both childhood and adult obesity is considered, it becomes clear that this problem has the potential to overwhelm the healthcare system. Just how extensive is the problem?

According to the National Center for Health Statistics at the Centers for Disease Control, approximately 32 percent of all Americans are obese. However, this is not just a problem for adults. Even more serious is the level of obesity in children. Trends are demonstrating increases in all age groups, including those aged 2 through 5. The prevalence for children between the ages of 6 and 11 has increased to almost 19 percent, and for those aged 12 to 19 it has increased to 17 percent.[3]

Although these numbers are startling in and of themselves, they also portend a number of serious health consequences. Overweight and obesity has been associated with an increased risk for hypertension, type 2 diabetes, coronary heart disease, stroke, arthritis, asthma, and even some cancers. In addition, childhood obesity can lead to psychosocial problems, including low self-esteem and social discrimination. These problems often exist even into adulthood. Preliminary studies also indicate that obesity may be associated with the premature onset of puberty. A recent study conducted by the Mott Children's Hospital at the University of Michigan indicated that obesity is associated with the onset of puberty occurring as early as nine years of age. Early onset of puberty has been associated with many other health outcomes, including teenage pregnancy, adult obesity, and cancer.[4]

Obesity is present in all socioeconomic groups in America. However, certain groups, and even certain states, seem to have greater incidence of this problem. For example, according to the Centers for Disease Control (CDC), several states, including Texas, Louisiana, Alabama, and Arkansas, have obesity rates of over 25 percent. Certain groups within the larger population also have different incidences of obesity. For example, approximately 37 percent of Mexican-American adults are obese, as compared to 30 percent of non-Hispanic white adults. The incident rate for non-Hispanic Black adults is 45 percent.

The CDC estimates the cost of obesity to exceed 9 percent of total medical costs in the United States. This includes direct costs for treatment of diseases related to these conditions and indirect costs, such as loss of productivity, absenteeism, and loss of income because of premature death.[5] Clearly, obesity affects the current delivery of health care, and certain groups have an increased incidence of this problem. If current trends continue, obesity, and particularly childhood obesity with its long-range consequences, could cause a major crisis for the healthcare system because of increased demand. It will most certainly affect the future cost of health care as the rate of obesity-related diseases continues to increase. What are the ethics concerns surrounding the epidemic of obesity in America?

First, consider the issue from a theoretical view. Utilitarianism seeks to provide the greatest good for the greatest number or, in the inverse, to prevent the greatest harm for the greatest number. What is its ethics position with respect to obesity? Treating the condition and preventing it in the future, especially among children, could provide the greatest benefit to the greatest number in terms of quality of life and cost to the system. Increased emphasis on lifestyle changes (e.g., diet, exercise, and stress management), changes in the food industry, and even an emphasis on school lunch programs will be required. However, the healthcare system is not designed for prevention on this scale. Where is the profit in prevention? Major changes in the basic orientation of the healthcare system may be required for it to function with a utilitarian view on this issue.

What about deontology? Obesity, like other lifestyle-related problems, carries a social stigma. This stigma cannot be a part of the deontology view because respect for patients irrespective of their condition is a mandate. It also is part of the concept of beneficence and should be an integral part of health care in general. As the prevalence of obesity increases, it will be easier and easier to ignore this basic tenant and blame the individual. Prejudice against the obese seems to be much more socially acceptable than prejudice against ethnic minorities. Education will be necessary to remind healthcare practitioners to function on a high level of deontology and beneficence and not to allow their own prejudices to impact the quality of their care.

The principle of autonomy must also be considered when thinking about the impact of the obesity epidemic. It is sometimes difficult for healthcare practitioners to understand why a person becomes obese. Their education, practice, and lack of cultural sensitivity often preclude an understanding of the individual's circumstances and health status. In addition, practitioners might place the total responsibility for treating this condition on the individual.

Although autonomy must honor an individual's ability to make choices, it does not mean that healthcare professionals have no responsibility to the patient. Healthcare providers are required to provide information and education so that the individual can make intelligent choices about how best to address his or her obesity. This implies that best practices have been identified for the treatment of obesity and can be communicated to the patient. Again, the healthcare system has not been designed for this type of chronic care treatment, so a major change in orientation may be required.

Autonomy also means that the patient has a choice not to adhere to the medical protocols that are prescribed for his or her care. Although this aspect of autonomy must be respected, it does pose a problem for the healthcare system. If the patient does not take any responsibility for his or her lifestyle, what is the system's ethical responsibility? This question might become a major one in the future if there is no intervention in the obesity epidemic. Can the system continue to pay for treatment of preventable conditions when the patient's actions actually exacerbate the condition? If the system should be responsible, how can this treatment be financed?

Finally, the principle of justice with respect to the obesity of epidemic merits consideration. What is just in this situation? Should those who have a more significant burden because of their social economic circumstances, ethnicity, or age be given greater attention? Should obese individuals have to assume greater financial and personal responsibility for their condition? Should there be a penalty for obesity, either through insurance copays or other financial mechanisms? The epidemic certainly raises many justice-type questions which need to be addressed in the immediate future.

Patient-Focused Care

It would seem logical that all health care would be patient-focused. However, because of many variables, including technology, patient-safety issues, and the educational experience of healthcare professionals, care has become much more centered on the professional rather than on the patient. However, emphasis on patient-focused care has been increasing because of the trend toward consumerism in health care and the work of the Planetree movement founded by Thieriot in 1978.[6] In addition, the increasingly higher utilization of the healthcare system by the baby boomers also promises a different set of expectations for the system and its providers.

It should be remembered that the patient's view of the healthcare system is not the same as the professional's view. For the professional, the system exists to enhance diagnosis, treatment, and to some extent, management of disease. The protocols associated with these functions are based on statistics and evidence. Following these protocols should yield efficient, cost-effective treatment that can effectively move patients through the system. A certain lack of emotional involvement is essential in maintaining objectivity and the successful provision of health care.

For patients, the experience of the healthcare system is entirely different. First, they are not even labeled as patients until they enter the system. Before this happens, they have made a number of efforts to treat their symptoms, including self-assessment, self-medication, and lifestyle changes. When these efforts have not been successful, the individual seeks the assistance of the professionals within the healthcare system. Once this contact is made and a diagnosis is given, the person becomes a patient. He or she is expected to assume the sick role, which includes compliance with the prescribed treatment regime, change in lifestyle behaviors, and a minimal amount of complaining.

Patients often experience more than a physical response to their illnesses. Depending on its severity, the illness can actually change the patient's entire life and relationships with family and friends. It is not surprising then that patients have a different expectation of the healthcare system. In general, they are looking for an environment that provides them with sufficient treatment and education to promote healing, not just a response to their diagnoses or symptoms. They have an expectation that professionals will act with beneficence and nonmaleficence. When this does not occur, they lose faith and trust in the system on which they must depend. An example of this loss of trust can be seen in the recent reports of substandard patient treatment of injured military personnel at Walter Reed Hospital and other centers.

Future changes in funding, legislation, and consumer power will certainly affect the need and demand for greater provision of patient-focused care. The challenge will be whether the system will be able to evolve rapidly enough to address this issue. Of course, such a difference in the orientation of the system can provoke its own set of ethical challenges.

One of the ethical challenges is centered on autonomy. In this case, the question becomes whose autonomy is the most important: the patient's or their clinician's? For the clinician, there is a need to be able to make patient treatment decisions based on superior knowledge and experience. Education, licensure, and continuing education provide the professional with the autonomy to decide what is best for the patient. Although this may be seen as paternalism, it is actually based in the desire to be both beneficent and to avoid harming the patient.

From the patient's view, the sanctity of their bodies and their feelings should be respected. They desire the ability to be a partner in their healthcare treatment rather than to submit without recourse. In addition, the number of patients who are likely to want a more autonomous role in their treatment is rising with the increased numbers of baby boomers seeking medical care. This creates a potential conflict between patient and clinician and presents a certain ethical challenge for the future.

In addition, the principle of justice should be considered in responding to the need for patient-focused care. What is fairness in response to this issue? Is it fair to address the patient's need to be treated with dignity and respect, or does this hinder efficient care? The answer on the surface seems to be "of course, we should respect the patient's rights." However, one also must consider the need to balance the benefit of cost-effective care against the burden of providing patient-centered care. Even though most of what patients require is not, at the surface, costly, the necessary shift in focus and treatment may create extra costs in training and design of delivery. Does this expense constitute an unnecessary burden on the healthcare system?

Protecting the Environment

In 2007, a film about the environment called *An Inconvenient Truth* won an Oscar. Although this film and its companion book are not without detractors, the recognition the work has attracted is indicative of an increased interest in the environment, especially global warming. What future ethics issues are presented by the changes in the environment?

The concern about the environment has grown from providing clean air, water, and safe housing. It has moved to the far more serious issue of sustaining the global environment itself. Sustaining the environment involves balancing what humans feel that they need to take from it with what it needs to support life for all species. Sustainability also involves taking environmental responsibility for the technologies that we create, whether they are found in new transportation or the latest communication device.

The use of the energy appears to be one of the main issues surrounding this responsibility and balancing act. As the world population grows and countries gain more wealth, demand for energy sources also increases. Because fossil fuels are currently the most inexpensive source of energy, there is increased concern about the excess demand and cost of supplying these fuels in a world market. Arguments are being made for increasing investment on a worldwide basis in alternative energy forms, including solar, wind, hydrogen, and hydroelectric power.

One must also consider the use of resources and the responsibility associated with their use. For example, the United States uses over 30 percent of the world's energy and each American consumes five times the average energy used in the world.[7] Because much of this energy comes from fossil fuels, people in the United States must be concerned about overuse of these irreplaceable resources and contribution to environmental problems, such as carbon dioxide emissions and smog. In addition, they must have the greatest concern for creating new sources of energy in order to be members of the environmental community.

The whole issue of sustainability of the environment is too large to be completely discussed here. However, ethical support certainly exists for caring about what happens to the world in which we all must live. For example, virtue ethics stresses practical wisdom and the ethical life. Is it is not an example of practical wisdom to do whatever we can to protect the world in which we live? Certainly, utilitarianism could also support the need to advance the knowledge and practices needed to sustain the global environment. It would seem logical that the greatest good for the greatest number is found in preserving the environment. Deontology could also support making every effort to preserve the environment as ethical duty. Certainly providing a livable environment passes the categorical imperative.

With respect to principles of ethics, the practice of justice seems appropriate. Because the United States consumes so much of the world's energy, it derives the greatest benefit from that energy. The justice principle of balancing benefits with burdens seems to indicate that the United States needs to take the lead in research, policy, and practice regarding sustainability of the environment. Although this is a highly charged political challenge, it certainly needs serious consideration, both now and in the future.

Ethical principles of beneficence, nonmaleficence, and autonomy should arguably be part of the consideration for sustainability. What greater kindness can be expressed than actions to preserve the environment in which we all must live? Because we are capable of causing great harm to the environment, we must constantly be aware of our actions and the potential harm they can cause. Such awareness should lead to actions that decrease environmental harm wherever possible. There are several ethical issues with respect to autonomy. How can we respect the autonomy of the individual, employer, and other members of society and still take action to protect the environment? This issue alone will be the source of future debate for both the United States and the larger global community.

Healthcare organizations cannot be ignorant of their responsibility for protecting the environment. Strategic planning efforts must include actions that decrease the amount of environmental damage caused by the institution. For example, healthcare facilities need to be conscientious about handling of waste products, recycling, and reusing materials. In addition, facilities, including hospitals, need to be much more aware of the practices associated with "green facilities."[8] These policies include water efficiency, the environmental impact of site location, construction materials, air quality, and waste reduction. Green hospitals also provide healthy food and education and use nonhazardous cleaning products in their daily operations. Although some administrators regard "greening" as a just a fad, communities served by hospitals and clinics are concerned about their environmental impact. Efforts at "greening" have received a favorable response and certainly warrant some thought from an ethical viewpoint.

CONCLUSION

The emerging issues presented in this chapter represent only a few of those that might be encountered in the twenty-first century. However, when the potential impact of these issues is considered, it becomes clear that they cannot be ignored. Each has the potential to affect dramatically how health care is practiced. In addition, if ignored, each could create a demand on the system that could prove difficult to meet clinically and financially. Finally, and some would argue most importantly, these issues will pose ethical concerns that must be part of future thinking and planning. Because knowledge is power, awareness of these issues should better prepare professionals to address them and practice health care in an ethics-based manner.

SUMMARY

This chapter summarizes the themes given each of the parts of this text. In addition, it presents four emergent issues that were not addressed, but are certainly part of healthcare ethics for the twenty-first century. The first issue of technology and its rapid evolution is one that challenges the industry both ethically and fiscally. The second issue of disease experience is also fraught with ethical concerns. For example, we will struggle with the ethical complexity and financial ramifications of childhood obesity for years to come.

The third issue of patient-focused care often surprises healthcare practitioners. We assume that we are in the patient care business and that we are always providing patient-focused care. However, this may not be the case from the patient's view. Ethics, especially concern for patient autonomy, must be at the center of the discussion about this issue. Finally, the idea of healthcare institutions as part of a larger global environment is presented. What is the responsibility of the healthcare system to its internal and external environment from an ethics viewpoint?

QUESTIONS FOR DISCUSSION

1. What ethical issues could be caused by the rapid change and increasing sophistication of technology? Do you think there will be an even greater gap between the "haves" and the "have nots"?

2. What is society's ethical responsibility in the issue of childhood obesity? What is the responsibility of the healthcare system?

3. Can you make an argument for patient-focused care from an ethics viewpoint? If this approach is ethical, why is it not the norm?

4. What is the healthcare system's ethical responsibility to the environment in which it exists?

5. What are the most important ethical lessons you learned from reading this text?

NOTES

1. For an excellent source on technology and ethics see, T. F. Budinger and M. D. Budinger, *Ethics of Emerging Technologies: Scientific Facts and Moral Challenges* (New York: John Wiley and Sons, 2006).

2. See S. Gottlieb, "The Future of Medical Technology," *The New Atlantis: A Journal of Technology and Society* 1 (2003): 79–87.

3. Check the CDC Web site (www.cdc.gov) for additional information and statistics on this issue.

4. For more information, see MSNBC.com, "Childhood Obesity Can Trigger Early Puberty," *MSNBC* (March 5, 2007). Available at www.msnbc.msn.com/id/17465229/.

5. Check the CDC Web site (www.cdc.gov) for additional information and statistics on this issue.

6. For an excellent resource on this topic, consult S. B. Frampton, L. Gilpin, and P. A. Charmel, *Putting Patients First: Designing and Practicing Patient-Centered Care* (San Francisco: Jossey Bass, 2003).

7. To gain greater understanding of impact of environment and ethics, see "Environmental Ethics" in T. F. Budinger and M. D. Budinger, eds., *Ethics of Emerging Technologies: Scientific Facts and Moral Challenges* (New York: John Wiley and Sons, 2006), 147–185.

8. For more information about green hospitals, consult K. Weller, "The Top 10 Green Hospitals in the U.S.: 2006," *The Green Guide* (Washington, D.C.: The National Geographic Society, 2007). Available at www.thegreenguide.com/doc/113/top10hospitals.

Glossary

This glossary includes words that may be confusing or not in common usage. It is designed to be a reference for understanding the concepts discussed in the text.

A priori. Term used to indicate knowledge that is based on experience.

Absolute difference (AD). Number obtained by subtracting the numerical measure of the health status of one group from that of another group.

Altered nuclear transfer technique (ANT). Scientists can use this technique to generate embryonic stem cells without first creating an embryo. This technique has been proposed as an ethical way to create stem cell lines.

Alternative fuel sources. Nonfossil-fuel-based sources of energy, including wind, hydrodynamic, hydrogen, and solar power.

Altruism. That a person is acting unselfishly or in the belief that his or her actions benefit others.

Amniocentesis. Procedure for taking a sample of amniotic fluid from the uterus; sample can then be used for genetic screening and detection of health conditions.

Antinomies. Two statements that appear to be correct, but do not agree. They create a paradox.

Artificial nutrition. Used for medical maintenance, a temporary form of providing nutrients in cases when a person cannot swallow.

Artificially inseminated by donor (AID) children. Children created by joining sperm and egg outside of the womb and then inserting them into a natural or surrogate mother.

Assisted death. Practices of voluntary active euthanasia and assisted suicide.

Assisted reproductive technology (ART). Any of a number of alternative ways to reproduce children. Cloning is one example of ART.

Assisted reproduction. Use of technologies, such as in vitro fertilization, artificial insemination, and cloning, to facilitate procreation.

Assisted suicide. Intentionally ending one's life through the assistance of a third party.

Autonomy. In ethics, the ability to act independently and to make decisions about actions, treatment, and health practices.

Beneficence. In ethics, to act with charity and kindness. It applies to both professionals and to organizations.

Best-off population. Method of computing the amount of inequality in population. In this case, those who are the best off in terms of health serve as the reference group for comparisons with the worst-off group.

Biological reductionism. A view that reduces human beings to the cellular level and assumes that one human can replace another.

Blastocyst. An embryo that is ready to be implanted in the wall of the uterus.

Bureaucratic parsimony. An organization's unwillingness to spend money or resources on programs.

Chorionic villi sampling (CVS). Process whereby a catheter is inserted into the uterus to collect a sample of fetal tissue from the developing placenta.

Cloning. Process of creating a plant or animal that is genetically identical to its parent through the use of asexual reproduction.

Clouded genetic heritage. Occurs when reproductive technologies are used and the genetic identity of the produced child is not known.

Collaborative reproduction. A type of social experiment that includes the use of surrogates, cloning, and other alternative reproductive options to produce a child.

Competency. The ability to understand the situation and make choices based on understood logic.

Decisional capacity. The ability to make decisions about one's personal life, including where one lives and receives care. It also includes decisions about the type of care received.

Decisional incapacity. The level of inability to make decisions about one's personal life, including where one lives and receives care. It also includes decisions about the type of care received.

Digital divide. Occurs when access to technology is not universal in a society, creating a group of "haves" and "have nots" with respect to technology use.

Disease experience. How patients see the disease process, which can be vastly different from the way professionals view it.

Disenfranchisement. When a person's rights to full participation in society appear to be limited; the individual does not feel that he or she has the right to benefits that others receive.

Domestic violence. A complex social problem that carries serious health care consequences especially for women.

Electronic medical records (EMR). Generic term for the creation, maintenance, and storage of a patient's medical record on a computer system.

Environmental sustainability. The ability of the local or global environment to maintain life for all species.

Ethical analysis. The application of ethical theory and principles to concrete clinical situations.

Ethical climate. The overall culture of an organization. The climate for the application of ethics to decision making can be one that is favorable or unfavorable.

Ethicist. A professional who typically has a doctoral degree in ethics, bioethics, and sometimes theology. He or she serves as a consultant on ethics issues for a hospital or ethics committee.

Ethics committee. A group of people that serves in an advisory capacity for ethics issues in a hospital or major clinic; membership varies depending on the committee's function.

Etiopathy. This term is used for the scientific study used to determine the causes of pathological changes in the body.

Eudaimonia. The translation of this term is "happiness" or "well-being." However, in Aristotle's philosophy it is different from mere pleasure in that it occurs when a person lives a rational life.

Family systems approach. An approach to psychotherapy that views the family as a unit and addresses problems within the system of the family.

Fetal biopsy. An invasive procedure for diagnosing disease or problems with fetal development.

Financially avoidable inequity. A term used to classify inequities in health care. It means that there are enough funds to correct the inequity.

Fungible. The ability to be interchanged or substitutable.

Futility. In general contexts, a term that means an action does not produce a valuable effect or that is useless. In medical situations, this is often difficult to determine, because it must define the medical limits of care. A definition of utility is used to balance benefit against harm.

Gender socialization. Process by which males and females learn their identities and roles in society.

Genetic mother. The female who provides the germ cells (egg) for the creation of a child; may or may not be the gestational mother.

Gestational mother. Female who carries the fertilized egg in her uterus; she may or may not be the genetic mother.

Gourmet children. Children who are special ordered for their genetic attributes (gender, height, intellect); also known as designer children.

Green hospitals. Facilities that make efforts to protect the environment through their internal and external actions.

Hackers. Individuals who use their expertise to break into a computer system; can be done for illegal purposes or just for their own amusement.

Hazard vulnerability analysis. Process involved in evaluating potential emergencies and their effect on hospitals and communities. Several areas are suggested for inclusion in such an analysis, including mitigation, response, and recovery operations.

Health inequality. Variations of health status across individuals within a population or a difference in the average or total health between two or more populations.

Health inequity. A difference in the health status of populations or individuals within populations that is judged to be morally unacceptable.

High-technology home care. Home-based health care where specific machinery is used to maintain life and/or quality of life.

Horizontal equity. The equal allocation of a resource across a population.

Hospitals in a box. Mobile or portable facilities that allow hospitals to expand their services in the event of an emergency.

Human-caused disaster. Situations of loss of life, property, and sense of safety that are created by the actions of humans rather than nature.

Human cloning. Process of creating a human being from a cell or other living tissue. Clones would have identical genetic makeup as their donors.

Hydatidiform mole. A tumor-like mass in the uterus that is often mistaken for a pregnancy.

Hydration. When fluids are artificially given to support medical treatment when the patient is unable to swallow.

Inerrant. Incapable of making a mistake.

Institutional review board (IRB). Committee made up of experts and concerned individuals whose mission is to assure protection of human subjects who are used in any research project.

Integrated ethics. An approach to ethics whereby ethics is part of the "business as usual" workings of an organization. Ethics is not segregated into an ethics committee or the chaplaincy.

Intergenerational problem. When a problem or condition affects patients of two or more generations. An example of an intergenerational problem would be domestic violence or alcoholism.

Intergenerational transmission of abuse. Process of passing the culture of abuse from one generation to another in families.

Inurement. The idea that charitable organizations must not operate for private interests or private gain. The IRS pays close attention to this with nonprofit organizations and monitors excessive benefit.

Mass casualty event. Natural or human-caused occurrences in which more than the expected number of deaths and injuries occur. Such events challenge hospitals and other healthcare systems.

Mass prophylaxis. Community preparedness for natural or human-caused disasters.

Medical paradigm. The logic used in traditional medical practice to assess and diagnose the patient's problems.

Medicalization of social problems. A philosophy of converting areas that used to be seen as social problems into medical ones. For example, alcoholism is now recognized as a disease and not just a social failing.

Medically fragile, technology-dependent (MF/TD) children. Individuals under the age of 18 who have medical conditions that make them dependent on technological assistance.

Mitigation. Organizational and individual efforts to lessen the impact of a disaster. Disaster planning is considered part of mitigation efforts.

Moral community. The group of people with whom we feel a moral affinity and for whom we assume an ethical obligation. Boundaries of the moral community are established by perception of who is a member and who is not.

Morally avoidable inequity. When an inequity is corrected, it must not violate other social values, such as violations of liberty or distributive justice.

Morning after pill. Contraceptives designed for use after sexual intercourse to prevent pregnancy.

Most socially advantaged population. Method of computing the amount of inequality in a population. In this case, the most socially advantaged group serves as a referent for comparison with other groups in the population.

Natural disaster. Situations where there is loss of life, property, and sense of safety that is caused by natural events such as floods, hurricanes, fires, and tornadoes.

Neonatal intensive care units (NICU). Specialized areas of a hospital designed to meet the needs of premature and severely ill infants. They require specialized technology and highly specialized professionals.

Networks. In the healthcare system, cooperative relationships between various types of healthcare organizations, including hospitals, clinics, long-term care facilities, and combinations of organizations.

Nonconsenting third party. With regard to reproductive technologies, it means the potential child created by these technologies. The child is acted upon without any possibility of consent.

Nonmaleficence. To refrain from causing harm or to prevent intentional harm from occurring.

Nonmarital third party. With regard to reproductive technologies, individuals who contribute to the procreation of a child, but who are not to be the parents of the child. Examples include egg and sperm donors.

Noumenal world. For Kant, the world as it exists within itself and not as we interpret it.

Palliative specialists. Healthcare professionals who specialize in providing care that reduces pain and suffering without eliminating the cause. Their expertise is particularly important for end-of-life care.

Partial birth abortion. This form of ending a pregnancy involves conducting procedures at the latest possible stage before live birth. It is banned in the United States except when it is necessary to save the mother's life.

Paternalism. An action taken by one person (usually a health professional) that limits the autonomy of another person. This infringement on autonomy is done to benefit the person or to protect him or her from harm. For example, paternalism occurs when a physician does not tell the patient the complete truth about his or her condition.

Patient-focused care. Delivery of healthcare services with the patient as the center of care. Elements of this care include information, patient-friendly environments, open medical records, and the use of care partners.

Patient Self-Determination Act (PSDA). Requires Medicare and Medicaid providers to provide written information about a person's rights to make healthcare decisions, including rights for accepting and/or refusing treatment.

Pediatric intensive care units (PICU). Areas of a hospital that are designed to treat severely ill infants. They often employ sophisticated technology and specialized medical care professionals.

Physician-assisted death. Active or passive euthanasia involving physician practice. In active euthanasia, the physician would directly support the death. In passive euthenasia, he or she would avoid practices that would prolong life. The physician might also use practices that would increase comfort but hasten death.

Plan B. Action by the FDA that made the morning after pill available to women over the age of 18 without a prescription.

Prehospital Advanced Directive (PHAD). Also called a living will, a document that is prepared by an individual before he or she becomes a patient. It specifies what should be done in end-of-life situations, including the actions of EMTs and emergency department personnel. It can also designate who can speak for the patient if he or she is unable to speak for him or herself. States vary in their laws regarding PHADs.

Prehospital do not resuscitate order (PHDNR). This document, prepared before one is a patient, specifies what is to be done in the event of a life-threatening or end-of-life situation. It spells out the patient's desire or lack of desire for cardiopulmonary resuscitation by EMTs or emergency department staff.

Prenatal diagnosis. Diagnosis of conditions or disease before birth.

Presymptomatic diagnosis. The ability to determine the presence of disease before actual symptoms are present; one of the potential benefits of genetic testing.

Prima facie. Term used to indicate that something is assumed to exist on initial examination. It is often assumed to be in place or assumed to be agreed upon by the staff.

Principle of subsidiary. Rationale for placing decision making at the level where the work is actually produced.

Psychic survival. Denial of feelings and formation of values in order to protect one from psychological harm.

Radio frequency identification tags (RFID). System for tracking patients and maintaining security that is currently used in some long-term care facilities.

Relative difference (RD). Number obtained by the division of the numerical measure of the health status of one group by that of another group.

Retraumatization. When a person suffers a trauma, such as domestic violence, he or she is often traumatized again by the processes used to gain information for treatment. The patient must relive the pain and psychological damage in order to obtain treatment. Retraumatization also occurs if the individual decides to press charges against the abuser.

Safety net. In health care, institutions that provide treatment to medically indigent patients who cannot obtain care from other sources. The emergency department of hospitals and public health clinics are examples of safety nets.

Second-trimester abortion. Ending of a pregnancy during the second trimester; a process that requires a modified surgical procedure, such as vacuum aspiration.

Selective abortion. Abortion performed for a special reason, such as when the fetus has the potential of a genetic disease.

Shelter in place. When a natural or human-caused disaster happens, it is sometimes necessary for people to remain in their homes, schools, or places of business until help is available.

Sine qua non. An essential condition or prerequisite.

Social mother. The female who cares for a child after birth; may or may not be the genetic and/or gestational mother.

Stakeholder theory. Used in healthcare management to denote the involvement of those who have an investment in the mission of an organization, including employees, board members, physicians, and others. Relationships are built on trust and facilitate the business practices of the organizations.

Stem cell line. A special type of cell that can develop into any kind of human tissue.

Stewardship. Management philosophy whereby one recognizes that one does not own resources. The manager, instead, protects the use of these resources in trust for the community or other stakeholders. Such a philosophy implies a high level of ethical awareness and application.

Subacute care. Care for conditions that are less severe than acute situations.

Summa Theologica. One of the primary works of St. Thomas Aquinas that includes his discourse on ethics.

Surge hospital. A facility that enables hospitals to expand their services quickly in the event of a disaster, such as convention centers, airport hangars, and schools.

Surrogate. In health care situations, one who makes decision for another, such as a surrogate for a nursing home resident.

Surrogate mother. With respect to reproductive technology, a woman who carries another woman's child in her womb.

Surveillance reports. In disaster planning, documents that provide information on potential natural or human-caused disasters. Various methods are used to obtain this information including weather reports, telephone monitoring, and tracking of suspicious individuals.

Systematic health inequality. A difference in health that consistently affects two or more populations that is not caused by random variation.

Technically avoidable inequity. An inequity in health care that can be corrected.

Technology bereft. A person who does not have access to or chooses not to use technology, including computers and/or the Internet.

Technology diffusion. When a technology becomes so common in a culture that it helps to define that culture and is expected by members of that culture.

Technology sophisticate. This term is used for a person who has a high level of knowledge about and/or use of technology, including computers and/or the Internet.

Teleological. Ethics theories that are based on explanations of ethics as related to a goal or result.

Total institution. Any type of facility that meets of the needs of an individual and where the meeting of those needs comes with restrictions; for example, a long-term care facility.

Total population average. Method of computing the amount of inequality in population; it examines the average of healthcare events in the population as a reference group to compare the same event with subpopulations.

Trauma theory. A recent addition to psychological theories, this research attempts to explain the effects of trauma as survival strategies or adaptations to life-shattering situations.

Unjust cause. One of the criteria for judging health inequities; health inequities that result from severe restrictions to lifestyle choices, unhealthy working conditions, and inadequate access to health services fall into this category.

Utilitarianism. A synonym for consequentialism, this term means that actions are ethical when they produce the greatest happiness or utility. The reverse is also true. Actions are good when they avoid producing the greatest harm.

Vertical equity. Allocation of different resources for different needs.

Voluntary active euthanasia. Patients freely choose to have a lethal agent directly administered to them by another individual, with a merciful intent.

Index